8/86

Date Due

PARENTS' GUIDE
TO NUTRITION

PARENTS' GUIDE TO NUTRITION

Healthy Eating From Birth Through Adolescence

Boston Children's Hospital

with

Susan Baker, M.D., Ph.D.

Roberta R. Henry, R.D.

Executive Editor

David Estridge

A Merloyd Lawrence Book

Addison-Wesley Publishing Company, Inc.

Reading, Massachusetts • Menlo Park, California
Don Mills, Ontario • Wokingham, England • Amsterdam
Sydney • Singapore • Tokyo • Madrid • Bogotá
Santiago • San Juan

Tables 2.5, 2.6, 2.13, 2.17, 2.24, 2.25, 2.27, 2.28, and 3.3 are adapted from Pennington, Jean A.T. and Church, H.N., *Bowes and Church's Food Values of Portions Commonly Used*, Fourteenth Edition, with the kind permission of J.B. Lippincott Company, Philadelphia, PA.

Table 2.10 is adapted from the American Dietetic Association *Handbook of Clinical Dietetics* with the kind permission of Yale University Press, New Haven, CT.

Table 6.2 is adapted from Young, E.A., "Perspectives on Fast Food," *Public Health Currents*, Vol. 21, No. 3(1981).

Library of Congress Cataloging-in-Publication Data

Baker, Susan.
  Parents' guide to nutrition.

  "A Merloyd Lawrence book."
  Bibliography: p.
  Includes index.
  1. Children—Nutrition.   I. Henry, Roberta R.
II. Children's Hospital (Boston, Mass.)   III. Title.
[DNLM: 1. Child Nutrition—popular works.   2. Nutrition
—in adolescence—popular works.   WS 115 B168p]
RJ206.B29 1986   649'.3   86-3435
ISBN 0-201-05729-8

Many of the designations used by manufacturers and sellers to distinguish their products are claimed as trademarks. Where these designations appear in the book and the authors are aware of a trademark claim, the designations have been printed with initial capital letters — for example, NutraSweet or Equal.

Cover design by Steve Snider
Text design by Kenneth J. Wilson
Set in 11 point Palatino by Compset, Inc., Beverly, MA
ISBN: 0-201-05729-8
First printing, March 1986
ABCDEFGHIJK-DO-89876

CONTENTS

FOREWORD

But sup them well,
and look unto them.

> William Shakespeare
> *The Taming of the Shrew*

Eating began with life on Earth; yet as a science, nutrition is relatively new. The amount of reliable information about food and health has increased enormously since the 1970s, and recommendations about diet continually change to reflect this rise. Unfortunately, half-truths and misinformation have grown just as explosively, and families often are confused by a bewildering mixture of fact and fiction, solid advice and sensational claims.

Parents who are curious about the soundness of their own nutrition beliefs may find it enlightening to take the nutrition quiz in Chapter 12 before reading further. It may come as a surprise to learn that many common beliefs about food are false while some of the most extreme statements actually contain a shred of truth.

We at The Children's Hospital of Boston believe that families will welcome a guide through this forest of fact and fiction. We want parents to understand the principles of child nutrition; how the body uses food; the links between nutrition and health; and successful ways to encourage children to eat food that is good for them. While it is true that more and more information about diet and health is available, most of it focuses on the needs and concerns of adults. We find this ironic because good nutrition during childhood is vital to a growing, developing body and a healthy adulthood. Although interest in child nutrition has increased in recent years, it has not yet received the full attention it deserves.

In this book we have tried to provide a practical alternative to the quick-remedy nutrition plans that are so abundant today. Many of these fad diets, which look and sound wonderful on paper, can actually be harmful, alienate children from their peers, or make caring parents doubt their own good sense. Instead, we emphasize that tasty, nourishing meals for children can be simple and inexpensive to prepare, and easily adaptable to the spectrum of individual tastes and lifestyles.

The skills and insights of a pediatrician and a registered dietitian, as well as the resources of The Children's Hospital of Boston, the largest pediatric health-care institution in the United States and the world's largest pediatric research center, have helped shape this book. We realize, of course, that one book cannot answer all questions about nutrition. We therefore encourage parents to use the resources and references listed at the end of this book. In addition, parents might wish to consult with their own pediatricians, family physicians, or registered dietitians.

Providing nourishing food is one of the most significant, lasting ways parents show their love for their children. With a sound diet, parents provide raw materials for growth and development—for active and alert children who grow physically, emotionally, and intellectually. By presenting that food in a warm, happy setting, parents nurture sensible eating habits that often last a lifetime. Feeding is caring, and feeding well is loving well.

1

THE MANY MEANINGS OF FOOD

I do not like the way you slide
I do not like your soft inside,
I do not like you lots of ways,
And I could do for many days
Without eggs.

Russell Hoban
Bread and Jam for Frances

A group of children, ranging in age from 3 to 7, were asked, "Why do you eat?" and "Why do you eat what you eat?" Their replies included:

"I eat because I'm hungry."

"I eat to grow."

"I want to get strong and beat up my brother."

"I eat because Mommy and Daddy tell me to."

"I don't know — I guess I eat because it's good for me."

"I eat because I like to."

"I eat peanut butter because I really *love* it."

"I don't eat beets because they're yucky."

Not surprisingly, hunger was the first and most frequent reason given for eating. Hunger is triggered by the body's need for six kinds of nutrients: protein, carbohydrates, fats, vitamins, minerals, and water. All these nutrients are needed for survival and growth. A lack of any one of them for a long period of time inevitably leads to health problems.

Infants and young children are especially sensitive to the hunger signals their bodies send out. Unless forced or strongly encouraged, they rarely eat more or less than they need. Even more remarkably, over the course of a few days, if presented with foods containing all the essential nutrients, children will adequately balance their diets.

In addition to filling the body's needs, food has rich cultural significance. This is immediately evident in the use of food-related words, often to signify emotions — sweetie, honey, apple pie, fruitcake, rotten egg, peach, spicy, salt of the earth, tart, and oily. People talk about "biting" comments, someone "stewing in his own juices," "eating her own words," "swallowing anger," or a controversy that people "can sink their teeth into."

This richness of meaning is also seen in the symbolic use of foods in many rituals and celebrations — turkey for Thanksgiving, horseradish for Passover, eggs at Easter, bread and wine in the Christian traditions, kosher foods in the Jewish, and yin and yang foods in the Zen. Special foods and festive eating rituals play important roles in birth celebrations, weddings, and funerals — the central events of people's lives.

The foods that people eat, when and how these foods are eaten, and even the size of a serving varies from country to country, as well as from neighborhood to neighborhood and house to house. Eating patterns, however, can be linked to several general trends — personal food preferences and family eating patterns; social roles and pressures; the larger culture; and environmental, technological, and economic factors affecting availability. Taken together, this complicated web determines whether a person eats rice and beans, steak and potatoes, or shredded cabbage and shrimp; six meals or three meals a day; uses fingers, chopsticks, gourd, or fork; and whether the meal satisfies hunger.

PERSONAL FOOD PREFERENCES AND FAMILY EATING PATTERNS

Individual eating patterns are formed by experiences, body type, psychological and emotional needs, and personal philosophies.

For the most part, personal food preferences are learned and developed at home throughout childhood. Beginning in infancy, children develop food preferences based on what they are fed. For example, children fed foods high in salt and sugar often continue to eat these throughout adulthood. A person fed hot peppers during childhood probably will grow up liking spicy foods.

Food preferences obviously are also influenced by what foods are around the house and eaten by others, and how members of the family react to various foods. One mother of three hated kale and never fixed it for her family. Her daughters grew up assuming they disliked this vegetable — even though they had never tasted it. In another family, the father got mad and announced he would not sit at the dinner table because beets were served. His young son, upset by the whole scene, never ate beets as an adult. The same boy, however, had an older brother who ate peanut-butter sandwiches for lunch almost every day. Following his big brother's example, peanut butter became the young boy's favorite too, and it remained a favorite after he grew up.

All these examples show that adults' diets often are similar to those they were fed as children, with additions and variations influenced by their environment. This profound and lasting impact of eating habits early in life is one reason well-balanced, wholesome diets for young children are so important.

Individual eating patterns change with age and physical condition. Young children have sensitive taste buds and, therefore, favor bland foods. Infants and adolescents, who both are growing rapidly, need far more to eat per pound of body weight than do adults (as any parent of a teenager knows all too well). Pregnant women and those who are breast feeding need to eat more than normal and require a number of special nutrients in larger-than-normal amounts; calcium and iron, for example, are particularly important during pregnancy.

Individual physical differences also play a major role in the way a particular person's eating habits vary from those of his or her family. People who are physically active require more calories a day than do sedentary people. Digestive ability, food allergies, and rate of metabolism (the complex chemical and physical processes that maintain human life) affect what and how much a person eats. Some children are unable to tolerate cow's milk, for example, and some are allergic to wheat. Special diets must be developed for these children (see Chapter 8).

Children sometimes use food and eating habits as a way to assert control, just as their parents do. A 2-year-old may refuse a cheese sandwich cut diagonally because of a strong need to assert independence. Similarly, teenagers are likely to use food as a way to demonstrate independence, especially in households where food has always been an important issue, or where the mother or father gains a great deal of control through the presentation of food.

Psychological and emotional states, which are particularly sensitive in adolescence, also affect how people eat. Some teenage girls, struggling for control and influenced by a culture that is preoccupied with slimness, suffer from eating disorders such as *anorexia nervosa* (becoming obsessed with food but eating very little because of imagined fatness) or *bulimia* (binging on large amounts of foods and feeling so guilty about it that vomiting is self-induced).

Physical and emotional factors often combine to affect appetite. A child who is exhausted or under stress may respond by eating less or more than usual. Anger, fatigue, joy, competitive feelings, and depression also can affect the way a child eats. Parents trying to feed their children well have to consider all these conditions. A child worn out after a long day of school and sports, for example, may need food quickly, but the family's usual heavy dinner may not be the answer. Scrambled eggs and toast may be all the weary child can manage.

Finally, knowledge of nutrition and personal philosophy deeply affect eating patterns. When people know about the body's needs for protein, carbohydrates, fats, minerals, and vitamins, and generally understand what foods meet those needs, they are more likely to pick out wholesome food and reject heavily advertised or sleekly packaged items that provide little nourishment. Personal beliefs affect how people use this knowledge. How people eat tells a lot about them. Boycotting grapes, savoring fine wines, choosing a vegetarian lifestyle, cooking large quantities of food for large numbers of people, eating only natural foods or organically grown fruits and vegetables — all these eating habits reflect the people's views, beliefs, and values, as well as how much information is available to them.

SOCIAL ROLES AND PRESSURES

Eating is a social activity involving family, friends, colleagues, or even enemies. How people relate or do not relate to other people — whom they love and what social lines they draw — is a big part of why they eat what they eat. Even eating alone is a situation that influences food choice.

At the most basic level, a person's sense of security, trust, love, and self-confidence is deeply affected by the amount of cuddling and loving received during infancy. Many studies point out the ill effects of feeding infants without giving them this kind of attention. In extreme situations, a child can fail to grow and thrive.

The bonding between mother and child that occurs during early feedings influences the emotional health of the infant for life. The guarantee of physical contact is one reason more and more doctors are recommending breast feeding. Bonding with the father, also important, is more likely if he participates in feedings when solids are introduced or if the baby is bottle fed. The emotional warmth of this physical connection is important for the mother and father, as well as the child.

As children grow, their parents continue to show concern and love by providing nourishing food. Preparing the family meal, making certain that children eat wholesome food, and encouraging sensible eating habits are all vitally important acts that children understand as signs of love and caring.

Shared family meals, therefore, are important times for children. Many remember meals as times of lively discussion, warmth, and fun. Memories of frequent arguments or criticism across the dinner table, however, can have harmful, subtle effects on a child's feelings about food.

Using food as a reward or punishment can have unfortunate consequences as well. Sweets should not be used as rewards, in part because this practice reinforces the belief that some foods are better than others. A child should never be punished by withholding a meal; this is as harmful an act as denying the child

sleep. Food denials can result in irritability, behavior problems, increased tension between parent and child, and eating
disorders.

Overfeeding a child may give the cook a sense of personal
satisfaction, yet this is another practice that can be harmful. In
addition to interfering with a child's natural sense of how much
is enough, overfeeding is manipulative and totally unnecessary
for good health and normal growth.

Food, indeed, is multifaceted. It is at the center of almost all
social life. Invitations to dinner reflect friendship, warmth, and
hospitality; the apple for the teacher, the teakettle on the stove,
and candy for Valentine's Day have special significance. Children learn these uses of food all too well; they even will share
certain foods with some friends but not others.

Social pressure strongly affects eating habits, both within
groups and as people move from one group to another. To most
children, neither coffee nor beer tastes good initially, but teenagers often are influenced by their peers to cultivate a liking for
them. In addition, many teenagers gather at the local pizzeria or
hamburger chain, urged there for social reasons more often than
the appeal of or desire for food.

Particular foods represent social status, taste, and wealth. Although such fashions vary in different parts of the country, Brie,
smoked salmon, sushi, or pasta primavera, for example, often
are considered sophisticated foods, while pork and beans may
be seen as a working-class dish.

Red meats historically have been considered status foods. As
people have increased their wealth and climbed the social lad-
der, many have increased their consumption of red meats — a
change, however, that has not benefited health. Most of the
high-grade red meats are fattier than the lower grades of meat,
or chicken, fish, and protein-rich grains and beans. Recently, as
these facts have become more widely known, the trend has begun to reverse itself: educated people of means are likely to limit
their consumption of red meats.

What we eat also reflects social roles and changing social patterns. As more women move into the work force, for example,
families are increasingly likely to eat food that is convenient,

quick, and easy to prepare. In addition, well-educated mothers are often more informed about the link between diet and health.

LARGER CULTURE

The larger culture, which includes the customs and accepted ways of the society in which a person lives, strongly influences eating habits. Cultural food differences are obvious among countries, religious groups, and ethnic groups within a country. The diets of the Chinese, the Iranians, the Nigerians, the French, the English, and the Americans are different, yet each supplies the essential raw materials. Foods acceptable to some are abhorrent to others. Some cultures, for example, consider roasted beetles or fried grasshoppers a delicacy; others treasure horsemeat; still others favor moldy, aromatic cheeses.

Culture also influences how often people eat, when they eat, and what kinds of food they choose. In some cultures, breakfast is the largest meal; in others, lunch or dinner. Some cultures encourage steak and potatoes for breakfast; others, coffee and a roll; still others, soup; and even others, orange juice and scrambled eggs. In general, Americans eat three meals a day; the British traditionally eat four. In some cultures foods are served separately, over several courses; in others they often are stewed together in one pot. In European countries, food is eaten with forks and spoons; in some Asian countries, it is eaten with chopsticks; in India, it is properly eaten with fingers.

Ancient food traditions often enhance nutritional value. For example, corn, extensively eaten by Latin Americans, traditionally is prepared by boiling it with powdered limestone before grinding to make tortillas. When people were asked why they added the limestone, they replied that it made the corn easier to manage. Recent information shows that limestone reacts chemically to make corn's B vitamins and protein more digestible and, therefore, more available to the body. Similarly, bitter manioc, a root popular in South America and Africa, is prepared by squeezing and cooking the pulp. This process releases poisonous cyanide from the root, thereby making it safe to eat.

The dietary laws of certain religions are based on a combina-

tion of knowledge, tradition, and superstition. Traditional orthodox Jewish laws forbidding the eating of shellfish and pork
probably are based on an understanding of the dangers of pol-
luted shellfish and undercooked pork. In addition, the pig was
a common food among the Jewish people's rival groups and may
have gained its negative image because of this. The Jewish law
that prohibits meat and milk from being eaten together is less
easily related to principles of health.

Hindus believe in reincarnation and hold that all life is sacred.
Thus, devout Hindus are vegetarians. Cows, in particular, are
considered most worthy of respect; therefore, any part of a cow
is forbidden food. Zen Buddhists divide foods into yin and yang
categories, while Peruvians and Indians believe different foods
have hot and cold properties that are unrelated to the food's actual temperature. In some cases, elaborate eating codes are
based on these beliefs. The highest level of the Zen macrobiotic
diet, for example, consists of only cereals and water, a diet that
may lead some to wisdom, according to belief, but also can lead
to severe malnutrition.

ENVIRONMENTAL, TECHNOLOGICAL, AND ECONOMIC FACTORS

The foods that people eat and how much they eat depend on
what is available and by their ability to obtain it. Availability is
largely a matter of terrain and climate. People living near bodies
of water, for example, are more likely to include seafood in their
diets than people living in landlocked regions. In farm country,
a drought or a flash flood can ruin a harvest, making less food
available. Rainy regions produce different foods than desert regions. Wheat grows well in some areas, coffee in others, and
apples in others. Soil in different regions varies in richness; possibilities for irrigation also play a major role in determining what
foods can be produced.

People have developed technologies of production, preservation, and distribution based on these basic realities of food
availability. Fertilizers, machines, and irrigation techniques
have increased the amount of food one person can produce, the
frequency with which it can be grown, and the places where it

can thrive. Former deserts, for example, have been turned into agricultural fruit baskets, and farms can now produce many times more wheat or corn than they could a century ago.

As agricultural technology has advanced — making it possible for one farmer to accomplish what it once took 20 to do — agribusiness has increasingly replaced small family farms. Changes in productive technology have gone hand in hand with changes in preservation technology. The ability to refrigerate, can, and freeze food safely has brought vast changes to the diet in developed nations. Instead of having to rely on root vegetables and dried meats, beans, and fruits for the long winter season, most food is available year round. Some fresh fruits and vegetables still are seasonal — many people look forward to strawberry, asparagus, or peach season — but most varieties of produce are available throughout the year, in fresh, canned, or frozen forms.

Distribution techniques are equally important to food availability. Refrigerated trains, trucks, ships, and planes now provide people in developed countries with fresh oranges, carrots, beef, chicken, broccoli, and lettuce all year. Countries lacking these distribution facilities are restricted to more limited seasonal diets.

Another strong influence on eating patterns is advertising and other forms of marketing. Sugared cereals, candy, and soft drinks sell so well in part because they are advertised on children's television programs. Americans today consume more refined carbohydrates such as those found in cookies and soft drinks than they do complex carbohydrate sources such as whole-grain flours, fruits, and vegetables. This is largely because sweets and snack foods are advertised heavily, while fruits and vegetables are not.

A country's history and political situation also play a role in eating patterns. Recent droughts in Africa have led to widespread famine in large part because during the last century colonial powers took the best land and used it for large export crop production: the growing of peanuts, cotton, and coffee for Europe and the United States. Not only was little usable land left for growing needs of the local population, but the plantations that grew crops for export overused soil to the point of depletion. When the colonial powers left Africa, the new African na-

tions were faced with increased technological requirements —
they now need trucks, for example, to move food from one part
of the country to another — and with large international debts.
Today, these African countries are forced to maintain the export
food crops, feeding nations in developed countries that have
their own food surpluses, despite the increased risk of hunger
and famine to their own growing populations.

Contemporary middle- and upper-class Americans and Europeans are fortunate to have the most extensive food selection
ever known. But this situation also has its unhappy consequences. Largely because of the excess fat and sugar that they
eat and the sedentary nature of their work and leisure activities,
many affluent people in these countries suffer high rates of obesity, heart attacks, high blood pressure, and strokes.

In addition to historical position, economic position plays a
significant role in food availability. Nationally, times of recession, depression, and inflation can affect the eating habits of
families, causing shoppers to cut back on extras and to buy less
expensive food that is wholesome. During the recession of the
late 1970s, for example, many families substituted chicken for
expensive steaks.

International economic position also influences eating habits
by affecting what foods are available and how they are produced. Roughly 25 percent of the world's population lives in affluent countries, and each person in these nations consumes an
average of one ton of grain each year. Less than 8 percent of this,
however, is consumed directly by people. Most is consumed by
animals that produce meat, milk, and eggs. In underdeveloped
countries, by contrast, each person consumes an average of only
418 pounds of grain each year, most of this directly.

In affluent countries, adults eat 100 grams or more of protein
daily, far more than is needed, and most of this comes from
animal sources. In the Third World, people eat approximately 50
grams a day, a figure close to the recommended amount, most
of it from vegetable sources.

Just as important as the larger economic picture is the particular financial position of the individual or family. In the United
States, some 20 million people — roughly one person in 12 —
suffer from hunger, and the number is growing, according to the

1985 *Hunger in America* report published by the Physicians' Task Force. Accompanying hunger are malnutrition and health problems, particularly among children and the elderly. Low-income areas show alarming rates of anemia and reduced levels of vitamin A, vitamin C, thiamin, and riboflavin. The same report found that among poor children there were high levels of growth retardation, greater risks of low birthweight and anemia, and higher rates of infant mortality and behavioral problems. The evidence indicates that current food subsidy programs in the United States are inadequate to meet the needs of the hungry.

Even at less dramatic levels, every shopper knows that food purchases vary with the amount of money available and with food costs. When the price of frozen orange juice goes down, many more people make it a part of their weekly shopping package. When the price of steak goes up, more people switch to hamburger or macaroni and cheese. When a paycheck shrinks, the food shopper buys fewer treats and concentrates more on staples of the family diet.

There are many ways to meet the body's needs for food. Knowledge of these needs, which will be outlined in the next chapter, permits families to adapt them to their personal and cultural preferences and to provide food to their children that enhances growth, good health, and mental and physical activity. Given the variety of tasty and economical ways to do this, parents can easily find a well-balanced eating pattern that fits into the family's lifestyle and that both children and parents will enjoy.

2

THE ESSENTIALS OF LIFE

And I would eat them in a boat.
And I would eat them with a
    goat . . .
And I will eat them in the rain.
And in the dark. And on a train.
And in a car. And in a tree.
They are so good, so good, you see!

Dr. Seuss
Green Eggs and Ham

A 4-year-old boy appeared in the kitchen, looked at the table, wrinkled up his face, and stuck out his tongue when he saw what awaited him for lunch. "Yuck!" "I hate tuna fish," and "I don't want to eat that green stuff." "I want root beer." This scene was familiar to his mother, who had become accustomed to his constant food refusals. Yet she remained calm about her son's limited diet, convinced that he got the things he needed to grow and develop — after all, he ate his chewable vitamin tablet every morning.

Growth and development, as well as health and survival, however, depend on more than just vitamins. In addition to vitamins, everyone needs protein, carbohydrates, fats, minerals, and water. These are nutrients — the body's fuel. The lack of any one of these in childhood will stunt a child's growth and, at any age, will lead to illness.

DAILY REQUIREMENTS

The Recommended Dietary Allowances (RDA) are the best reference for anyone interested in knowing the nutritional needs of healthy people. Developed by the Food and Nutrition Board of the National Academy of Sciences' National Research Council, the RDA outline the amounts of 17 nutrients that people need according to age. The RDA can be met by eating a variety of food that is affordable and enjoyable — without the addition of vitamin-mineral or other supplements.

As Table 2.1 shows, recommendations made for each group are based on averages of weight, height, physical activity, and normal health. Most people will not fit neatly into these categories. In addition, many recommendations are higher than the requirements; therefore most children and adults can thrive with something less than the recommended level.

Some essential vitamins and minerals, however, are not listed in the RDA because there is insufficient information to make a firm recommendation. For those, the Estimated Safe and Adequate Daily Dietary Intakes of Selected Vitamins and Minerals (shown in Table 2.2) can be used as a guideline. The upper levels for the trace elements should not be exceeded for long periods of time because large amounts can be toxic. These figures, like the RDA, are developed and published by the National Research Council of the National Academy of Sciences.

Processed foods often are labeled with nutritional information. The labels indicate the percentage of the U.S. Recommended Daily (as opposed to dietary) Allowances (USRDA) in the product, per serving. As shown in Table 2.3, these figures are *not* the same as the RDA. The Food and Drug Administration established the USRDA using the highest values in the 1973 RDA as the basis for each USRDA category. This information provides a much rougher guide to daily requirements than the current RDA. Thus, for children and women in particular, these figures are unnecessarily high; both groups can safely eat less.

Baby foods and vitamin-mineral supplements for infants and young children have a different USRDA, which provides information relevant to all children from birth to 4 years of age. Again, the figures are high and provide for widely varying needs. Finally, vitamin-mineral supplements for pregnant and

Table 2.1
FOOD AND NUTRITION BOARD, NATIONAL ACADEMY OF SCIENCES, NATIONAL RESEARCH COUNCIL: RECOMMENDED DAILY DIETARY ALLOWANCES,[a] REVISED 1980
(Designed for the maintenance of good nutrition of practically all healthy people in the U.S.A.)

	Age (years)	Weight (kg)	Weight (lb)	Height (cm)	Height (in)	Protein (g)	Vitamin A (μg RE)[b]	Vitamin D (μg)[c]	Vitamin E (mg α-TE)[d]
Infants	0.0–0.5	6	13	60	24	kg × 2.2	420	10	3
	0.5–1.0	9	20	71	28	kg × 2.0	400	10	4
Children	1–3	13	29	90	35	23	400	10	5
	4–6	20	44	112	44	30	500	10	6
	7–10	28	62	132	52	34	700	10	7
Males	11–14	45	99	157	62	45	1000	10	8
	15–18	66	145	176	69	56	1000	10	10
	19–22	70	154	177	70	56	1000	7.5	10
	23–50	70	154	178	70	56	1000	5	10
	51+	70	154	178	70	56	1000	5	10
Females	11–14	46	101	157	62	46	800	10	8
	15–18	55	120	163	64	46	800	10	8
	19–22	55	120	163	64	44	800	7.5	8
	23–50	55	120	163	64	44	800	5	8
	51+	55	120	163	64	44	800	5	8
Pregnant						+30	+200	+5	+2
Lactating						+20	+400	+5	+3

[a]The allowances are intended to provide for individual variations among most normal persons as they live in the United States under usual environmental stresses. Diets should be based on a variety of common foods in order to provide other nutrients for which human requirements have been less well defined.

[b]Retinol equivalents. 1 retinol equivalent = 1 μg (microgram) retinol or 6 μg β carotene.

[c]As cholecalciferol. 10 μg cholecalciferol = 400 IU of vitamin D.

[d]α-tocopherol equivalents. 1 mg d-α tocopherol = 1 α-TE.

Table 2.1
Continued

	Age (years)	Weight (kg)	Weight (lb)	Height (cm)	Height (in)	Water-soluble Vitamins Vitamin C (mg)	Thiamin (mg)	Riboflavin (mg)	Niacin (mg NE)[e]	Vitamin B6 (mg)	Folacin[f] (µg)	Vitamin B12 (µg)
Infants	0.0–0.5	6	13	60	24	35	0.3	0.4	6	0.3	30	0.5[g]
	0.5–1.0	9	20	71	28	35	0.5	0.6	8	0.6	45	1.5
Children	1–3	13	29	90	35	45	0.7	0.8	9	0.9	100	2.0
	4–6	20	44	112	44	45	0.9	1.0	11	1.3	200	2.5
	7–10	28	62	132	52	45	1.2	1.4	16	1.6	300	3.0
Males	11–14	45	99	157	62	50	1.4	1.6	18	1.8	400	3.0
	15–18	66	145	176	69	60	1.4	1.7	18	2.0	400	3.0
	19–22	70	154	177	70	60	1.5	1.7	19	2.2	400	3.0
	23–50	70	154	178	70	60	1.4	1.6	18	2.2	400	3.0
	51+	70	154	178	70	60	1.2	1.4	16	2.2	400	3.0
Females	11–14	46	101	157	62	50	1.1	1.3	15	1.8	400	3.0
	15–18	55	120	163	64	60	1.1	1.3	14	2.0	400	3.0
	19–22	55	120	163	64	60	1.1	1.3	14	2.0	400	3.0
	23–50	55	120	163	64	60	1.0	1.2	13	2.0	400	3.0
	51+	55	120	163	64	60	1.0	1.2	13	2.0	400	3.0
Pregnant						+20	+0.4	+0.3	+2	+0.6	+400	+1.0
Lactating						+40	+0.5	+0.5	+5	+0.5	+100	+1.0

[e] 1 NE (niacin equivalent) is equal to 1 mg of niacin or 60 mg of dietary tryptophan.

[f] The folacin allowances refer to dietary sources as determined by *Lactobacillus casei* assay after treatment with enzymes (conjugases) to make polyglutamyl forms of the vitamin available to the test organism.

[g] The recommended dietary allowance for vitamin B$_{12}$ in infants is based on average concentration of the vitamin in human milk. The allowances after weaning are based on energy intake (as recommended by the American Academy of Pediatrics) and consideration of other factors, such as intestinal absorption.

Table 2.1
Continued

Age (years)	Weight (kg)	Weight (lb)	Height (cm)	Height (in)	Minerals Calcium (mg)	Phosphorus (mg)	Magnesium (mg)	Iron (mg)	Zinc (mg)	Iodine (μg)
Infants										
0.0–0.5	6	13	60	24	360	240	50	10	3	40
0.5–1.0	9	20	71	28	540	360	70	15	5	50
Children										
1–3	13	29	90	35	800	800	150	15	10	70
4–6	20	44	112	44	800	800	200	10	10	90
7–10	28	62	132	52	800	800	250	10	10	120
Males										
11–14	45	99	157	62	1200	1200	350	18	15	150
15–18	66	145	176	69	1200	1200	400	18	15	150
19–22	70	154	177	70	800	800	350	10	15	150
23–50	70	154	178	70	800	800	350	10	15	150
51+	70	154	178	70	800	800	350	10	15	150
Females										
11–14	46	101	157	62	1200	1200	300	18	15	150
15–18	55	120	163	64	1200	1200	300	18	15	150
19–22	55	120	163	64	800	800	300	18	15	150
23–50	55	120	163	64	800	800	300	18	15	150
51+	55	120	163	64	800	800	300	10	15	150
Pregnant					+400	+400	+150	h	+5	+25
Lactating					+400	+400	+150	h	+10	+50

[h]The increased requirement during pregnancy cannot be met by the iron content of habitual American diets nor by the existing iron stores of many women; therefore the use of 30–60 mg of supplemental iron is recommended. Iron needs during lactation are not substantially different from those of nonpregnant women, but continued supplementation of the mother for 2–3 months after parturition is advisable in order to replenish stores depleted by pregnancy.

Table 2.2
ESTIMATED SAFE AND ADEQUATE DAILY DIETARY INTAKES OF SELECTED VITAMINS AND MINERALS[a]

Vitamins

	Age (years)	Vitamin K (µg)	Biotin (µg)	Pantothenic Acid (mg)
Infants	0–0.5	12	35	2
	0.5–1	10–20	50	3
Children and adolescents	1–3	15–30	65	3
	4–6	20–40	85	3–4
	7–10	30–60	120	4–5
	11+	50–100	100–200	4–7
Adults		70–140	100–200	4–7

Trace Elements[b]

	Age (years)	Copper (mg)	Manganese (mg)	Fluoride (mg)	Chromium (mg)	Selenium (mg)	Molybdenum (mg)
Infants	0–0.5	0.5–0.7	0.5–0.7	0.1–0.5	0.01–0.04	0.01–0.04	0.03–0.06
	0.5–1	0.7–1.0	0.7–1.0	0.2–1.0	0.02–0.06	0.02–0.06	0.04–0.08
Children and adolescents	1–3	1.0–1.5	1.0–1.5	0.5–1.5	0.02–0.08	0.02–0.08	0.05–0.1
	4–6	1.5–2.0	1.5–2.0	1.0–2.5	0.03–0.12	0.03–0.12	0.06–0.15
	7–10	2.0–2.5	2.0–3.0	1.5–2.5	0.05–0.2	0.05–0.2	0.10–0.3
	11+	2.0–3.0	2.5–5.0	1.5–2.5	0.05–0.2	0.05–0.2	0.15–0.5
Adults		2.0–3.0	2.5–5.0	1.5–4.0	0.05–0.2	0.05–0.2	0.15–0.5

	Age (years)	Electrolytes		
		Sodium (mg)	Potassium (mg)	Chloride (mg)
Infants	0–0.5	115–350	350–925	275–700
	0.5–1	250–750	425–1275	400–1200
Children and adolescents	1–3	325–975	550–1650	500–1500
	4–6	450–1350	775–2325	700–2100
	7–10	600–1800	1000–3000	925–2775
	11+	900–2700	1525–4575	1400–4200
Adults		1100–3300	1875–5625	1700–5100

aBecause there is less information on which to base allowances, these figures are provided here in the form of ranges of recommended intakes.
bSince the toxic levels for many trace elements may be only several times usual intakes, the upper levels for the trace elements given in this table should not be habitually exceeded.

(From Food and Nutrition Board, National Academy of Sciences — National Research Council: Recommended Dietary Allowances. 9th ed. Washington, D.C., 1980.)

Table 2.3
UNITED STATES RECOMMENDED DAILY ALLOWANCES (USRDA)[a]

	Unit[b]	Infants (birth–12 mo.)	Children under 4 yrs.	Adults and children 4 or more yrs.	Pregnant or lactating women
Protein[c]	g	25	28	65	—
Protein[d]	g	18	20	45	—
Vitamin A	IU	1500	2500	5000	8000
Vitamin D	IU	400	400	400	400
Vitamin E	IU	5	10	30	30
Vitamin C	mg	35	40	60	60
Folic acid	mg	0.1	0.2	0.4	0.8
Thiamin (B$_1$)	mg	0.5	0.7	1.5	1.7
Riboflavin (B$_2$)	mg	0.6	0.8	1.7	2.0
Niacin	mg	8	9	20	20
Vitamin B$_6$	mg	0.4	0.7	2.0	2.5
Vitamin B$_{12}$	µg	2	3	6	8

Biotin	mg	0.05	0.15	0.3	0.3
Pantothenic acid	mg	3	5	10	10
Calcium	g	0.6	0.8	1.0	1.3
Phosphorus	g	0.5	0.8	1.0	1.3
Iodine	µg	45	70	150	150
Iron	mg	15	10	18	18
Magnesium	mg	70	200	400	450
Copper	mg	0.6	1.0	2.0	2.0
Zinc	mg	5	8	15	15

[a]The USRDA are nutrient standards set by the Food and Drug Administration in 1973 using the Recommended Dietary Allowances of the National Academy of Sciences, National Research Council. The USRDA are established for four age–sex groups. Generally, the highest values in the RDA table were selected for use within each USRDA category. The nutritional information on food labels is expressed as percent of the USRDA.

[b]g = Grams; IU = International Units; mg = Milligrams; µg = Micrograms.

[c]Protein efficiency ratio less than casein.

[d]Protein efficiency ratio greater than or equal to casein.

Adapted from the FDA consumer memo, "Nutrition Labels and U.S. RDA." 81-2146, 1981.

lactating women have separate USRDA figures.

The RDA, Estimated Safe and Adequate Daily Dietary Intakes, and USRDA are general and tend to overestimate needs. Although they should not be considered requirements, they do provide guidelines and can be used with the knowledge that erring somewhat on either side of the recommendation generally will not be harmful. The requirements are easily met by providing children with a balanced and varied diet.

The rest of this chapter is intended to inform parents about the six nutrient groups, the foods that contain them, and how to meet the daily recommendations for each. This information underlies the dietary suggestions presented in the next two chapters for feeding children from conception through adolescence.

PROTEIN

Everyone needs protein for growth, normal body functioning, and disease prevention. It is especially important during periods of rapid growth — infancy, childhood, and adolescence — and during pregnancy. Some of the ways the body uses protein are:

building new tissues;

repairing and replacing tissues;

making antibodies, which help fight infection;

transporting nutrients and oxygen both in the blood and in and out of cells;

regulating the balance of water, acids, and bases; and

regulating the chemical and physical processes in the body, called metabolism.

Protein is made up of amino acids, which carry nitrogen, an element needed for human life. A total of 22 amino acids are found in living tissue. All but nine (or possibly ten) of them can be manufactured by the body. These nine or ten are called the essential amino acids because they *must* be absorbed from food.

They are: methionine (plus cystine), threonine, tryptophan, iso-leucine, leucine, lysine, valine, phenylalanine (plus tyrosine), and histidine. Taurine, according to recent research, also may be an essential amino acid.

Life cannot be sustained without these essential amino acids. Because they cannot be stored and are used within a few hours of eating, all of them must be supplied daily. Deficiencies over time will result in serious health problems.

Further, to ensure good health, these essential amino acids must be eaten in the right proportion. The protein in food varies according to its amino acid composition. In other words, the quality of any protein depends on the proportion or balance of the amino acids it contains. The quality of the protein in turn dictates how much of certain foods must be eaten to fulfill daily nutritional requirements. Quality and quantity of proteins, therefore, are important.

Proteins, even in small amounts, will be used efficiently if their amino acid composition provides the daily requirement for each amino acid. If an essential amino acid is missing from the diet of a well-nourished person, the body fails to use the other amino acids, except as a source of calories. If an essential amino acid is present in a very small amount and large quantities of the protein must be eaten to supply an adequate amount of that amino acid, the protein will not be used efficiently.

It is not difficult to plan meals with an adequate amino-acid balance on a daily basis. The protein found in milk and eggs has approximately the right proportion of amino acids; meat, fish, and poultry also have amino acids in the right proportion. These foods from animal sources, therefore, are referred to as complete or high-quality protein sources. Small quantities of these will meet daily protein requirements. For example, one egg and three ounces of meat will provide more than the 23 grams that a toddler needs in a day (see Table 2.5 for more specifics).

The protein found in nonanimal sources — grains, legumes, nuts, seeds, and, to a lesser extent, vegetables (especially the dark green, leafy variety) — lack certain amino acids and, there-fore, are called incomplete or low-quality proteins. It is possible, however, to improve the quality of protein from these nonanimal sources by adding small amounts of high-quality protein to them — cheese to macaroni, for example, or hamburger to spaghetti sauce, or sliced eggs to potato salad. Nonanimal products also can be combined to achieve high-quality protein. (The guidelines for combining protein are presented in Table 7.2.)

The quantity of protein a person needs is determined by age, physical condition, and the quality (amino acid distribution) of the protein. More protein per pound of body weight is needed during infancy than at any other period of life. Besides the need for protein during periods of growth, extra protein is needed for repair after surgery or during periods of injury, illness, or stress.

While the greatest need for protein in relation to weight occurs during infancy, the absolute need for protein increases rather than decreases as children get older. Stated another way, an infant needs 1 gram of protein per pound while an adolescent girl needs only .39 gram per pound; however, the infant weighing 13 pounds needs only 13 grams of protein a day, while the

Table 2.4
DAILY RECOMMENDED DIETARY ALLOWANCES FOR PROTEIN

	Age	Protein/lb.	Average Daily Protein Requirement
Infants	0–6 mo.	1 gm/lb.	13 gm
	6–12 mo.	.90 gm/lb.	18 gm
Children	1–3	.81 gm/lb.	23 gm
	4–6	.68 gm/lb.	30 gm
	7–10	.55 gm/lb.	34 gm
Males	11–14	.45 gm/lb.	45 gm
	15–18	.39 gm/lb.	56 gm
Females	11–14	.45 gm/lb.	46 gm
	15–18	.39 gm/lb.	46 gm
Adults	Over 19	.36 gm/lb.	44–56 gm
	Pregnant	.62 gm/lb.	74 gm
	Lactating	.53 gm/lb.	64 gm

teenager weighing 118 pounds needs 46 grams of protein. Table 2.4 illustrates this and shows both the RDA for children of average weight and the decreasing needs per pound of body weight.

Eating an adequate amount of protein is not difficult for most people. Table 2.5 lists the more common sources of high-quality protein and their protein content. Table 2.6 lists the protein content of other foods. Using these figures in conjunction with Table 2.4 will help parents provide their children with the recommended protein level.

For example, based on the RDA, a child who is 5 years old and weighs 41 pounds should eat 28 grams of protein a day (41 pounds × .68 grams of protein per pound). Using the information provided in Tables 2.5 and 2.6, this amount can be provided in a number of ways:

3 ounces chicken	21 grams
¼ cup cottage cheese	7 grams
Total	28 grams protein

OR

2 cups milk	16 grams
1 egg	7 grams
2 slices whole-wheat bread	5 grams
Total	28 grams protein

OR

½ cup plain yogurt	6 grams
1 tablespoon peanut butter	4 grams
2 slices raisin bread	4 grams
2 ounces fish	14 grams
Total	28 grams protein

OR

3½ ounces meat	28 grams
Total	28 grams protein

Table 2.5
COMMON SOURCES OF HIGH-QUALITY PROTEIN

Food	Serving Size	Average Protein (gm)
Egg — large	1	6
Milk — whole, skim, lowfat, buttermilk	1 cup	8
Milk — protein fortified	1 cup	10
Yogurt — low-fat, fruit flavored	1 cup	9
low-fat, plain	1 cup	12
Meat — beef, veal, lamb, pork, poultry	1 oz.	7
Fish — fresh or canned	1 oz.	7
Ice cream or ice milk	1 cup	8
Cheese, hard or soft	1 oz.	7
Cottage cheese	¼ cup	7

(Adapted from Pennington, Jean A. T., and Church, H. N., *Bowes and Church's Food Values of Portions Commonly Used*, Fourteenth Edition. Philadelphia: J. B. Lippincott Company, 1985.)

Table 2.6
PROTEIN CONTENT OF OTHER SELECTED FOODS

Food	Serving Size	Average Protein (gm)*
Lentils, cooked	⅔ cup	8
Peanut butter	2 tbsp.	8
Peanut	1 oz.	7
Sunflower seeds	1 oz.	7
Breads	1 slice	2 (average)
Pumpernickel	1 slice	3
Whole wheat	1 slice	2
American rye	1 slice	2
Raisin	1 slice	2
White	1 slice	2
Cereals	1 cup (1 oz.)	2 (average)
Life	⅔ cup (1 oz.)	5
All Bran	⅓ cup (1 oz.)	4
Cheerios	1¼ cup (1 oz.)	4
Apple Jacks	1 cup (1 oz.)	2
Cap'n Crunch	¾ cup (1 oz.)	2
Corn Flakes	1 cup (1 oz.)	2
Froot Loops	1 cup (1 oz.)	2
Crazy Cow, chocolate	1 cup (1 oz.)	1
Boo Berry	1 cup (1 oz.)	1

Table 2.6
Continued

Food	Serving Size	Average Protein (gm)*
Rice, white	1 cup	2
brown	½ cup	3
Vegetables	½ cup	2 (average)
Green beans, canned	⅔ cup	1
Corn, frozen	½ cup	3
Cauliflower	⅔ cup	2
Mushrooms, raw	10 small	3
canned	⅓ cup	1
Peas, frozen, tiny	½ cup	5
canned	½ cup	2
Carrots, raw	1 large	1
canned	1 cup	1
Lettuce	3½ oz.	1
Fruit	½ cup	1 or less (average)
Apple, medium	1 each	less than 1
Banana, medium	1 each	1
Cantaloupe	1 cup (pieces)	1
Cherries, sweet	10 each	1
Fruit cocktail, canned	½ cup	less than 1
Grapefruit, medium	½ each	1
Orange	1 each	1
Sugars (honey, table sugar, molasses, brown sugar)		0
Butter, margarine, oils		0

*All protein figures have been rounded to the nearest whole number.

(Adapted from Pennington, Jean A. T., and Church, H. N., *Bowes and Church's Food Values of Portions Commonly Used*, Fourteenth Edition. Philadelphia: J. B. Lippincott Company, 1985.)

The effect of portion size on the protein (and all other nutrients) content of the diet should be immediately obvious and is extremely important. Adding just one additional ounce of meat adds 7 grams of protein.

Many people, often under the mistaken assumption that meat is the only source of protein, eat too much of it. Two-thirds of the nation's protein comes from animal sources and one-third from vegetable; in 1909, half came from animal sources and half from vegetable. For several reasons, this change in America's dietary habits is unfortunate and undesirable. Although red meats are a good source of dietary iron, many varieties are high in fat and, therefore, calories. Chicken and fish are lower in fat and are good substitutes for red meats.

Meat protein is the most expensive protein to produce. Cows must be fed 21 pounds of vegetable protein to produce one pound of usable meat protein. An acre of cereals can produce five times more protein than an acre devoted to meat production. An acre of legumes produces ten times more, and an acre of leafy vegetables produces 15 times more.

Thus, while eating red meat is one way to get protein, other food should be considered as well. Feeding children less red meat can benefit their health, as long as the required amounts of protein and iron are supplied from other foods.

CARBOHYDRATES

Carbohydrates are often considered to be less than nutritious, undesirable, or fattening. In fact, carbohydrates are essential in the diet to provide energy. This in turn permits proteins to be used for growth and maintenance of body cells. Carbohydrates are essential and should never be drastically cut from the diet.

Carbohydrates are named for their chemical composition: carbon, hydrogen, and oxygen. Through a highly complex mechanism involving the sun, air, and soil (photosynthesis), plants store energy in the form of carbohydrates. Carbohydrates make up the supporting tissue of plants and are an important food for all animals, including humans.

When people eat cereal grains, fruits, and vegetables — rich sources of carbohydrates — they obtain energy directly at the rate of 4 calories per gram; when animals eat plants, humans benefit indirectly by eating meat. Carbohydrates from cereal grains represent the primary source of energy for many nations of the world.

Carbohydrates, in their digested form — glucose — are the body's main energy source. In addition to providing general energy needs, glucose is a necessary source of energy for the brain and is required for nerve tissue and the liver to function.

There are three classifications of carbohydrates: monosaccha-

Table 2.7
MONOSACCHARIDES

Glucose (also known as dextrose, corn sugar, and grape sugar)
The most important end product of di- and polysaccharide digestion
The type of carbohydrate circulating in the blood
Used for energy by body tissues

    Food sources: sweet fruits (e.g., grapes); sweet vegetables
    (e.g., sweet corn); certain roots (e.g., rutabaga)

Fructose (also known as fruit sugar or levulose)
Is the sweetest sugar (70 percent sweeter per gram than other sugars)
Is not easily crystallized
Is an end product of the breakdown of sucrose

    Food sources: honey, ripe fruits, and many vegetables

Galactose
Is not available in nature
Is the result of the breakdown of lactose (milk sugar)

---

rides (single sugars), disaccharides (double sugars), and poly-saccharides (multiple sugars).

Monosaccharides are simple carbohydrates. They are more or less sweet, water soluble, diffusable, crystallizable, and are not affected by digestive enzymes. Glucose, fructose, and galactose are monosaccharides (see Table 2.7).

Disaccharides are of varying sweetness, water soluble, diffusible, crystallizable, and, perhaps most important, are broken down to monosaccharides during digestion. Sucrose, maltose, and lactose are disaccharides (see Table 2.8).

Polysaccharides are complex carbohydrates. They are not sweet, are not crystalline, are generally insoluble, and are digested with varying degrees of completeness. Starch, glycogen, and cellulose are polysaccharides (see Table 2.9).

Carbohydrates, as previously mentioned, often are undervalued as a food source; yet they generally are rich in valuable vitamins and minerals, especially the B-complex vitamins, and many are low in calories. A medium-sized potato, for example, without butter and not cooked in fat, contains an average of 110 calories. It is rich in vitamins and minerals, and provides some protein. Bread also provides vitamins as well as carbohydrates

Table 2.8
DISACCHARIDES

Sucrose (also known as table sugar)
Is the most common disaccharide

> Food sources: sugar cane and beets, sugar maple sap,
> sorghum cane, many fruits and vegetables

Maltose (also known as malt sugar)
Is the intermediate product in the digestion of starch to glucose

> Food sources: germinated grain (usually barley) fermented
> to produce malted products of cereal, beer, and other
> liquors

Lactose (also known as milk sugar)
Is less sweet than other sugars
Is produced only by mammals

---

and, alone, is not high in calories. (An average slice of bread contains approximately 65 calories.) Combinations of carbohydrate-rich rice and cooked dried beans can supply all the necessary protein cheaply and without many calories.

Fiber and sugar, both types of carbohydrates, have been the focus of much debate in recent years. Basically the cry is that sugar is bad, fiber is good. As in many areas of nutrition, debate and research continue; the answers are not yet clear. Certain facts, however, are known and worthwhile to review.

Fiber

Fiber, also called roughage or nature's broom, is the undigestible portion of edible plants that ends up in the large intestine after the body has digested and absorbed protein, fats, carbohydrates, vitamins, minerals, and water from these foods. Several types of fiber are found in foods: cellulose, hemicellulose, lignin, cutins, pectin, gums, mucilages, and algal substances.

Dietary fiber is important to both children and adults. Whole-grain breads and cereals, fruits, and vegetables — good sources of fiber — provide the necessary bulk that helps eliminate solid waste matter. In its role as a natural laxative, fiber absorbs water, softening the stool and making it easier to pass.

Table 2.9
POLYSACCHARIDES

Starch
Eventually is broken down to glucose

> Food sources: cereal grains, seeds, roots, potatoes

Glycogen (also known as animal starch)
Is the form in which animals and humans store carbohydrates (in the liver)

> Food sources: diet ordinarily contains none

Cellulose (one type of dietary fiber)
Is nondigestible in humans
Provides necessary bulk to the diet
Absorbs water (therefore has a laxative effect)

> Food sources: skins of fruits and vegetables, coverings of seeds and whole grains, legumes, and nuts

---

Fiber also is thought to be somewhat effective as an aid in weight loss. By absorbing water, fiber tends to make people feel full. In addition, fiber helps slow down the speed at which the stomach empties, so the full feeling lasts for a while. There also is some speculation that high-fiber foods require a lot of chewing, so people take more time to eat and therefore eat less.

The foods highest in fiber include whole grains, brown rice, legumes, seeds and nuts, and fruits and vegetables, as shown in Table 2.10. Cooking, canning, or freezing these foods does not significantly affect fiber levels. Foods that do *not* contribute fiber to the diet include meat, fish, eggs, milk and dairy products, fats, sugars, and most beverages.

There is no RDA for fiber; nor is there an Estimated Safe and Adequate Daily Dietary Intake level. Many physicians and registered dietitians, however, advise people to eat between 25 and 50 grams of dietary fiber daily, which is more than twice the average 10 to 20 grams that people in developed countries currently eat each day.

Although the benefits of fiber are many, adding too much fiber too fast can create problems. Excess fiber can cause gas, cramps, bloating, and diarrhea. The discomfort usually is temporary, however, as the body can adjust well to higher fiber lev-

Table 2.10
APPROXIMATE DIETARY FIBER CONTENT OF SELECTED FOODS

Food	Serving Size	Dietary Fiber (gm)
Fruits		
Apple, with peel	1 medium	2.41
Banana	1 medium	1.75
Grapefruit, canned	½ cup	0.53
Peaches, with skin	1 medium	2.28
Pears, with skin	1 medium	4.14
Strawberries, raw	10 large	2.12
canned	⅜ cup	1.00
Nuts		
Brazils	¼ cup	2.71
Peanuts	1 tbsp.	0.84
Peanut butter	1 tbsp.	1.13
Vegetables		
Broccoli, tops, boiled	½ cup	2.99
Brussels sprouts	½ cup	2.00
Cabbage	½ cup	2.07
Carrots, young, boiled	½ cup	2.78
Cauliflower	½ cup	1.13
Corn, sweet, cooked	1 medium ear	4.74
canned	½ cup	4.72
Legumes		
Beans, baked, canned	⅓ cup	6.18
Peas, frozen	½ cup	5.66
canned	½ cup	5.26
Lettuce, raw	½ cup	0.84
Onion, raw	one 2¼"	2.10
Peppers	½ cup	0.63
Potato	one 2¼"	3.51
Tomatoes, fresh	1 small	1.40
canned	½ cup	1.02
Turnips, raw	⅔ cup	1.89
Breads		
White	1 slice	0.63
Brown, Boston	1 slice	1.79
Whole wheat	1 slice	1.96

Table 2.10
Continued

Food	Serving Size	Dietary Fiber (gm)
Breakfast Cereals		
All Bran	¾ cup	11.20
Corn Flakes	¾ cup	2.09
Grape-nuts	¾ cup	5.88
Rice Krispies	¾ cup	0.94
Puffed Wheat	¾ cup	1.39
Shredded Wheat	1 biscuit	2.70
Special K	¾ cup	0.65
Weetabix	¾ cup	5.34

(Adapted from American Dietetic Association, *Handbook of Clinical Dietetics*, Yale University Press, New Haven, CT., 1981.)

els. A more serious problem with excessive amounts of fiber is that fiber can bind with iron, zinc, copper, magnesium, calcium, and chromium, preventing the body from absorbing these essential minerals. These problems do not occur with great frequency because of the low level of fiber in the average diet.

As a rule, gradually increasing the amount of fiber in the diet usually is a good idea. As Chapter 7 shows, however, going overboard with a high-fiber diet can cause problems for both children and adults.

Sugar

Sugar, today more than ever before, is the cause of great concern. In many respects, the concern is justified.

In recent years, honey, brown sugar, raw or crude sugar, and blackstrap molasses, have all been touted as being superior to regular white, cane, or beet sugar. The truth is that while impurities in these products may contribute some minerals to the diet, the amounts are not significant and hardly justify the higher cost of these sweeteners. Table 2.11 outlines the pros and cons of using these alternatives.

The advantages and disadvantages of concentrated forms of sugar, as shown in Table 2.12, apply to brown sugar, honey, raw

Table 2.11
ALTERNATIVE SWEETENERS:
Are They Really Superior to White Sugar?

Brown sugar	Made by adding a small amount of molasses to white sugar; *nutritionally equal to white sugar*
Honey	Sweeter, stickier, more expensive than white sugar; *nutritionally equal to white sugar*
Raw sugar	Darker, larger grounds, and much more expensive than white sugar; *nutritionally equal to white sugar*
Molasses	Formed as a byproduct of sucrose production; light molasses (first extraction) *is nutritionally equal to white sugar;* medium molasses (second extraction) contains 1.2 milligrams of iron in each tablespoon; and blackstrap molasses (third extraction) contains 2.3 grams of iron in each tablespoon

Table 2.12
CONCENTRATED SWEETS — GOOD AND BAD

Advantages	*Disadvantages*
• contribute carbohydrate calories to the diet • are a relatively inexpensive source of calories • are rapidly converted to glucose	• contribute only trace amounts (if any) of the other essential nutrients (thus, the term "empty calories" is frequently applied) • contain no bulk or fiber • contribute to tooth decay, which can directly affect overall health • are frequently consumed in excess, to the exclusion of essential nutrients such as protein, vitamins, and minerals

Sources: Candies, jellies, jams, marmalades, table sugar, brown sugar, raw sugar, honey, table syrup, maple syrup, molasses

sugar, and molasses, as well as white sugar. Like all forms of carbohydrate, sugar and all other sources of concentrated sweets provide 4 calories per gram.

Sugar is a major ingredient in many baked goods and desserts. Some, such as frosting or fudge, contain almost all sugar, while others, such as custard, muffins, or pies, contain sugar plus various combinations of milk, eggs, whole-grain flours, or fruits, which contribute some protein, fat, fiber, or essential vitamins and minerals to the diet.

Given these facts, parents must decide if and when sugars are appropriate additions to their children's diets. If children learn to enjoy wholesome food early in life, sweets might be added legitimately. In any event, they never should be added as a reward or bribe because children may reject foods that are good sources of vitamins, minerals, fiber, and protein in favor of sweets that are high in calories and low in nutrients.

Table 2.13 lists the sugar content of selected foods. The information is, at best, interesting; however, a wise parent will evaluate other nutrients provided by specific foods to determine their value in a child's diet. Most fruits, for example, consist of a high level of natural sugar; yet they also provide essential vitamins, minerals, and fiber. As a result these high-sugar fruits should be included in every diet every day.

FATS

Fats are another essential part of the diet. They are the most concentrated source of calories, providing 9 calories per gram. As a result they provide twice as much energy as protein and carbohydrates. Additionally, they provide and carry the fat-soluble vitamins — A, D, E, and K — and supply the essential fatty acids. Food sources of fat include butter, margarine, shortening, oil, salad dressings, and meats. Excess proteins and carbohydrates, which are not used by tissues, are rapidly converted to fat and stored as adipose (fat) tissue.

Basically, fats are divided into two categories: saturated and unsaturated. Saturated fats are those that generally harden at room temperature and almost always harden in the refrigerator.

Table 2.13
SUGAR CONTENT OF SELECTED FOODS

Food	Serving Size	Sugar (gm)	Sugar (tsp.)
Beverages			
Cola-type soft drinks	12 fl. oz.	40.7	10.2
Ginger ale	12 fl. oz.	29.0	7.25
Orange soda	12 fl. oz.	45.8	11.5
Kool-aid	8 fl. oz.	24.2	6.1
Lemonade, canned, frozen, mix	8 fl. oz.	22.5	5.6
Tang, orange	3 tsp. in 6 fl. oz. water	21.7	5.4
Candy and Candy Bars			
Chocolate chips	1 oz.	17.0	4.25
Chocolate-flavored chips	1 oz.	7.6	1.9
Milk chocolate	1.07 oz. bar	17.0	4.25
Milk chocolate, almonds	1 oz.	14.0	3.5
Peanut butter cups	1.6 oz.	21.0	5.25
Jelly beans	10	26.4	6.6
Lifesavers	1 each	2.4	0.6
Chewing gum	1 stick	2.4	0.6
Salt-water taffy	1 piece	2.4	0.6
Bubble gum	1 piece	4.0	1.0
Marshmallows	4 large	21.2	5.3
Cereals (all cup sizes are 1 ounce of cereal)			
Boo Berry	1 cup	13.0	3.25
40% Bran	¾ cup	5.0	1.25
Cheerios, regular	1¼ cup	1.0	0.25
Honey Nut	¾ cup	10.0	2.5
Cocoa Krispies	¾ cup	12.0	3.0
Corn Flakes	1 cup	2.0	0.5
Crazy Cow, choc./straw.	1 cup	12.0	3.0
Frankenberry	1 cup	13.0	3.3
Froot Loops	1 cup	13.0	3.3
Kaboom	1 cup	6.0	1.5
Puffed Rice or Wheat	1 cup	0.0	0.0
Raisin Bran	¾ cup	12.0	3.0
Rice Krispies	1 cup	3.0	0.75
Shredded Wheat	1 biscuit	0.0	0.0
Sugar Smacks	¾ cup	16.0	4.0
Total	1 cup	3.0	0.75
Trix	1 cup	12.0	3.0
Wheaties	1 cup	3.0	0.75

Table 2.13
Continued

Food	Serving Size	Sugar (gm)	Sugar (tsp.)
Desserts			
Pudding, instant, choc., lemon, vanilla	½ cup	26.5	6.6
Pudding pops, average for all flavors	1 pop	14.4	3.6
Toaster pastry	1 each	15.0	3.8
Twinkies	1 each	19.2	4.8
Fruits and Fruit Juices			
Apple	3½ oz.	9.9	2.5
Banana	3½ oz.	14.0	3.5
Blueberries	3½ oz.	5.8	1.45
Cantaloupe/honeydew	3½ oz.	11.1	2.78
Grapes	3½ oz.	13.6	3.4
Grapefruit	3½ oz.	6.8	1.7
Orange	3½ oz.	8.2	2.1
Peach	3½ oz.	6.7	1.68
Strawberries	3½ oz.	5.2	1.3

(Adapted from Pennington, Jean A. T., and Church, H. N., *Bowes and Church's Food Values of Portions Commonly Used*, Fourteenth Edition. Philadelphia: J. B. Lippincott Company, 1985.)

Table 2.14 provides a list of the most common sources of saturated fat in the average diet.

Unsaturated fats are further divided into monounsaturated and polyunsaturated fats. Of these, polyunsaturated fats are the most important. Polyunsaturated fats are from vegetable sources and are usually liquid at room temperature. Unlike saturated fats, polyunsaturated fats actually help the body get rid of excess, newly formed cholesterol.

Table 2.15 provides a list of the common sources of polyunsaturated fat in the diet.

Saturated fats tend to raise blood cholesterol levels.

Table 2.14
SATURATED FAT SOURCES

Animal sources	Meats — beef, veal, lamb, pork, ham
	Dairy products — butter, whole milk, cream, cheese made from whole milk or cream
Other sources	"Hydrogenated" (hardened) fats, such as most margarines and shortening, coconut oil, cocoa butter, palm oil, palm kernel oil

Table 2.15
POLYUNSATURATED FAT SOURCES

Vegetable oils	Safflower, sunflower, corn, soybean, cottonseed
Note:	Peanut oil and olive oil are not high in polyunsaturated fats

Polyunsaturated fats tend to lower blood cholesterol levels

Wise shopping is the key to buying the best oils and margarines. LABELS MUST BE READ CAREFULLY. Labels of many hydrogenated fats will declare they are low in cholesterol. While this is true, the process used to harden them puts them into the saturated-fat category. Some margarine labels will state, "partially hydrogenated." This may be acceptable if they contain *twice* as much polyunsaturated fat as saturated fat. Preference should be given to cooking fats, margarines, and salad dressings made from the recommended polyunsaturated oils. Table 2.16 compares the polyunsaturated and saturated fat content of vegetable oils.

Parents who are in doubt about the polyunsaturated content of the oil they use may want to try the refrigerator test:

THE REFRIGERATOR TEST

Place a small amount of cooking oil in a glass and place this in the refrigerator for at least an hour. The portion that solidifies represents the saturated fat in that type of oil. If more than half has solidified, think about switching from the oil you commonly use to one that has a higher percentage of polyunsaturated fat.

As mentioned previously, fats also provide essential fatty acids. Although there are three essential fatty acids (linoleic, linolenic, and arachidonic), only linoleic cannot be made by the body. Linoleic acid is absolutely necessary; when deficiencies arise, growth retardation, dermatitis, and faulty use and deposition of fats occurs.

Adults require approximately 1 to 2 percent of their daily calories from linoleic acid, which is found in corn, safflower, and soybean oils. Babies especially require sufficient quantities of linoleic acid to prevent growth retardation and skin problems. Human milk, the standard for nutritional values for infants, contains 7 percent of its calories as linoleic acid, while most formulas contain 10 percent and cow's milk contains 1 percent. This low level of linoleic acid in cow's milk is one of the important reasons infants should not be fed unmodified cow's milk alone. Also, skim and low-fat milk do not provide adequate linoleic acid and should not be given to children younger than 2 years.

In addition to providing calories and linoleic acid, dietary fats serve vital functions in growing children. Because fats are absorbed slowly, children may not feel hungry too quickly after a meal that contains fats. Other nutrients eaten at the same time will pass slowly through the gastrointestinal tract and will be available for absorption for a prolonged period of time. Including fats in the breakfast may lead to a feeling of satiety throughout the morning. When a child is fed a breakfast with no fats, such as cereal with skim milk, hunger probably will set in again within a few hours.

Body fat is the storage depot for energy. Thus, body fat is available as a source of energy when there is little food or during serious illness. In addition, body fat supports and cushions vital organs; provides insulation from heat and cold; provides oils to

Table 2.16
COMPARISON OF COMMON COOKING OILS

Vegetable Oil	Polyunsaturated Fat Content (%)	Saturated Fat Content (%)	Ratio P:S
The Best			
*Safflower oil	74	9	7.1:1
Sunflower oil	64	10	5.8:1
*Corn oil	58	13	4.3:1
*Soybean oil	58	15	3.9:1
Mediocre			
Cotton seed oil	52	29	1.8:1
Peanut oil	35	20	1.8:1
Olive oil	15	16	0.9:1
The Worst			
Palm oil	2	81	0.1:1
Coconut oil	2	86	0.1:1

*Best sources of the essential fatty acid linoleic.

skin and hair; and functions in the transport and absorption of fat-soluble vitamins.

Cholesterol

Cholesterol, often thought of as a fat, is not a fat itself. It is, however, related to fats. Cholesterol, found in dairy products, egg yolks, and red meats, is not in itself bad. In fact, it is involved in converting vitamin D to a useful form, and it is required for normal body function. It is an important structural part of all cells, especially brain and nerve cells, and is an intermediary in the synthesis of many hormones. The liver manufactures cholesterol; therefore, it does not have to be eaten. Most people in developed countries, however, eat more than 600 milligrams of cholesterol a day, even though 300 milligrams has been suggested as the maximum daily requirement. Saturated fat or cholesterol in excess can accumulate in the arteries and lead to heart attacks and strokes.

Although studies show that infants fed on breast milk have higher cholesterol levels in their blood than children fed formulas, by 3 or 4 years of age their cholesterol levels are the same.

Several studies have further indicated that moderate — not low — intakes of cholesterol in babies help develop regulatory mechanisms for cholesterol metabolism in adulthood. For these reasons, *cholesterol should not be restricted in the diets of infants, and only moderately restricted in young children's diets.* By the time a child has reached adolescence, however, cholesterol should be limited to 300 milligrams daily. Table 2.17 shows the amount of cholesterol in common foods.

CALORIES

The ability of the body to do work and operate all its systems is dependent upon energy production. Just as a light bulb will not burn without electricity, a body cannot function without energy. The energy for the body is supplied by calories.

Calories are units of heat measurement. A calorie is scientifically defined as the amount of heat required to raise the temperature of one gram of water one degree centigrade at sea level. Calories are a measure of the amount of energy available from the food people eat. Calories from food provide the energy the body needs for smooth functioning of the muscles, brain, nerves, and the production of tissue, blood, and bones.

As Table 2.18 shows, calories, or energy, come only from the three nutrients discussed above — protein, carbohydrates, and fats. Vitamins, minerals, and water contain no calories.

The number of calories infants, children, adolescents, and adults require each day varies according to a number of factors:

AGE: children of all ages need more calories per pound of body weight than adults because the energy requirement for growth is substantial;

SIZE: larger people require more total calories;

SEX: men, in general, need more calories than women;

HEALTH: people need more calories during certain illnesses, when they have a fever, or after surgery;

PHYSICAL ACTIVITY: when more energy is expended, as during growth or strenuous activity, more calories are required;

PREGNANCY: pregnant women and women who are nursing require additional calories.

Table 2.17
CHOLESTEROL COMPARISONS OF SELECTED FOODS

Food	Serving Size	Cholesterol (mg)
Egg, chicken, whole	1 each	275
Egg substitute, frozen	¼ cup	1
Milk, whole (3.5% fat)	1 cup	34
low fat (2% fat)	1 cup	18
(1% fat)	1 cup	10
skim	1 cup	4
buttermilk	1 cup	9
Cheese		
Cheddar	1 oz.	30
Cottage (4% fat)	½ cup	16
(2% fat)	½ cup	10
(1% fat)	½ cup	5
Cream cheese	2 tbsp.	31
Ricotta, part skim	½ cup	38
American	1 oz.	27
American, cheese food	1 oz.	18
Yogurt, plain, whole milk	1 cup	29
low-fat	1 cup	14
skim	1 cup	4
Butter	1 tbsp.	36
Margarine	1 tbsp.	0
Ice cream, vanilla (10% fat)	1 cup	59
Ice milk, vanilla	1 cup	18
Cream, heavy, whipping	1 tbsp.	21
medium	1 tbsp.	13
light	1 tbsp.	10
half and half	1 tbsp.	6
sour	1 tbsp.	5
Beef, lean	3 oz.	60
Veal	3 oz.	77
Pork	3 oz.	60
Ham, smoked, cooked	3 oz.	51
Chicken, turkey (without skin)	3 oz.	79
Liver, chicken	3 oz.	540
calf, fried	3 oz.	375
Hot dog, beef (30% fat)	1 each	22
Bologna, beef	1 oz. (1 slice)	13
Canadian bacon	1 oz.	12

Table 2.17
Continued

Food	Serving Size	Cholesterol (mg)
Fish	3 oz.	40
Shellfish		
Lobster	3 oz.	171
Shrimp	3 oz.	130
Tuna, canned, light, in water	3 oz.	51

(Adapted from Pennington, Jean A. T., and Church, H. N., *Bowes and Church's Food Values of Portions Commonly Used*, Fourteenth Edition. Philadelphia: J. B. Lippincott Company, 1985.)

Table 2.18
CALORIE CONTENT OF NUTRIENTS

1 gram of protein	= 4 calories
1 gram of carbohydrate	= 4 calories
1 gram of fat	= 9 calories
Vitamins	= 0 calories
Minerals	= 0 calories
Water	= 0 calories

Table 2.19 provides guidelines for caloric intake. These guidelines are based on *average* weights for each age group and assumed energy expenditure. *Any individual child may vary normally from these averages.*

One pound of body fat equals 3,500 calories. If a person eats fewer calories than needed for daily activity, then the body draws energy from the fat cells. If 3,500 calories are taken from the fat cells, the result is a one-pound weight loss. Conversely, if a person eats more calories than needed for activity, these extra calories are stored as fat cells. For every 3,500 calories stored the body gains one pound of fat.

Table 2.19
RECOMMENDED CALORIE INTAKE

	Age (years)	Weight (lbs)	Height (in)	Calorie Needs	
				Average	Range
Infants	birth–½	13	24	690	570–870
	½–1	20	28	945	720–1215
Children	1–3	29	35	1300	900–1800
	4–6	44	44	1700	1300–2300
	7–10	62	52	2400	1650–3300
Males	11–14	99	62	2700	2000–3900
	15–18	145	69	2800	2100–3900
	19–22	154	70	2900	2500–3300
	23–50	154	70	2700	2300–3100
	51–75	154	70	2400	2000–2800
	76+	154	70	2050	1650–2450
Females	11–14	101	62	2200	1500–3000
	15–18	120	64	2100	1200–3000
	19–22	120	64	2100	1700–2500
	23–50	120	64	2000	1600–2400
	51–75	120	64	1800	1400–2200
	76+	120	64	1600	1200–2000
Pregnant				+300	
Lactating				+500	

(Adapted from *Recommended Dietary Allowances*, "Mean Heights and Weights and Recommended Energy Intake," Food and Nutrition Board, National Academy of Sciences — National Research Council, Washington, D.C., 1980.)

VITAMINS

Vitamins are organic (i.e., carbon-containing) compounds that are found in both plants and animals; therefore, they occur in all foods. Only small amounts are needed to regulate the body's metabolism — the complex chemical and physical processes that maintain human life. Vitamins have no caloric value, yet they are essential for normal body functions, growth, and good health. In addition to regulating metabolism, they are active in the conversion of fat and carbohydrates to energy, and they help to form bones and tissues. Vitamins always work together with other food elements; they are *not* substitutes for protein, carbo-hydrates, or fats.

Vitamins, which occur in such minute concentrations that they were not named as a separate food component until 1912, are divided into two groups: fat-soluble vitamins (A, D, E, and K) and water-soluble vitamins (the eight B vitamins and vitamin C). Fat-soluble vitamins need dietary fat and bile salts (excreted from the liver and gall bladder to break down fat into a form that permits its absorption) so that they can be absorbed through the wall of the intestine and then be distributed and stored in the body. Because they can be stored in body fat, fat-soluble vitamins do not have to be eaten daily. This also means that if too much of these vitamins are taken, they can accumulate and cause illness. Vitamins A and D, in particular, are harmful if taken in excess. (See Chapter 7 for further discussion of the potentially dangerous effects of megavitamin dosages.)

Any disorder that interferes with the absorption of the fat-soluble vitamins can lead to deficiencies. For example, diseases that prevent the proper digestion of fat or a lack of bile salts can cause fat-soluble vitamins to go unabsorbed. In addition, excessive intake of mineral oil can lead to fat-soluble vitamin deficiencies. Table 2.20 reviews the functions and sources of, as well as the risks involved in taking, fat-soluble vitamins.

Water-soluble vitamins are not stored in body tissues and rarely are found at dangerously high levels. Excess amounts of water-soluble vitamins are excreted in the urine. These vitamins must be provided in the diet on a daily basis. Water-soluble vitamins are more likely to be destroyed by overprocessing and improper preparation and storage of foods than are the fat-soluble vitamins. For example, water-soluble vitamins leach out into cooking water and often are poured down the drain. In addition, extreme heat and light can destroy the water-soluble vitamins. Table 2.21 reviews the functions and sources of, as well as the risks involved in taking, the water-soluble vitamins.

Vitamin deficiencies are rare in this country. Foods rich in vitamins are milk fortified with vitamins A and D; eggs; dark green, leafy vegetables; fruits; and, for the B vitamins especially, whole-grain and enriched cereals and breads. Any child eating such foods regularly should be receiving enough vitamins.

Table 2.20
THE FAT-SOLUBLE VITAMINS

				Risks	
Vitamin	RDA	Best Food Sources	Needed For	Too Little, Too Long	Too Much, Too Long
A	Infants: 400–420 μg RE* Children: 400–1000 μg RE Adults: 800–1000 μg RE	Eggs; liver; yellow fruits and vegetables; dark green, leafy vegetables; butter; fish-liver oils	Healthy skin; night and color vision; proper bone growth; tooth development; growth and repair of tissues	Night blindness; retarded growth; rough, dry skin; dry eyes	Hair loss; dry skin; headaches; fatigue; irritability; joint and bone pain; abnormal growth in children; liver damage
D (the "sunshine" vitamin)	Infants and children: 10 μg or 400 IU** Adults: 5–10 μg or 200–400 IU	Fortified milk; egg yolk; fish-liver oils; butter; tuna; salmon; sardines; shrimp	Regulation of calcium and phosphorus absorption; proper bone mineralization; proper tooth formation	Rickets in children; osteomalacia (bone softens and shortens, increasing the likelihood of fractures and stooped posture) in adults; muscular weakness; muscle twitching	Calcium deposits in kidneys and high blood calcium levels in infants; widespread calcium deposits; nausea; vomiting; anorexia; high blood pressure; high cholesterol

E (alpha tocopherol)	Infants: 3–4 mg αTE*** or 4.5–6 IU Children: 5–10 mg αTE or 7.5–15 IU Adults: 8–10 mg αTE or 12–15 IU	Vegetable oils; margarine; wheat germ; whole-grain cereals and breads; soy beans; raw or sprouted seeds; sweet potatoes; nuts	Formation of muscles, red blood cells and other tissues; prevents oxygen injury to tissues	Deficiency extremely rare in people	Headache, skin rash, blurred vision, fatigue and weakness reported, but no definite symptoms of excess are known
K (antihemorrhaging vitamin)	No RDA Estimated safe and adequate intake: Infants: 10–20 μg Children: 15–100 μg Adults: 70–140 μg	Green leafy vegetables; (this vitamin is made in the human intestine, except in newborns)	Blood clotting; maintenance of normal bone metabolism	Hemorrhages (especially in newborn infants)	Jaundice in babies because of breakdown of red blood cells

*RE = Retinal Equivalents

**IU = International Units

***αTE = Alpha Tocopherol Equivalents

Table 2.21
THE WATER-SOLUBLE VITAMINS

Vitamin	RDA	Best Food Sources	Needed For	Risks	
				Too Little, Too Long	Too Much, Too Long
B₁ (Thiamin, the antiberiberi vitamin)	Infants: 0.3–0.5 mg Children: 0.7–1.4 mg Adults: 1.0–1.5 mg	Whole-grain and enriched cereals and breads; brewer's yeast; nuts and seeds; liver; soybeans	Breakdown of carbohydrates for energy; growth and repair of tissue; maintenance of nervous system, heart, muscles, and intestines	Confusion; muscle weakness; leg cramps; swelling of the heart (disease called beriberi)	None known
B₂ (Riboflavin)	Infants: 0.4–0.6 mg Children: 0.8–1.7 mg Adults: 1.2–1.7 mg	Liver; brewer's yeast; milk, cottage cheese, yogurt; eggs; whole-grain and enriched cereals and breads	Breakdown of carbohydrates, proteins, and fats for energy; growth and repair of tissue	Skin disorders, including cracks around lips and corners of the mouth; sensitivity to light	None known
B₃ (Niacin, the antipellagra vitamin)	Infants: 6–8 mg NE* Children: 9–18 mg NE Adults: 13–19 mg NE	Liver; whole-grain and enriched cereals and breads; potatoes; brewer's yeast; brown rice; peanut butter	Breakdown of carbohydrates, proteins, and fats for energy (in conjunction with thiamin and riboflavin)	Skin disorders; diarrhea; confusion; irritability; mouth swelling, smooth tongue (pellagra)	Duodenal ulcer; elevated blood-sugar levels; gouty arthritis; abnormal heart beats; "flushing" or burning, itching skin

Vitamin	Amounts	Sources	Functions	Deficiency symptoms
B₆ (Pyridoxine)	Infants: 0.3–0.6 mg Children: 0.9–2.0 mg Adults: 2.0–2.2 mg	Whole-grain (not enriched) cereals and breads; bananas and other fruits; seeds and nuts	Carbohydrate, protein, and fat absorption and metabolism; absorption of vitamin B₁₂; formation of red blood cells	Skin disorders — dermatitis, eczema; sore mouth, lips and tongue; dizziness; nausea; anemia; convulsions; insomnia; cramps; tingling; numbness	Nervous-system disorders; high-dose dependency can occur — when reduced to normal levels, deficiency symptoms can occur
B₁₂ (Cobalamin)	Infants: 0.5–1.5 μg Children: 2.0–3.0 μg Adults: 3.0 μg	Liver; milk; yogurt; eggs; cottage cheese	Carbohydrate, protein, and fat metabolism; red blood cell production; formation of genetic material (RNA and DNA)	Pernicious anemia	None known

Table 2.21
Continued

Vitamin	RDA	Best Food Sources	Needed For	Risks — Too Little, Too Long	Risks — Too Much, Too Long
Biotin	No RDA Estimated safe and adequate intake: Infants: 35–50 µg Children: 65–200 µg Adults: 100–200 µg	Liver; egg yolks; nuts; dark green, leafy vegetables	Formation of fatty acids; release of energy from carbohydrates	None known, except where large amounts of *raw* egg whites (which can destroy biotin) are consumed — in these cases, loss of appetite; nausea; pallor; anemia; eczema; fatigue; confusion; depression; and hair loss may result	None known
Folic acid (Folate or folacin)	Infants: 30–45 µg Children: 100–400 µg Adults: 400 µg	Wheat germ; avocado; fruits; eggs; cheese; milk; dark green, leafy vegetables	Formation of genetic material (RNA and DNA) with vitamin B_{12}; red blood cell formation; protein metabolism	Anemias: macrocytic and megaloblastic; large red blood cells; smooth tongue; diarrhea; poor growth; impaired absorption of all nutrients; pernicious anemia during pregnancy	None known

Vitamin	RDA / Intake	Best Sources	Functions	Deficiency Symptoms	Toxicity / Excess
Pantothenic acid	No RDA Estimated safe and adequate intake: Infants: 2–3 mg Children: 3–7 mg Adults: 4–7 mg	Liver; cabbage; cauliflower; avocado; eggs; whole-grain cereals and breads; nuts and seeds	Release of energy for carbohydrates, proteins, and fats; formation of hormones; nerve function; synthesis of cholesterol, steroids, and fatty acids	None known, except in experiments: fatigue; abdominal cramping; muscular weakness; insomnia; muscle cramps; tingling or burning feet	None known
C (ascorbic acid)	Infants: 35 mg Children: 45–60 mg Adults: 60 mg	Fruits and vegetables: guava, black currants, red pepper, broccoli, brussels sprouts, green pepper, cantaloupe, strawberries, mango, cauliflower, tomatoes, oranges, grapefruit, potatoes, dark green, leafy vegetables	Formation of collagen (substance that holds cells together); strengthening all connective tissue, skin, bones, teeth, muscles, tendons, cartilage, and capillaries; protecting vitamins A, E, B_1, B_2, pantothenic acid, and folic acid from combining with oxygen	Scurvy: weakness; bleeding gums; fatigue; bleeding into joints and skin; aching bones, joints, muscles; poor wound healing; irritability; poor appetite, weight loss	Dependency on high doses (especially in infants if megadoses are taken during pregnancy); withdrawal symptoms mirror scurvy; may induce B_{12} deficiency

*NE = Niacin Equivalents   1 NE = 1 mg of niacin

Parents should not give infants or children vitamin supplements without consulting a pediatrician, for they usually are not required. Vitamin supplements should not be used as substitutes for vitamins that can be obtained from food. (Contrary to belief, when vitamin supplements are recommended, taking them before meals will *not* stimulate the appetite; nor will they curb hunger.) Some situations in which a physician may recommend supplementation include:

Vitamin D supplements of 400 IU are often prescribed for breast-fed infants up to the age of 6 months, as breast milk contains little vitamin D. After 6 months, other foods that contain vitamin D — e.g., fortified milk — usually are added to the diet. A significant source of vitamin D for all children is sunlight, which can be relied upon as an adequate source after 1 year of age. Because too much vitamin D can be toxic (see Table 2.20), supplements should be given only if the child is not receiving vitamin D elsewhere.

Vitamin B_{12} supplements are essential if parents insist that their children follow a vegetarian diet that excludes meat, milk, eggs, and all other food from animal sources. This type of diet is inadequate and dangerous for growing children; parents should not place their children on such a strict vegetarian diet (see Chapter 7 for further discussion). B_{12} is necessary to prevent pernicious anemia, a disorder resulting in faulty red blood cell formation.

Vitamin C (ascorbic acid) supplements may be needed by infants fed an evaporated milk formula. Much has been written about the powers of large amounts of vitamin C to prevent and cure the common cold; no conclusive evidence yet exists to support or refute those theories.

One potential danger of taking megadoses of vitamin C is that the body becomes accustomed to excreting the excess. When less is taken, the body continues to excrete large amounts and becomes deficient in vitamin C. Pregnant women should not take megadoses of vitamin C because it is transferred to the infant, who then becomes deficient after birth when no longer receiving large quantities.

B_1, thiamin, is required in extra amounts during periods of physical and mental stress, fever, exercise, and pregnancy. The amount needed generally increases when more carbohydrates are eaten.

B_6 is needed in increased amounts as more protein is eaten because it aids in metabolism.

Vitamin E is needed when more polyunsaturated fats are eaten because it helps to prevent the oxidation of polyunsaturated fatty acids.

In general, the way to provide children with adequate vitamins is to provide them with a varied diet. Overcooking should be avoided, particularly when cooking in water. Steaming vegetables is a good way to retain vitamins. Refrigeration and freezing also preserve vitamins in many fruits and vegetables. (See Chapter 10 for specific information on how to prepare and store food to preserve vitamin content.)

MINERALS

Minerals are inorganic (non-carbon-containing) substances which, like vitamins, are required in relatively small amounts and yet are vitally important to good health. The major minerals (macrominerals) — calcium, phosphorus, magnesium, sulfur, sodium, potassium, and chloride — comprise 4 to 5 percent of the body's weight.

Microminerals, or trace minerals or elements — iron, zinc, iodine, copper, manganese, fluoride, chromium, selenium, molybdenum, and cobalt — make up only 0.01 percent of the total body weight. Only a few milligrams or micrograms of these are needed each day. In addition, tin, nickel, arsenic, vanadium, silicon, and cadmium may be essential trace minerals, but insufficient information is available to establish appropriate levels. Although macrominerals are needed in far greater amounts and compose a larger percentage of body weight, microminerals are equally important to growth and good health.

Most of the details parents need to know about individual minerals — what their function is, how much is required, and in what foods they are found — are included in Tables 2.22 and 2.23.

Some minerals and some mineral groups, however, require additional discussion.

Calcium, Phosphorus, and Magnesium

Together these three minerals compose 98 percent of the body's mineral content. Although their functions vary, as Table 2.22 shows, they are essential in the formation and maintenance of bones and teeth.

Calcium is particularly important for growing children, adolescents, and pregnant or nursing mothers. Calcium is required throughout life because bone calcium is replaced approximately every five years, and because this mineral is important for maintenance of body fluids, nerves, and muscle cells. The richest sources of calcium are milk and other dairy products, as Table 2.24 shows.

For children who have allergies to milk, or adults who cannot drink or do not like milk and dairy products, calcium is available from other sources. These are listed in Table 2.25.

When the dietary supply of calcium is insufficient, calcium will be released from bones to maintain correct blood levels. This process causes rickets in children and contributes to osteoporosis (bone loss) in elderly people.

When food cannot meet calcium needs, such as when breast feeding and eating insufficient amounts of dairy products, or when children refuse to eat most dietary sources of calcium, a physician may recommend calcium supplements. While supplements should not replace dietary sources, they often are used to enhance or increase the level of daily calcium. There are several different calcium supplements on the market that contain various amounts of calcium. Most supplements contain calcium carbonate, calcium lactate, or calcium gluconate. Calcium carbonate, which contains about 40 percent calcium, has the most calcium per tablet, and calcium gluconate, which contains only 9 percent calcium, has one of the lowest calcium levels. The body, however, absorbs all these forms of calcium equally well, so the type of supplements should depend on how much cal-

Table 2.22
THE MACROMINERALS

Mineral	RDA	Best Food Sources	Needed For	Risks		
				Too Little, Too Long	Too Much, Too Long	
Calcium	Infants: 360–540 mg Children: 800–1200 mg Adults: 800 mg	Dairy products; sardines and salmon with bones; collards (see Tables 2.23 and 2.24)	Building and maintaining bones and teeth; normal growth; absorption of vitamin B_{12}; blood clotting; muscle contractions	Children: distorted bone growth (rickets) Adults: osteoporosis (porous, fragile bones)	Impaired absorption of iron, zinc, and manganese; calcium deposits throughout the body; fatigue	
Phosphorus	Infants: 240–360 mg Children: 800–1200 mg Adults: 800 mg	Brewer's yeast; calves' liver; milk, cheese, yogurt; seeds and nuts; tofu; bran	Building bones and teeth; carbohydrate, fat, and protein metabolism; growth and repair of tissue; storage and release of energy; transmitting nerve impulses and maintaining healthy nerves	Rare, however, loss of appetite; weakness; malaise; poor bone and teeth formation; muscle cramps, joint pain may occur if deficiency is prolonged	Imbalance of calcium-phosphorus ratio can lead to calcium deficiency	
Magnesium	Infants: 50–70 mg Children: 150–400 mg Adults: 300–350 mg	Whole grains; nuts and seeds; dark green, leafy vegetables	Building bones; transmission of nerve impulses; regulation of body temperature; use of vitamins B, C, and E; metabolism of calcium, phosphorus, sodium, and potassium	Muscle tremors or twitching; muscle weakness or cramps; insomnia; irregular heartbeat; abnormal calcium deposits	Especially in people with kidney disease: disturbed nervous-system function from unbalanced calcium-magnesium ratio	

Table 2.22
Continued

Mineral	RDA	Best Food Sources	Needed For	Too Little, Too Long	Too Much, Too Long
					Risks
Sulfur	No RDA No estimated safe and adequate intake	Meat, fish, poultry; eggs, milk; legumes, nuts	A component of thiamin and biotin; proper function of enzymes; detoxification of compounds that may otherwise be toxic to the body	Very rare	None known
(The Electrolytes) Sodium	No RDA Estimated safe and adequate intake: Infants: 115–750 mg Children: 325–2700 mg Adults: 1100–3300 mg	Table salt (sodium chloride); foods processed with sodium (see Tables 2.25 and 2.26)	Proper fluid and electrolyte balance (with potassium); maintaining proper calcium and phosphorus for proper heart function; regulation of acid-base balance	Nausea; muscular weakness; muscle cramps; headache; low blood pressure; seizures; coma (may be experienced when excessive loss occurs as in excessive sweating, diarrhea, or certain kidney disorders)	Swelling of hands, feet and other areas of the body (edema); muscle cramps (as a result of potassium loss); high blood pressure; heart disease

Potassium	No RDA Estimated safe and adequate intake: Infants: 350–1275 mg Children: 550–4575 mg Adults: 1875–5625 mg	Fruits and vegetables, especially baked potato, cantaloupe, avocado, lima beans, soybeans, banana, mango, broccoli; whole grains; blackstrap molasses; brewer's yeast; seeds and nuts; meats; dairy products	Proper fluid and electrolyte balance; muscle contraction; transmission of nerve impulses; release of energy for carbohydrates, protein, and fat; maintaining normal heartbeat	Abnormal heart rhythm; muscular weakness; cramps; fatigue; insomnia; indigestion or constipation (may be experienced when excessive loss occurs as in diarrhea, certain kidney disorders)	High blood potassium levels causing muscular paralysis, and/or abnormal heart rhythm
Chloride	No RDA Estimated safe and adequate intake: Infants: 275–1200 mg Children: 500–4200 mg Adults: 1700–5100 mg	Table salt	Balance of body fluids, acids, and bases; activation of enzyme in saliva; production of necessary stomach acid (hydrochloric acid)	Very rare	Disturbed acid-base balance

Table 2.23
THE TRACE MINERALS

Mineral	RDA	Best Food Sources	Needed For	Risks	
				Too Little, Too Long	*Too Much, Too Long*
Iron	Infants: 10–15 mg Children: 10–18 mg Adults: 10–18 mg	Liver; red meat; tofu; brewer's yeast; blackstrap molasses; dark green, leafy vegetables; dried fruits	Formation of hemoglobin (iron-containing part of red blood cell that carries oxygen to lungs)	Anemia with fatigue, weakness, paleness, and shortness of breath; lowered resistance to infection	Toxic iron buildup in heart, liver, and pancreas
Fluoride	No RDA Estimated safe and adequate intake: Infants: 0.1–1.0 mg Children: 0.5–2.5 mg Adults: 1.5–4.0 mg	Fluoridated water; any foods grown or cooked with fluoridated water; seafoods	Formation of strong, decay-resistant teeth; maintenance of strong bones	Excessive tooth decay; osteoporosis (porous, brittle bones)	Mottled teeth; brittle bones
Copper	No RDA Estimated safe and adequate intake: Infants: 0.5–1.0 mg Children: 1.0–3.0 mg Adults: 2.0–3.0 mg	Oysters; nuts and seeds; legumes; oatmeal; mushrooms; milk	Allows iron to be absorbed and used for hemoglobin formation; protein metabolism	Unknown; however, may result in anemia because of poor iron absorption; loss of hair; skeletal defects	Nausea, vomiting, diarrhea; headache; weakness; metallic taste (cooking acidic foods in unlined copper pots can lead to excess)
Zinc	Infants: 3–5 mg Children: 10–15 mg Adults: 15 mg	Wheat germ; liver; eggs; nuts; whole grains; oatmeal; ricotta cheese; chickpeas; lentils	Formation of RNA and DNA; is part of many, many enzymes; absorption of B vitamins and use of vitamin A; normal bone formation and development of the fetus	Fetus: abnormal brain development Children: growth failure; failure to mature sexually; loss of appetite; delayed wound healing; skin rash; diarrhea	Nausea, vomiting, abdominal pain; fever; premature birth; stillbirth; may cause atherosclerosis; copper deficiency; iron deficiency; increased need for vitamin A

Mineral	Recommended intake	Food sources	Function	Deficiency symptoms	Excess symptoms
Iodine	Infants: 40–50 µg; Children: 70–150 µg; Adults: 150 µg	Seafood; iodized table salt	Production of thyroid hormones (thyroxine and triiodothyronine) which regulate metabolism, energy production, and growth rate	Adults: goiter (enlarged thyroid and reduced hormone production) Newborns (whose mothers were deficient): retarded growth; mental retardation; protruding abdomen; swollen features	Not known, but iodine poisoning may occur
Chromium	No RDA Estimated safe and adequate intake: Infants: 0.01–0.06 mg; Children: 0.02–0.2 mg; Adults: 0.05–0.2 mg	Whole-grain breads and cereals; cheese; brewer's yeast; meat; dried beans; peanuts	Metabolism of glucose	Possibility of abnormal sugar metabolism	Not known
Manganese	No RDA Estimated safe and adequate intake: Infants: 0.5–1.0 mg; Children: 1.0–5.0 mg; Adults: 2.5–5.0 mg	Wheat germ; fruits; oatmeal; nuts; brown rice	Nervous system function; normal bone structure; reproduction; lactation; vitamin B_{12} activation; cholesterol formation (part of many enzymes that metabolize carbohydrates, protein, and fat)	Not known in humans, but in animals retarded growth; abnormal bone development; digestive disturbances; birth defects	Adverse effects to central nervous system — weakness, blurred speech, spastic gait

Table 2.23
Continued

Mineral	RDA	Best Food Sources	Needed For	Risks	
				Too Little, Too Long	*Too Much, Too Long*
Molybdenum	No RDA Estimated safe and adequate intake: Infants: 0.03–0.08 mg Children: 0.05–0.3 mg Adults: 0.15–0.5 mg	Whole grains; legumes; liver; kidney	Mobilization of iron for the liver (as part of the enzyme xanthine oxidase)	Not known in humans	Goutlike symptoms; copper deficiency; diarrhea; anemia; slowed growth
Selenium	No RDA Estimated safe and adequate intake: Infants: 0.01–0.06 mg Children: 0.02–0.2 mg Adults: 0.05–0.2 mg	Seafoods; liver; whole grains; meats; egg yolks; garlic	Preventing breakdown of fats and other body chemicals (works closely with vitamin E)	Cardiomyopathy (disease of heart muscle); abnormal white blood cell function	Stiffness; hair loss; blindness; abdominal pain; depression; lung disease; garlic odor to breath
Cobalt (a constituent of vitamin B_{12})	No RDA No estimated safe and adequate intake (See vitamin B_{12} Table 2.21)	Liver; poultry; milk; eggs; yogurt	See vitamin B_{12}, Table 2.21	See vitamin B_{12}, Table 2.21	See vitamin B_{12}, Table 2.21

Table 2.24
CALCIUM-RICH FOODS

Food	Serving Size	Calcium (mg)
Milk, whole (3.5% fat)	8 oz.	288
2% fat, protein fortified	8 oz.	352
1% fat, protein fortified	8 oz.	349
2% fat	8 oz.	297
1% fat	8 oz.	300
skim (nonfat)	8 oz.	302
Yogurt, plain, low-fat (with nonfat dry milk)	1 cup	415
whole milk	1 cup	274
fruit flavored	1 cup	314
Cottage cheese (2% fat)	1 cup	155
Cheese		
Ricotta (part skim)	½ cup	337
American	1 oz.	174
Cheddar	1 oz.	204
Ice cream (10% fat/ice milk)	½ cup	88

(Adapted from Pennington, Jean A. T., and Church, H. N., *Bowes and Church's Food Values of Portions Commonly Used*, Fourteenth Edition. Philadelphia: J. B. Lippincott Company, 1985.)

cium is needed, how many tablets must be taken daily, how well they can be tolerated, and their price. Table 2.26 provides more information on the various types of calcium supplements.

Vitamin D is required for calcium absorption and is added to some supplements as well as most pasteurized milks. The absorption of calcium also is enhanced by vitamin C. Moreover, when the body needs more calcium, it absorbs it more efficiently.

Other conditions prevent the efficient absorption of calcium: too much fat, particularly saturated fats; too much protein; oxalic acid, found in spinach, chard, beet greens, and rhubarb; lack of exercise; and stress. Extra calcium may be necessary when any of these factors exists.

Phosphorus is required in amounts approximately equal to calcium. If large quantities of phosphorus are consumed, more

Table 2.25
ALTERNATIVE CALCIUM SOURCES

Food	Serving Size	Calcium (mg)
Sardines, with bones	3 oz.	372
Salmon, fresh, cooked	3 oz.	355
Collards, raw	½ cup	179
Collards, frozen	½ cup	149
Tofu, calcium sulfate processed	4 oz.	145
Bok choy	½ cup	126
Turnip greens, fresh	½ cup	126
Oysters, raw	7–9	113
Kale, raw	½ cup	103
Shrimp, canned	3 oz.	99
Turnip greens, frozen	½ cup	98
Mustard greens	½ cup	97
Beans, dried, cooked	1 cup	90
Kale, frozen	½ cup	79

(Adapted from Pennington, Jean A. T., and Church, H. N., *Bowes and Church's Food Values of Portions Commonly Used*, Fourteenth Edition. Philadelphia: J. B. Lippincott Company, 1985. Also from Adams, Catherine F., and Agricultural Research Service, U.S. Department of Agriculture, *Nutritive Values of American Foods: In Common Units, Handbook 456*. Washington, D.C.: Government Printing Office, 1975.)

calcium is needed. Generally, phosphorus is readily available and deficiencies are rare. In milk, calcium and phosphorus are found in almost equal amounts, and phosphorus is found in many protein-rich foods such as meat, eggs, and legumes.

Magnesium is required in lesser amounts than calcium and phosphorus. An adequate amount is available in foods commonly eaten: milk, meat, green vegetables, whole-grain cereals, and legumes. Eating large amounts of calcium, protein, vitamin D, and alcohol increases the requirement for magnesium, as does physical or psychological stress.

Sodium, Potassium, and Chloride

In combination, sodium, potassium, and chloride are necessary for the balance of fluids, acids, and bases inside and outside

Table 2.26
A COMPARISON OF CALCIUM SUPPLEMENTS

Source of Calcium	Percentage of Calcium (by weight)	Comments
Calcium carbonate (synthetic or natural, such as oyster shell and egg shell; found in some over-the-counter antacids)	40	Can cause gas and constipation at high levels
Calcium chloride	36	Can irritate stomach lining; generally not a good supplement
Bone meal	31	Can be contaminated with lead, mercury, and other heavy metals
Calcium phosphate	31	Good if calcium and phosphorus are both needed, but phosphorus increase may be undesirable
Dolomite	22	May be contaminated with heavy metals such as lead or mercury
Calcium lactate	13	Should be avoided by persons who are lactose intolerant
Calcium gluconate	9	Low calcium content per tablet, so many tablets may be needed to meet daily requirements

of cells, and normal functioning of muscles. These substances, when dissolved in water, separate into positively and negatively charged particles called ions. Ions conduct the minute electrical current necessary for smooth function of the body's systems. Sodium, potassium, and chloride, therefore, are known as electrolytes.

Getting enough sodium, potassium, and chloride is not a problem; getting too much of them, particularly sodium, can be. Table salt, which is 40 percent sodium (60 percent chloride) is eaten by most Americans in large quantities. The amount of sodium found in foods is usually expressed in milligrams or grams (1,000 milligrams = 1 gram).

1 teaspoon table salt = approximately 2,300 milligrams (2.3 grams) sodium

For many adults excess salt is associated with high blood pressure, which is associated with strokes, heart attacks, and kidney disease. Many experts believe that a child's intake of salt will affect his or her health as an adult, although this has not been proved conclusively. Controversy exists over the exact amount of salt that can be safely consumed; however, moderation in salt consumption is strongly urged. Excess dietary sodium is rarely necessary. Table 2.27 shows the amount of sodium in common foods.

Breakfast cereals, which often are criticized for their high sugar contents, are surprisingly high in sodium, and this may be even greater cause for concern. Some of the cereals that are thought to be the best sources of vitamins, minerals, and fiber, in fact, contain more sodium than some of the most sugary cereals. Table 2.28 shows the sodium content of some cereals.

Although salt is thought to enhance flavors, many people have discovered wonderful, natural flavors when salt is eliminated from the table and in cooking. Adequate amounts of sodium are present in a balanced diet. There is no need to salt foods and, in most instances, efforts should be made to limit foods high in sodium.

Table 2.27
SODIUM CONTENT OF SELECTED FOODS

Food	Serving Size	Sodium (mg)
Table salt	1 tsp.	2300
Soups	1 cup	1000 (average)
Chicken noodle/water	1 cup	1107
Chicken rice/water	1 cup	814
Clam chowder, Manhattan	1 cup	1808
Clam chowder, New England/milk	1 cup	992
Minestrone/water	1 cup	911
Cream of potato/milk	1 cup	1060
Tomato/milk	1 cup	932
/water	1 cup	872
Vegetable, vegetarian	1 cup	823
/beef/water	1 cup	957
Bouillon, canned	1 cup	782
/package/water	1 cup	1358
Cheese, natural		
Cheddar	1 oz.	176
Cottage, creamed	½ cup	457
dry curd, low fat	½ cup	459
Cream cheese	2 tbsp.	84
Ricotta, part skim	½ cup	155
Cheese, processed		
American	1 oz.	406
Swiss	1 oz.	388
Cheese products		
Cheese food		
American	1 oz.	337
Swiss	1 oz.	440
Cheese spread		
American	1 oz.	381
Milk	1 cup	130
Breads	1 slice	150
Meats, unprocessed beef, veal, lamb, chicken, turkey, pork, fresh ham	1 oz.	15

Table 2.27
Continued

Food	Serving Size	Sodium (mg)
Ham, cured	1 oz.	205
Hot dog	1 each	500
Bologna	1 slice	230
Bacon	2 slices	228
Peanut butter	1 tbsp.	75
Rice, noodles, pasta (cooked without salt)	1 cup	10
Salad dressings	1 tbsp.	200
Vegetables, canned	½ cup	220
frozen	½ cup	less than 50
fresh	½ cup	less than 25
Butter, salted	1 tsp.	41
unsalted	1 tsp.	1
Margarine, salted	1 tsp.	44
unsalted	1 tsp.	1
Oil	1 tbsp.	0
Fruits and fruit juice		negligible
Raisins	1 oz.	10
Tomato or vegetable juice	1 cup	490
Pickles		
Bread and butter	4 slices	168
Dill	½ large (1¾ oz.)	714
Kosher	1 large (2 oz.)	581
Sour	½ large (1¾ oz.)	677
Sweet	½ large (1¾ oz.)	286
Olives, green	2 medium	312
Snacks		
Corn chips	1 oz.	218
Popcorn, unsalted	1 cup	trace
Potato chips	1 oz.	210
Pretzels, regular	1 oz.	451

(Adapted from Pennington, Jean A. T., and Church, H. N., *Bowes and Church's Food Values of Portions Commonly Used*, Fourteenth Edition. Philadelphia: J. B. Lippincott Company, 1985.)

Table 2.28
SODIUM CONTENT OF CEREALS

Cold Cereals

Product	Serving Size	Sodium (mg)
Grape-nuts	½ cup	394
Kaboom	1 cup	370
Wheaties	1 cup	354
Total	1 cup	352
Rice Krispies	1 cup	340
Corn Flakes	1 cup	300
Cap'n Crunch	1 cup	284
Kix	1 cup	226
Alpha Bits	1 cup	219
Boo Berry	1 cup	210
Cocoa Puffs	1 cup	205
King Vitamin	1 cup	174
Granola, Nature Valley	1 cup	174
Sugar Smacks	1 cup	100
Shredded Wheat	1 biscuit	0
Puffed Wheat	1 cup	0
Puffed Rice	1 cup	0

Cooked, Hot Cereals
(serving size = ¾ cup)

Product	Salt Added: (cooked according to label instructions) Sodium (mg)	No Salt Added Sodium (mg)
Farina	576	1
Wheatina	433	4
Corn grits, regular, quick	405	0
Ralston	357	3
Cream of Wheat, quick	347	104
Cream of Rice	317	1
Oatmeal, regular	280	1
Cream of Wheat, instant	273	5
Cream of Wheat, regular	252	2
Malt-O-Meal, plain/ chocolate	243	2
Maypo	194	6
Maltex	142	7

Table 2.28
Continued

Instant Hot Cereals
(serving size = 1 packet)

Product	Sodium (mg)
Corn grits	344
Oatmeal, plain	286
cinnamon and spice	280
maple and brown sugar	280
bran and raisins	247
raisin and spice	225
apple and cinnamon	222
Cream of Wheat, mix and eat	241

(Adapted from Pennington, Jean A. T., and Church, H. N., *Bowes and Church's Food Values of Portions Commonly Used*, Fourteenth Edition. Philadelphia: J. B. Lippincott Company, 1985.)

There are exceptions, of course. Salt should be added to the diet during strenuous physical activity or in hot weather, when sweating can mean an excessive loss of needed sodium. (One gram — 1,000 milligrams — of sodium is lost for every quart of sweat.) The body, however, will begin to conserve sodium if strenuous exercise in heat is prolonged — after about a week of such exercise, the body loses only one-half to one-third the normal amount. Also, recent studies have shown that pregnant women may need additional salt — contrary to common belief. A pregnant woman should discuss this issue with her physician.

Overconsumption of salt occurs for two major reasons: (1) most Americans add salt to their food when cooking and at the table to enhance flavor; (2) because salt is an excellent preservative, large quantities are added to processed foods such as soups, American cheese, and cottage cheese.

When checking labels for sodium, consumers should look not only for salt but also for sodium additives such as sodium phosphate (in cheeses); sodium nitrate (a preservative often added to meats); baking soda, or sodium bicarbonate; baking powder; sodium ascorbate; sodium saccharin; and monosodium glutamate

(MSG). Additives such as these, however, account for less than one-tenth of the sodium found in processed foods. Table salt continues to be the primary source of sodium in the diet. The Food and Drug Administration will require the sodium content of foods to appear on labels beginning in July 1986. This information will be a valuable aid to consumers in making food choices.

HOW MUCH SALT?

1 Take a paper towel or a napkin.
2 Sit at the table as though you were about to eat.
3 Take the salt shaker and shake it onto the paper towel as though you were normally salting a meal, item by item.
4 Pour the salt from the paper towel or napkin into a teaspoon.

How full is it? Surprised? This is only for 1 meal, and it does not include the sodium in processed foods, or that added in the kitchen. (*Remember:* 1 teaspoon table salt = 2,300 mg sodium)

In addition, when choosing food, the following bits of information might be useful:

Canned soups and bouillon are high in sodium.

Regular canned vegetables are higher in sodium than the fresh, frozen, or low-sodium canned varieties.

Salad dressings contain a significant amount of sodium.

Preseasoned rice, noodles, potatoes, and stuffing mixes are high in sodium.

Instant hot cereals contain more sodium than regular or quick-cooking varieties.

Cold cereals may vary widely in their sodium content.

If a food tastes salty, it probably is very high in sodium.

One way to reduce the amount of sodium in the diet is to limit the amount of salt used in cooking. A variety of herbs and spices

can be used to bring out and add flavors to foods that are normally salted. Table 2.29 is a list of flavoring aids that can make
salt-free cooking more exciting.

Iron

Iron, a trace element, is especially important in the formation
of red blood cells and muscle protein. Iron deficiency causes
anemia. For this reason, iron is particularly important during
periods of growth, when additional red blood cells are formed.
Infants, adolescents, and pregnant and lactating women require
high amounts of iron. Menstruating women lose blood and require more iron than men.

Iron is more readily absorbed when vitamin C and calcium are
present. A greater percentage of dietary iron is absorbed during
periods of growth or when there is a deficiency. Animal sources
of iron are more readily absorbed than vegetable sources. Of the
supplementary forms available, ferrous salts are better absorbed
than ferric salts.

Although iron is found in many foods, iron deficiency is a
common problem for women and children. Parents should attempt to include iron-rich foods (see Table 2.30) in a child's diet.

It may reassure parents to learn that many of children's favorite foods are fairly good sources of iron. Table 2.31 provides the
amount of iron in some of these foods.

If a child refuses to eat iron-rich foods, iron supplements may
be necessary. Supplementation, however, should be tried only
after the child's pediatrician has been consulted.

Parents should NEVER give their children iron supplements
without advice from a physician.

Babies are born with enough body iron to last for approximately six months; iron-deficiency anemia is most likely to occur
between 6 months, when the original supply runs out, and 18
months, when the child is well launched on an iron-rich diet.
Breast milk supplies adequate iron that is relatively well ab-

Table 2.29
FLAVORING WITHOUT SALT

Meat, Poultry, and Fish

Beef	Crushed bay leaves, mustard powder, cumin, ginger, pepper, marjoram, thyme, sage, nutmeg, curry, coriander, oregano, onion powder
Veal	Crushed bay leaves, pepper, ginger, marjoram, curry, sage, mint, tarragon, dill, oregano
Lamb	Curry, rosemary, mint, tarragon, sage, garlic powder, cumin, savory
Pork	Garlic powder, onion powder, sage, rosemary, savory, fennel, cumin
Poultry	Oregano, curry, ginger, marjoram, sage, parsley, paprika, lemon peel, thyme, garlic powder, sesame seeds
Fish	Crushed bay leaves, lemon peel, orange peel, dill, parsley, thyme, paprika, curry, mustard, marjoram, tarragon

Vegetables

Asparagus	Garlic powder, lemon peel, rosemary, savory, marjoram, dill, onion powder
Beans	Pepper, cayenne, cumin, chili powder, garlic
Broccoli	Tarragon, lemon peel, pepper, mustard
Brussels sprouts	Lemon peel, caraway seeds, garlic powder, onion powder
Carrots	Dill, mint, thyme, basil, parsley powder, minced onion, onion powder, dry mustard
Corn	Onion powder, minced onion, basil, oregano
Cucumbers	Dill, lemon peel, garlic powder, chives, onion powder
Green beans	Lemon peel, marjoram, curry, dill, nutmeg, caraway seeds, sesame seeds
Peas	Sage, onion powder, garlic powder, pepper, savory
Potatoes	Parsley, paprika, dill, pepper, caraway seeds, curry, mace, onion powder, garlic powder
Squash	Ginger, nutmeg, allspice, onion powder, basil

Other Foods

Eggs	Basil, pepper, onion powder, garlic powder, paprika, parsley, dry mustard, tarragon, crushed bay leaves
Pasta dishes	Oregano, garlic powder, thyme, onion powder, cayenne pepper, crushed bay leaves, chives, basil

Table 2.29
Continued

Other Foods (continued)

Rice	Saffron, curry, basil, oregano, onion powder, chives
Salads	Dill, chervil, parsley, lemon peel, tarragon, marjoram, basil, chives
Soups	*Chowders:* pepper, peppercorns, bay leaves, dill, paprika, marjoram, thyme, tarragon. *Vegetable, beef, or chicken stock:* thyme, basil, curry, garlic powder, onion powder, dill, oregano, bay leaves, pepper

---

sorbed (see Chapter 3, Feeding Infants). The iron in cow's milk, the basis for most infant formulas, is less well absorbed. It is recommended that babies fed on formula be started on an iron-fortified formula at 4 months and move to iron-fortified cereal by 6 months. Breast-fed babies should begin eating iron-fortified cereals by 6 months of age. Iron-fortified cereals contain 7 milligrams of iron in every 4-tablespoon serving. Children who weigh from 10 to 15 pounds require five milligrams of iron daily, and 15- to 20-pound children need 10 milligrams.

Any vitamin containing iron should be kept out of the reach of children. Chronic iron overdose can interfere with zinc absorption, lead to abnormalities in the heart, liver, and pancreas, and can be fatal. An acute iron overdose also can be fatal.

Fluoride

All children should receive fluoride, an important trace element. The best source is fluoridated water; if the local water supply is not fluoridated, fluoride supplements should be given.

Evidence indicates that a child who consumes fluoride from birth or, if breast fed, from 6 months, and continues to drink fluoridated water throughout life will have 50 to 65 percent fewer cavities in his or her permanent teeth than a child who receives little or no fluoride. Fluoride also contributes to stronger bones. Too much fluoride, however, can lead to an un-

Table 2.30
IRON-RICH FOODS

Meats	Especially liver, kidney, red meats, liverwurst
Fish	Especially clams, oysters, shrimp, sardines
Poultry	Especially turkey, chicken livers
Dark green, leafy vegetables	Especially spinach, chard, kale, greens
Dried fruits	Especially raisins, apricots, dates, figs, peaches, prunes
Breads and cereals	Especially whole-grain or enriched breads, iron-fortified cereals, oatmeal, bran flakes, wheat germ
Cooked dried beans	Especially lentils, soybeans, peas
Nuts	Especially almonds, cashews, Brazil, pecans
Other iron-rich foods	Blackstrap molasses, table syrup, egg yolks, brewer's yeast

Table 2.31
APPROXIMATE IRON CONTENT OF CHILDREN'S FAVORITE FOODS

Food	Serving Size	Iron Content (mgs)
Hamburger, small	1	3.0
large	1	5.2
Big Mac	1	4.3
Quarter Pounder	1	5.1
Spaghetti with meatballs	1 cup	3.3
Frankfurters and beans	1 cup	4.8
Pork and beans	1 cup	5.9
Raisins	⅝ cup	3.5
Cereals, fortified	1 serving	4.5–17.8
Nuts	1 cup	5.0–7.0
Seeds, sunflower	3½ oz.	7.1
Chili con carne	1 cup	3.6
Beef burrito	1 medium	4.6
Beef tostado	1 medium	3.4
Cheese pizza	2 slices	3.0
Cheese pizza with beef	2 slices	4.8

(*Source:* Nutrition Services, Department of Nutrition and Food Service, Children's Hospital, Boston.)

sightly, though harmless, tooth discoloration. Large amounts of fluoride — 20 to 80 milligrams a day over a number of years — can be seriously toxic and should be avoided.

Breast milk contains little or no fluoride; therefore, breast-fed babies may be given fluoride supplements, although there is no evidence that babies who are breast fed for the first six months of life without fluoride supplements develop more cavities than those who are given the supplement.

Babies fed a concentrated or powdered formula mixed with water need not have a supplement if the drinking water contains one milligram fluoride per liter, or one part per million, as is the case in many communities. The water department of a local town can provide information on fluoridation of public water. Parents need this information to make a wise decision about fluoride supplements.

Children on ready-to-feed formulas will need a supplement because most of these kinds of formulas do not contain fluoride. In communities that have fluoridated water, supplementation should continue until the child begins drinking water, juices made with water, and foods cooked in water.

In communities without fluoridated water, supplementation should be continued at least until permanent teeth are present (usually 6 to 12 years of age). Supplementary fluoride should not exceed .25 milligrams a day, even though many supplements contain .5 milligrams.

Although there is controversy about whether infants younger than 6 months old need supplements, most experts agree that after 6 months of age children should receive them. There also is controversy about whether fluoride supplements taken during pregnancy help children's tooth development. Most specialists agree that fluoride is not available to the fetus, and that such supplementation is, therefore, useless.

WATER

Water is often forgotten in discussions of nutrition. It contains no calories, and by itself contains limited nutrients. In fact, however, in addition to fluoride, most drinking water carries small amounts of numerous minerals. Without water, humans would

Table 2.32
APPROXIMATE WATER CONTENT OF FOODS

Fruits and vegetables	80 to 95 percent water
Meat, poultry, fish	50 to 75 percent water
Milk	87 percent water
Bread	36 percent water

die quickly. While survival for several weeks without the other nutrients is possible, people can live only a few days without water. Even a small loss of water in the body can be serious: a 5-percent loss makes the skin shrink and the muscles weak; a 10-percent loss causes major medical problems; and a 20-percent loss is associated with death.

Adults are composed of roughly 66 percent water; newborns are 85 percent water. Water is found in every part of the body: blood, muscles, bones, brain. For good health, all the water used in a day for respiration, perspiration, and urination must be replaced each day. Adults should consume on average 2½ to three quarts a day, and even more in hot weather. This is accomplished not only by drinking liquids, but also by eating foods that contain water. As Table 2.32 shows, foods contain a large percentage of water.

In addition to comprising such a large proportion of the body, water serves many vital roles. It transports nutrients in the blood; plays an important part in digestion, nutrient absorption, and elimination of body wastes in urine and sweat; dissolves other elements needed in metabolism; maintains body temperature through sweating; lubricates joints and other body tissues; provides a cushion for the fetus; aids in growth and body repair; and helps eliminate solid waste.

Replacement of water on a daily basis is essential. Generally, the body provides adequate thirst signals, and most children will consume enough water to satisfy their needs. Parents, however, may need to pay attention to their child's water consumption on hot days. Because fever and diarrhea greatly increase the need for fluids, parents also should be certain to provide extra water in those circumstances. (See Chapter 8 for further discussion of diet during illness.)

PUTTING IT ALL TOGETHER

At this point, parents may be saying, "I now know about the nutrients, how much of each my child needs, and some food sources, but am I supposed to keep track of and calculate my child's intake of calories and nutrients every day?" The answer is, obviously, "No." Not only is diet calculation tedious and time consuming, but the results of even the most careful calculations will only be approximate and are unnecessary. Fortunately, there is an easy-to-follow practical approach to this seemingly overwhelming problem: Use the Basic Four Food Groups.

Almost all the foods people eat can be grouped with relative ease into one of four major categories — meat, milk, bread and cereal, vegetable and fruit — according to the nutrients they provide and their overall usefulness to the body. As the following discussion illustrates, each group in the Basic Four is important. Each provides essential nutrients to the diet.

Meat Group

The meat group provides protein of high quality. It also provides iron, the B vitamins, phosphorus, zinc, and other trace elements. Vegetarians can satisfy these requirements by combining high-protein nonmeat foods — grains, legumes, nuts and seeds, dairy products, and vegetables. Little meat is required to satisfy the protein requirement: two to three ounces twice a day will suffice. Americans can cut back on their usual half-pound or pound servings and probably improve their overall diet and health.

Milk Group

The milk group provides most of the calcium and phosphorus needed by children and adults. It also contributes significant proportions of high-quality protein and carbohydrate, as well as riboflavin, and vitamins A and D, if the milk is fortified. In addition, whole milk (approximately 4 percent fat), 2-percent milk, and 1-percent milk provide fat. The amount of milk needed varies significantly for each age group — children, adolescents, and pregnant and lactating women have particularly high requirements. People who do not like milk can substitute cheese, yogurt, cottage cheese, and custards.

Table 2.33
BASIC FOUR FOOD GROUPS

Meat group	Meat (lean); poultry; fish; eggs; dried cooked beans, peas, lentils; peanut butter; cheese
Milk group	Milk (whole, low fat, skim, buttermilk, evaporated, dry/reconstituted); ice cream and ice milk; yogurt; cheese
Vegetable and fruit group	All fruits; all vegetables, except those listed in the meat group
Bread and cereal group	All breads; all cereals; pasta (noodles, macaroni, spaghetti); rice

Bread and Cereal Group

The bread and cereal group provides important carbohydrates, protein, fiber, B vitamins (especially thiamin and niacin), iron, zinc, and other trace minerals.

Vegetable and Fruit Group

The vegetable and fruit group primarily provides carbohydrates, fiber, vitamins (especially A and C, but also the B vitamins), folic acid, iron, and other minerals. It is important to eat at least one fruit high in vitamin C and at least one vegetable or fruit high in vitamin A each day.

Other Foods

In addition to these four groups, fats should be eaten for additional calories. Eliminating fats entirely from the diet stops children's growth and leads to essential fatty acid deficiency. A tablespoon of margarine, butter, or mayonnaise each day usually will provide a sufficient amount of fat. Table 2.33 outlines some of the foods in each of the four groups.

For parents who are curious or concerned about certain nutrients and their content in specific foods, there are three valuable references:

Labels — See Chapter 10 for how to interpret the information provided on food labels.

Bowes and Church's Food Values of Portions Commonly Used, by Jean A. T. Pennington and H. N. Church, Fourteenth Edition. (Philadelphia: J. B. Lippincott Company, 1985). This book, available in many bookstores or by special order, provides reliable nutrient data for common foods in household measures.

The U.S. Department of Agriculture's *Handbook 456* provides reliable data for household measures and market units of approximately 1,500 foods.

If either of the two reference books are used, parents would be well advised to read the explanations provided regarding how to interpret data. For example, in *Handbook 456*, dashes (—) are frequently used. Readers could easily assume that this means the food does not contain any of the nutrient in question. In fact, in this book, a dash denotes lack of reliable data for a nutrient believed to be present in measurable amounts.

NUTRIENT CONTENT OF FOODS: A WORD TO THE WISE

The nutrient content of foods provided in this book and other reliable references (see the Useful Reading section at the end of this book) should be used as a *guideline* only. Most nutrient figures are *average* values. Individual foods, however, often have a wide range of values. Variations in food values are the result of soil content, season, processing, method of preparation, and the method used to analyze the nutrients.

All the nutrients children need to grow and develop are found among the foods in the four groups. Using the Basic Four Food Groups as a method of planning meals for children is the easiest way to provide a nutritious, well-balanced diet. In the next two chapters, this Basic Four approach is used to give parents practical guidelines for feeding their children from conception through adolescence.

3

LET'S EAT!
CONCEPTION THROUGH
INFANCY

. . . and when, at the age of a month,
he had gained only a third of an
ounce, his mother was so worried
she sent for the doctor. . . . Everything seemed to be all right, and Mrs.
Little was pleased to get such a good
report.
"Feed him up!" said the doctor cheer-
fully as he left.

E. B. White
Stuart Little

The fetus, growing and devel-
oping inside the womb, depends entirely on its mother to supply all nourishment necessary to bring a new, healthy life into
the outside world. After birth, infants continue to depend on
others to fulfill all their needs. This absolute dependency places
upon parents the responsibility of feeding their children well —
to ensure their survival and to safeguard their health and well-
being. This role must be taken seriously.

A mother should begin by being careful of her own diet
throughout pregnancy. Later on, she should continue to eat well
herself and to feed her newborn wisely. If a mother is poorly
nourished during pregnancy or if an infant receives a diet

deficient in essential nutrients, lifelong health problems may develop.

Pregnant women and new parents normally have many questions about how best to fill the nutritional needs of the baby, both before and after birth. Should pregnant women stop drinking coffee? Take vitamins? Drink alcoholic beverages? Is it best for a mother to breast feed or bottle feed her newborn? When should an infant begin to eat solid foods? And, what are the best first foods?

Although there are always areas of controversy, this chapter is intended to eliminate much of the uncertainty about diet from conception through the first year. In this chapter we move from a discussion of diet during pregnancy to the pros and cons of breast feeding and bottle feeding, to the introduction of solid foods, and, finally, to a discussion of the appropriate foods for infants younger than 1 year of age.

MEALS DURING PREGNANCY

Good nutrition begins even before conception. Eating well before conception prepares the mother's body for the physically demanding period of pregnancy. The mother's pre-pregnancy health, therefore, can affect the fetus's health, development, and chance of survival. If a woman is eating poorly and a pregnancy begins, she must promptly improve her diet to compensate for nutrients not present at the time of conception.

After conception the mother's diet is crucial to the development of a healthy baby. In fact, contrary to previous theories, malnutrition affects the child more severely than it does the mother. In evolutionary terms, this makes sense: a baby born to a nutritionally depleted mother does not have a good chance of surviving. Therefore, with few exceptions, the mother's nutritional needs are met first, followed by the needs of the fetus.

Both the quantity and the quality of the mother's diet affect the fetus, in many ways — birth weight, and the risks of malformation, spontaneous abortion, mortality, or retardation. Table 3.1 outlines the developmental stages of the fetus. Because organs develop from the very beginning, the mother's diet matters right from the start. Fetal growth itself is rapid throughout pregnancy, particularly in the last trimester.

Table 3.1
DEVELOPMENTAL STAGES OF THE FETUS

Three Weeks
⅕", .0001 oz.   Embryo's brain, spinal cord, heart, and blood
                       vessels begin to develop.

One Month
¼", .001 oz.   Embryo's nervous and circulatory systems begin to
                       form. Kidneys start to develop. Tissues for
                       muscles and bones, digestive tract and the eyes,
                       ears, and mouth begin to develop. The crude
                       heart beats regularly. Baby possesses the
                       beginnings of all major organs.

Six Weeks
½", .01 oz.   Face takes shape. Buds for arms, legs, backbone,
                       and liver begin to form. Upper and lower jaws
                       develop.

Two Months
1", ⅟₃₀ oz.   Fetus has clearly defined eyes, ears, nose, and
                       arms. The hands have fingers and the feet have
                       toes. Cartilage forms, and bones begin to
                       distinguish themselves. The fetus moves, but
                       the mother cannot yet feel these movements.

Three Months
3", 1 oz.   Tooth buds begin to form inside the jaw. Vocal
                       cords start to take shape, and all organs become
                       better defined, more precise, and functional.
                       Fingernails and toenails form. Nostrils close,
                       eyelids fuse shut. Liver begins to produce red
                       blood cells. Sex organs become defined.

Four Months
6½", 4 oz.   Fetus's movements become more pronounced and
                       mother may feel a slight flutter. Fetus swallows
                       and excretes amniotic fluid. Early fecal matter,
                       called meconium, collects in fetus's intestinal
                       tract. Nearly all organs are formed. Fine hair
                       covers body. Obstetrician can detect a heartbeat
                       using amplified stethoscope.

Five Months
12", 1½ lbs.   Fetus develops hair, eyebrows, lashes, facial
                       expressions, and begins to move vigorously and
                       frequently. Mother can feel definite fetal
                       movements. Most organ systems function, first

Table 3.1
Continued

Five months (continued)

sucking responses appear, fetus grips with hands. Eyelids are still fused shut, but blinking-like movements begin. Bones in the ear begin to harden.

Six Months
15", 2½ lbs.

Fetus's skin, nails, and hair take on adult form. Fat cells begin to form and vernix — the oily substance that protects the baby from the amniotic fluid — develops. Nostrils reopen, and the baby begins to make muscular breathing motions. The fetus demonstrates brain-wave patterns, and crude hearing and vision systems are present.

Seven Months
16½", 4 lbs.

Fetus's eyes are completely formed and can perceive light. The eyelids reopen. Taste buds on tongue are functional. Organs continue to mature. Nerve cells mature, fetus continues to lay down fat cells.

Eight Months
18", 5½ lbs.

Nervous system undergoes further development. Fatty sheath, called myelin, forms around nerve fibers. Fetus continues to grow in length, weight, and strength.

Nine Months
20", 7½ lbs.

Lungs prepare to function independently. Fetus continues to grow in length, weight, and strength.

The nutritional needs of pregnant women increase dramatically both because of the rapid fetal growth and because of changes in the mother's body necessary to nourish the fetus and promote breast milk production. Pregnant women, therefore, need more calories overall and more of each nutrient.

Current understanding of how much weight should be gained during pregnancy contradicts theories in vogue before 1970. For the past several centuries, many doctors have encouraged women to restrict weight gain while pregnant to a maximum of

18 pounds. At the time, this advice made sense: the mortality rate of women at birth was high, and smaller babies were more easily delivered. Now, however, it is recognized that somewhat larger babies — from 6 pounds 10 ounces to 9 pounds 14 ounces — are more likely to survive and have fewer complications at birth.

Women whose weight is normal prior to conception should gain between 22 and 28 pounds during pregnancy. Women who are underweight before conception can gain up to 30 pounds, and obese women should gain approximately 16 pounds. A minimum of 15 pounds should be gained because studies show that infant mortality rates double when maternal weight gain is inadequate.

The baby itself accounts for only one-third or less of the total weight gain; a quarter goes to tissues surrounding the baby — placenta, amniotic fluid, and uterus; and slightly less than half is needed by the mother. The mother's blood supply increases during pregnancy, from approximately 8½ to 11 pints, as she supplies blood to the placenta and the baby. During pregnancy, fatty tissue increases and is redistributed in the abdomen, back, and upper thighs in preparation for the demands made by the rapid growth of the baby during the last trimester and the high energy expenditure at the time of delivery and while breast feeding.

Most of the baby's growth occurs during the final trimester. The mother gains little weight during the first trimester, generally only 1½ to three pounds. Beginning with the second trimester, however, mothers should gain approximately one pound every seven to nine days. In general, a mother's low weight gain during the last trimester will mean a smaller baby, with smaller organs — smaller brain, heart, kidney, and liver.

Women should not go on reducing diets while pregnant.

Dieting during pregnancy is generally unwise. Not only does dieting deprive the baby and the mother of energy and nutrients needed for healthy development, but dieting can permanently harm the fetus. Weight loss during pregnancy is associated with increased fetus and infant mortality. Women who have worked hard to maintain a slim figure must realize that weight gain and a bigger waist measurement go hand in hand with a normal pregnancy. Slimness can be and should be restored gradually with proper exercise and sensible diet — but only after the baby is born.

In addition to the need for more calories, other needs increase during pregnancy as follows (see also the Recommended Dietary Allowances in Table 2.1):

Protein: 75 grams a day is needed on average. Extra protein is needed for increases in breast and uterus size and in blood volume, for construction of the placenta and amniotic fluid, and for fetal growth. Lack of protein can lead to growth delays or mental retardation in the baby. Excessive protein intake, however, is unnecessary. (See Chapter 2 for more information on protein.)

Iron: 60 milligrams of supplemental iron often is recommended throughout pregnancy and for two to three months after the baby is born to replenish stores depleted by pregnancy. Iron is one of the few nutrients that the fetus will take from the mother if needed. Maternal anemia is common and is usually the result of too little iron. An anemic mother is less able to tolerate the blood loss at birth and is more vulnerable to infection after the birth. Vitamin C enhances the absorption of iron; however, too much vitamin C taken by the mother can lead to vitamin C deficiency in the infant after birth. Tea, antacids, and calcium phosphate prevent optimal iron absorption. Even when iron supplements are taken, iron-rich foods such as organ meats, red meats, and dark green, leafy vegetables should be eaten frequently and regularly. (See Chapter 2 for more information on iron.)

Folic Acid: 0.8 milligrams is recommended because folates are needed for the production of hemoglobin and the formation of DNA and RNA, the central building blocks of life. Because folic acid is often limited in the normal diet, supplements are prescribed frequently. (See Chapter 2 for more information on folic acid.)

Calcium: At least 1,200 milligrams are needed each day, especially during the last trimester of pregnancy, when the baby's bones and teeth are forming and growing. Calcium, like iron, will be taken by the baby from the mother's stores if she does not consume enough, thus creating the potential for maternal deficiency. Vitamin D, although toxic if consumed to excess, enhances the absorption of calcium; enough vitamin D for this purpose is found in the daily quart of milk recommended for pregnant women. If a pregnant woman is unable to consume calcium from dairy products, calcium supplements may be recommended by the obstetrician. (See Chapter 2 for information on calcium and calcium supplements.)

Sodium: 2 to 3 grams of sodium are recommended because the normal fluid retention somewhat increases the body's sodium needs. Contrary to previous medical theory, very-low-salt or salt-free diets are not advisable. (See Chapter 2 for more information on sodium.)

Fluoride: Debate continues about how useful fluoride is to the fetus. It is, however, useful to the mother for strong bones and teeth. In communities where the water is not fluoridated, fluoride supplements often are prescribed. (See Chapter 2 for more information on fluoride.)

Fiber: Needs increase because constipation can occur during pregnancy, when the digestive system slows down. (See Chapter 2 for more information on fiber.)

In order to get the nutrients needed, pregnant women should add 300 calories a day to their diets and follow the Basic Four Food Guide for Pregnant Women outlined in Table 3.2.

Caffeine in excess may be damaging to the fetus. It is best to eliminate caffeine entirely from the diet. Coffee, tea, and many soft drinks (especially cola-type drinks) contain caffeine and should be eliminated. Table 3.3 provides a closer look at the caffeine content of foods. Herbal teas should be considered with caution because some contain chemicals that may be harmful to the fetus (see Table 7.4). Also, some decaffeinated coffees, prepared with methylene chloride or formaldahyde, may be harm-

Table 3.2
BASIC FOUR FOOD GUIDE FOR PREGNANT WOMEN
(1,900 to 2,700 calories a day)

Food Group	Recommended Servings Each Day	Average Serving Size
Milk group (or equivalent)	4	
Milk, whole, low-fat, skim		1 cup
Buttermilk		1 cup
Powdered milk		4 tbsp.
Evaporated milk		3 oz.
Cheese		1½ oz.
Cottage cheese		1 cup
Yogurt		1 cup
Tofu (soybean curd)		1 cup
Meat, fish, poultry (or equivalent) (liver is desirable once a week)	3	2–3 oz.
Eggs		2 whole
Peanut butter		¼ cup
Cooked dried peas or beans		1 cup
Luncheon meat		2–3 slices
Tofu		1 cup
Nuts and seeds		½ cup
Cheese		2 oz.
Vegetables and fruits	4	½–¾ cup
Citrus fruits (vitamin C source)	1 or more	
Orange, mango, guava		1 medium
Grapefruit, cantaloupe		½ medium
Orange or grapefruit juice		½ cup
Strawberries		1 cup
Tomatoes or tomato juice		½ cup
Yellow or green vegetable or fruit (vitamin A source)	1 or more	
Broccoli		½ cup
Spinach		½ cup
Carrots		½ cup
Squash		½ cup
Cantaloupe		½ fruit
Apricots		10 halves
Other fruits and vegetables	2	
Fresh, frozen, canned fruits and vegetables		½ cup
Potato, turnip, most whole vegetables		1 medium

Table 3.2
Continued

Food Group	Recommended Servings Each Day	Average Serving Size
Apple, banana, most whole fruits		1 medium
Breads and cereals (whole grain or enriched)	4	
Bread		1 slice
Dry cereal (unsweetened)		¾ cup
Cooked cereal		½ cup
Rice, noodles, pasta		½ cup
Roll		1 medium
Bagel		½ medium
Crackers		4 whole
Muffins		1 medium
Other Foods		
Fats and oils	3–6	
Butter, margarine, mayonnaise		1 tbsp.
Vegetable oil		1 tbsp.
Salad dressing		1 tbsp.
Sour cream		1 tbsp.
Olives		5 small
Nuts		6 medium
Avocado		⅛ medium
Liquids (in addition to milk)	6 or more	
Water		8 oz.
Fruit juice		8 oz.
Vegetable juice		8 oz.
Seltzer water, club soda		8 oz.
Caffeine-free soft drinks		8 oz.
Desserts and snacks	as needed	
Pudding		½ cup
Ice cream or ice milk		1 cup
Custard		1 cup
Dried fruits		3 oz.
Cookies		2–3 medium
Cake		1 oz.
Pie		1½ oz.
Sugar, honey, molasses, jam, jelly, preserves		2 tbsp.

Table 3.3
CAFFEINE* CONTENT OF SELECTED PRODUCTS

Product	Serving Size	Caffeine (mg)
Coffee	5 fluid oz.	
Automatic drip		137
Percolated		117
Instant		60
Instant, decaffeinated		3
Tea	5 fluid oz.	
American Black		
One-minute brew		28
Three-minute brew		42
Five-minute brew		46
Green		
One-minute brew		14
Three-minute brew		27
Five-minute brew		31
Soft Drinks**	12 fluid oz.	
Colas, diet colas, Dr. Pepper types		30–46
Caffeine-free		trace
Chocolate		
Milk chocolate	1 ounce	1–15
Dark sweet	1 ounce	5–35
Cocoa, prepared	6 fluid oz.	2–8
Chocolate milk	8 fluid oz.	2–7

*Caffeine is naturally present in coffee, tea, chocolate, and cocoa.

**There is no caffeine in regular or diet club soda, ginger ale, grape soda, lemon-lime sodas, orange soda, root beer, seltzer, sparkling water, tonic water, 7-Up, Sprite, Teem, Fanta sodas, or Fresca.

(Adapted from Pennington, Jean A. T., and Church, H. N., *Bowes and Church's Food Values of Portions Commonly Used,* Fourteenth Edition. Philadelphia: J. B. Lippincott Company, 1985.)

ful. In all these cases the caffeine and the chemicals are absorbed by the fetus.

Alcohol is extremely dangerous to the baby. As little as two drinks a day can cause low-birthweight babies and developmental and learning difficulties. Chronic excessive drinking can lead to Fetal Alcohol Syndrome, which involves extensive mental and physical defects. Most experts, therefore, recommend that alcohol be avoided during pregnancy.

Cigarette smoking can depress the appetite and is associated with low-birthweight infants. Furthermore, nicotine is harmful to the fetus, and carbon monoxide from cigarette smoke reduces the oxygen supply to the baby's red blood cells by constricting the blood vessels in the placenta. Abstention from smoking during pregnancy, therefore, is also strongly advised.

During pregnancy, some women experience nausea — often called morning sickness, even though it can continue throughout the day. This can lead to a decline in appetite, which can be harmful to the baby, who needs the same nourishment no matter how the mother feels. Many women find relief from nausea by drinking fluids an hour before and after meals and eating dry foods (crackers, melba toast, cereals, baked potatoes); eating crackers before getting out of bed in the morning; or eating small, frequent meals. Various approaches should be tried because it is important for pregnant women to continue eating a balanced diet.

Heartburn is another problem for some pregnant women. In most cases, heartburn occurs because the enlarged uterus presses on the stomach and pushes partially digested food back up the esophagus. Eating smaller amounts more frequently has helped many women with this problem as well.

Barring morning sickness or relentless heartburn, most pregnant women do not have to make an effort to consume extra calories; they simply get hungrier and eat accordingly. Their emphasis should be on making sure the calories they eat are from a variety of protein-, vitamin-, and mineral-rich foods.

FEEDING INFANTS

Most infants double their birth weight in the first four months of life, and triple it by one year. Consequently, during this period of rapid growth it is crucial that babies get the proper nourishment for normal growth and development. On average, babies need 45 to 50 calories for each pound of weight. For example, an 8½-pound baby needs 383–425 calories a day; a 10-

pound baby needs 450–500 calories a day. In the first four months a third of this is for growth and two-thirds for maintenance. After four months, as growth slows and activity increases, only one-tenth is used for growth.

Infancy is the only time when the Basic Four Food Guide does not apply. For the first four to six months after birth, a child receives all the basic nutrients and calories from breast milk or formula. Until age 4 to 6 months, infants should be fed only breast milk or formula.

Unmodified cow's milk will *not* provide infants with the nutrients needed; it should *not* be offered.

Parents are advised to decide before the child is born whether to breast feed or bottle feed their baby. Pediatricians and registered dietitians generally agree that breast milk is preferable but that a properly composed formula is acceptable. The decision to breast feed or bottle feed should be based on the parents' feelings after weighing the pros and cons of each.

Breast Feeding

There are many advantages of breast feeding human milk over bottle feeding formula. These advantages are listed in Table 3.4.

The composition of human milk varies from one mother to another, with the stage of lactation, the time of day, the time of sampling during a single feeding, the mother's health, and the emotional state of the mother. Despite these variations there are identifiable stages of human milk production. They are colostrum, transition milk, and mature milk.

Colostrum, a thick, yellow secretion (the yellow color is caused by carotene, the same substance that produces the yellow-orange color in carrots, squash, and other fruits and vegetables), is produced for approximately the first five days after delivery. Colostrum has a higher content of minerals, protein, and fat-soluble vitamins than mature milk. Since it has a lower content of fat, it has fewer calories per ounce. Colostrum is rich in proteins that help prevent infection. It also contains cells that

Table 3.4
NUTRITIONAL ADVANTAGES OF BREAST MILK

Protein	Contains ideal amount for human infants — far less than cow's milk Higher percentage of whey and casein than most formulas — more easily digested
Carbohydrate	Greater percentage; more lactose
Fat	Higher fat content; greater percent as unsaturated; provides essential fatty acid (linoleic acid)
Cholesterol	Content sufficient for babies (formulas do not contain cholesterol)
Calcium	Content less than formulas, but more efficiently absorbed

Vitamins and Minerals

Other Advantages of Breast Milk
• Sterile
• Rarely allergenic
• Provides immunity against disease
• Encourages bonding between mother and child
• More economical
• More convenient (no bottles, cans, or bags)
• Aids maternal weight loss
• Enhances contraction of the uterus
• Delays menstruation and fertility
• Less problem with infant constipation; softer, more frequent stools

are thought to offer protection against infection. Colostrum helps the infant pass meconium, the first stools.

Transition milk is produced from approximately 6 to 15 days after delivery. The concentration of total protein in transition milk is less than that in colostrum, and the concentration of proteins that are protective against infection also decreases. Lactose, fat, and total calories increase. Water-soluble vitamins (such as the B vitamins) increase, and fat-soluble vitamins (vitamins A, D, E, and K) decrease.

Mature breast milk appears thin with a bluish tinge. Its composition is highly variable and, because most analyses of human milk have been performed on a limited number of samples, they do not take this variation into account. Nevertheless, human milk differs markedly from cow's milk and infant formulas that are based on cow's milk. Not all the subtleties of human milk composition are appreciated. As the comparison below indicates, however, most components of human milk have advantages from an evolutionary point of view, as might be expected.

The major components of milk are water, fat, protein, carbohydrates, and minerals. Most of the calories in human milk are derived from fat and reflect the fat composition of the mother's diet. Cholesterol is present in human milk but not in infant formulas. Its value to infants remains unclear, but some experts have suggested it is necessary for proper development of the nervous system.

The main carbohydrate in both human milk and cow's milk is lactose, a sugar. Breast milk, however, contains a slightly higher concentration of lactose than cow's milk.

The protein content of human milk is less than that of cow's milk and formulas and differs in its composition. The protein of human milk is composed of approximately 60 percent lactalbumin (whey), slightly less than 40 percent casein (curd), and small amounts of other compounds, as well as antibodies. Cow's milk, conversely, is approximately 80 percent casein, which is more difficult for the human infant to digest. Further, the amino acid composition of casein in human milk differs from that of cow's milk. The whey in human milk is different from cow's milk and formulas in that it contains lactoferrin, a protein that aids iron absorption and is thought to protect against some infections. Disease-fighting agents called immunoglobulins are present in breast milk and provide protection against infection by preventing viruses and bacteria from invading the gastrointestinal tract. Lysozymes, enzymes that destroy bacteria, also are present in human milk.

In addition, the protein content and the level of most minerals, including calcium, phosphorus, sodium, and potassium, in breast milk is lower than that of cow's milk or infant formula. This is an advantage because less waste must be excreted. The newborn kidney is immature and cannot concentrate wastes. Therefore, the baby loses more water with cow's milk or formula than with breast milk. While most infants can tolerate this, infants with fever, diarrhea, or other problems sometimes have difficulty maintaining an adequate level of body water. The additional need to excrete water with wastes when cow's milk is used places these babies at risk of dehydration.

There are very few physical conditions that would make breast feeding inadvisable. If a woman has a condition for which a drug is prescribed, she should ask her physician or pharmacist whether the drug(s) in question are transferred to breast milk or will have an effect on the baby. Maternal medication is not necessarily a reason to discontinue breast feeding, if the physician can determine the degree to which the medication enters breast milk.

Chief among the advantages of breast milk is the physical closeness between the mother and child. Holding and cuddling are important parts of infant development, and breast feeding helps to insure that it will happen at every feeding. The bonding that develops between mothers and newborns is greatly enhanced by the experience of breast feeding.

Among its other advantages is the fact that breast-fed babies are less likely to overeat. Since breastfeeding mothers do not know exactly how much their babies eat, they are less inclined to force down a few extra ounces. Further, breast feeding is cheaper and, in many ways, more convenient. There are no bottles to clean, no formulas to make up or buy, no concerns about sterility or about clean water, no extra supplies to take along when traveling, and errors in formula preparation cannot occur.

Breast feeding enhances the contraction of the uterus, and it often delays menstruation and a return to fertility. Nevertheless, *no mother should count on nursing to prevent pregnancy*. Breast feeding also helps the mother lose weight more quickly after birth, as nursing requires extra energy (calories) and consumes the fat gained during pregnancy. One very weight-conscious mother described the intervals during which she breast fed her children as the "most pleasurable times of my life." She ate the foods she liked and still lost weight. By the time her children were weaned, she was back to her pre-pregnant weight.

Breast feeding does mean a continuing responsibility to maintain a well-balanced diet that remains high in nutrients. A mother who is breast feeding should continue to eat as she did while pregnant and to consume three quarts of liquid a day, including one quart of milk. People who eat no animal products must take a supplement of vitamin B_{12} when nursing. Table 3.5, the Basic Four Food Guide for Nursing Mothers, shows what types of food and how much of these foods nursing women should eat each day.

Caffeine and alcohol are excreted in breast milk, so nursing mother should reduce or eliminate these substances from their diets. Mothers who are breast feeding also should refrain from smoking because nicotine and several other chemicals accumulate in breast milk. In addition, smoking has been found to limit the amount of milk that a woman produces.

Breast milk can transfer environmental contaminants, such as certain pesticides and some drugs, to the infant. Industrial chemicals called PCBs (polychlorinated biphenyls) and insecticides such as DDT (dicholo-diphenyl-trichloroethane) have received much publicity because traces of these contaminants have been found in the breast milk of most women. Despite this, breast feeding remains the best method of feeding. For most women, only minute amounts of these chemicals are present in breast milk, and such small amounts pose few health risks to infants. The advantages of breast feeding far outweigh any possible risks, for most infants.

Women who have worked directly with toxic chemicals, have eaten a large quantity of fish taken from contaminated waters, or live in areas where they are continuously exposed to high levels of environmental pollutants may want to have their breast milk tested. (Public health departments should be able to supply information about where to send samples.)

Breast Feeding and Working Mothers: Many women continue to breast feed after returning to work. To provide adequate nourishment during the work day while she is away, a mother can supplement the baby's diet with prepared infant formulas and continue to breast feed when she returns home. Instead of using formula, however, many women prefer to express breast milk while at work and give their baby mother's milk exclusively. Supplementing with either formula or expressed breast milk is

Table 3.5
BASIC FOUR FOOD GUIDE FOR NURSING MOTHERS
(2,100 to 2,900 calories a day)

Food Group	Recommended Servings Each Day	Average Serving Size
Milk group (or equivalent)	5	
Milk, whole, low fat, skim		1 cup
Buttermilk		1 cup
Powdered milk		4 tbsp.
Evaporated milk		3 oz.
Cheese		1½ oz.
Cottage cheese		1 cup
Yogurt		1 cup
Tofu		1 cup
Meat, fish, poultry (or equivalent)	4	2–3 oz.
Eggs		2 whole
Peanut butter		¼ cup
Cooked dried peas or beans		¼ cup
Luncheon meat		2–3 slices
Tofu		1 cup
Nuts and seeds		½ cup
Cheese		2 oz.
Vegetables and fruits	4	½–¾ cup
Citrus fruits (vitamin C source)	1 or more	
Orange, mango, guava		1 medium
Grapefruit, cantaloupe		½ medium
Orange or grapefruit juice		½ cup
Strawberries		1 cup
Tomatoes or tomato juice		½ cup
Yellow or green vegetable or fruit (vitamin A source)	1 or more	
Broccoli		½ cup
Spinach		½ cup
Carrots		½ cup
Squash		½ cup
Cantaloupe		½ fruit
Apricots		10 halves
Other fruits and vegetables	2 or more	
Fresh, frozen, canned fruits and vegetables		½ cup
Potato, turnip, most whole vegetables		1 medium

Table 3.5
Continued

Food Group	Recommended Servings Each Day	Average Serving Size
Apple, banana, most whole fruits		1 medium
Breads and cereals (whole grain or enriched)	4	
Bread		1 slice
Dry cereal (unsweetened)		¾ cup
Cooked cereal		½ cup
Rice, noodles, pasta		½ cup
Roll		1 medium
Bagel		½ medium
Crackers		4 whole
Muffins		1 medium
Other foods		
Fats and oils	6	
Butter, margarine, mayonnaise		1 tbsp.
Vegetable oil		1 tbsp.
Salad dressing		1 tbsp.
Sour cream		1 tbsp.
Olives		5 small
Nuts		6 medium
Avocado		⅛ medium
Liquids (in addition to milk)	6 or more	
Water		8 oz.
Fruit juice		8 oz.
Vegetable juice		8 oz.
Seltzer water, club soda		8 oz.
Caffeine-free soft drinks		8 oz.
Coffee, tea		in moderation
Desserts and snacks	as needed	
Pudding		½ cup
Ice cream or ice milk		1 cup
Custard		1 cup
Dried fruits		3 oz.
Cookies		2–3 medium
Cake		1 ounce
Pie		1½ ounce
Sugar, honey, molasses, jam, jelly, preserves		2 tbsp.

fine. No mother need feel guilty about supplementing with formula. Successful mothering is never measured by the number of times a mother supplies her infant with expressed breast milk.

Depending on the mother's job and the attitude of co-workers, expressing can be simple and natural. Too often, society considers breasts objects of sexual excitement rather than organs that nourish infants. In time, as increasing numbers of women choose to breast feed, a more relaxed attitude toward breasts may develop.

Some women find that before returning to work it is helpful to speak with their supervisors and explain confidently that they are breast feeding, and that they plan to do so even after returning to work. They can ask for suggestions about finding a private location — preferably not a bathroom — where they can express breast milk. A quiet corner of a lunchroom or a borrowed office might be acceptable places. Expressing milk can be performed during morning and afternoon coffee breaks as well as at lunchtime. No one should be shocked, disgusted, or make embarrassing remarks. If someone displays such a negative attitude, an effective way to handle this is to simply explain that the best food for a baby is mother's milk. Bear in mind, however, that there is no need to make co-workers uncomfortable. A private place is usually best.

Before returning to work, a small supply of breast milk should be expressed each day and frozen. It usually is not a problem in the first several months after birth to obtain extra milk. This extra supply assures that there will be breast milk available if, for some reason, a mother finds it impossible to express.

Expressing milk should be done at approximately the same time every day. It can be performed by hand or with a handheld or an electric pump. Handheld pumps are common but some women find using them uncomfortable. Electric pumps, which exert intermittent pressure, are gentle and thorough and are readily available from rental agencies.

Probably the least cumbersome method is hand expression. After thorough hand washing, the nipples should be washed with water and the breast supported with one hand. The thumb and the forefinger of the other hand are placed at the edge of the areola, and gentle pressure is applied in the general direction of the nipple. A few drops will dribble out, and when the let-down reflex occurs, the milk squirts out. A clean container is used to catch the milk. Expression continues until only a few drops of milk appear; then the other breast is expressed. A second expression of the first and then the second breast should then be performed. The milk bottle is capped and placed in a refrigerator. Breast milk should be used within a day after it is refrigerated. It will stay fresh up to two weeks in the freezer.

Support from other nursing mothers is invaluable. The Nursing Mothers Council or La Leche League can provide information and names of experienced counselors on breast feeding (see Resources at end of book for address). In addition, obstetric nurses, whom the mother may meet at the time of delivery, can provide assistance.

Often the best part of a mother's working day is nursing the baby just before leaving for work or just after returning home. A quiet time for nursing can be arranged by having the husband, older children, or someone else help prepare breakfast and dinner.

Stress and fatigue, the biggest problems associated with breast feeding while working, can directly affect the quantity of milk a mother expresses. For a day or so, a mother may be unable to express enough milk to satisfy her baby. If this occurs, the baby can be fed formula supplement or expressed breast milk that has been frozen. Breast milk usually returns to full volume within a few days with extra rest and less stress.

Formula Feeding

Although breast feeding has special advantages, formula feeding can be an acceptable way to nourish infants. Infant formula manufacturers constantly are improving the composition of formulas, always trying to approximate human milk, the gold standard for infant nutrition. Even though cow's milk is the basis of most formulas, formula manufacturers have been able to modify cow's milk to duplicate most of the qualities of human milk. The percentages of whey and casein used in formula manufacture resemble the composition of human milk, so formulas are easily digested. Vegetable oils are added to provide the required amount of unsaturated fat, with its requisite linoleic acid.

Vitamins and minerals are added to meet the needs of the infant and, in some instances, formulas may even provide more iron and vitamin D than breast milk. Formulas contain no cholesterol and contain more protein than breast milk.

Formulas must be chosen and/or made with care. Commercial formulas are available in three forms: powders and concentrates, which must be mixed with water, and ready to feed, which do not require dilution and tend to be more expensive. All are equally nutritious.

It is important that all formula labels be read carefully. *Concentrated and powdered formulas must be diluted with water.* The standard dilution is 1 : 1. For example, to every 13 ounces of water, add 13 ounces of concentrate. Failure to carefully follow the directions provided on the can or by a pediatrician can be extremely dangerous to the baby. If too little water is added, dehydration, kidney stones, and other serious medical problems can result. If too much water is added, the baby will not receive the necessary nutrients unless larger volumes of formula are consumed. For babies with lactose intolerance or an allergy to cow's milk, soy-based or other specialized formulas are available and often prescribed. (See Chapter 8 for suggestions on feeding babies with allergies and other food-related problems.)

Skim milk, 2-percent, or 1-percent milk never should be the basis of baby's formula. They contain too much protein and too little fatty acid, vitamin E, and vitamin C. Unmodified cow's milk alone also is not suitable for infants, for the reasons mentioned above in the discussion of breast feeding. These problems include: (1) The high protein content of cow's milk could make it difficult for the infant to excrete the products of protein digestion, thereby leading to excess water loss. In small infants this can cause dehydration because their immature kidneys cannot concentrate wastes. (2) Infants who are sensitive to cow's-milk protein (see Chapter 8) may lose some blood because of certain reactions that can occur in the digestive tract. Excessive blood loss can lead to iron deficiency anemia in some sensitive infants.

Parents often assume that their infants prefer warm liquids. Many infants, however, readily accept and prefer formula or expressed breast milk at body temperature, room temperature, or even slightly cooler. It is a good idea to experiment to determine what is the most readily accepted temperature for an infant. Hot liquids, obviously, should never be fed to infants.

All formula, expressed breast milk, or any other food should be temperature tested before it is fed to an infant.

Although microwave ovens have become popular, time-saving tools for heating bottles, they must be used with caution because the formula can become very hot even though the bottle feels cool. In addition, when tightly closed bottles are heated in the microwave the water turns to steam. When the steam builds inside a closed container, the increasing pressure can cause the bottle to explode. A 1-week-old Illinois baby, in fact, spent two weeks in the hospital with second-degree burns when the plastic liner of a bottle exploded several seconds after it was removed from a microwave oven.

Old-fashioned bottle-warming methods remain the safest and most reliable way to heat formula or expressed breast milk. The five simple steps to warm a bottle are outlined in Table 3.6.

Nipples and bottles must be clean. Parents should watch for contamination, which can occur easily if formulas are prepared or stored carelessly. In the past, the need for sterilization of bottles and all equipment used to prepare formula was emphasized. Times, however, have changed, and fewer pediatricians insist that babies need this degree of cleanliness. If, however, parents want to sterilize utensils (e.g., the can opener, measuring and mixing equipment), bottles, and nipples, using one of three methods outlined in Table 3.7 will assure optimum cleanliness.

It is important that mothers who bottle feed spend time holding and cuddling their babies during feedings. The emotional bonding and feelings of security that result from these times are of critical importance to the child's developing sense of self.

FEEDING SCHEDULES

For a number of social reasons, until the 1960s and 1970s it was advised that babies be fed according to a strict schedule. During the days when whole families worked together to make

Table 3.6
WARMING INFANT FORMULAS OR EXPRESSED BREAST MILK

1 Place the bottle in a pan of hot (not boiling) tap water or hold the bottle under hot running tap water for a few minutes.

2 When the bottle begins to feel warm, shake it gently.

3 Place the bottle back into the pan of hot water or under the hot tap water.

4 Test the temperature of the formula by shaking a few drops on the underside of the wrist. The liquid should feel lukewarm to slightly warm.

5 If the liquid feels too warm, let the bottle sit at room temperature for several minutes to cool. Always retest the temperature before feeding the infant.

Table 3.7
STERILIZING BABY BOTTLES

Method 1:
• All the equipment is boiled for 20 minutes before the bottles are filled.
• The water to be used in the formula is boiled for five minutes.
• The bottles then are filled carefully and refrigerated. They must be used within 48 hours.

Method 2:
• The formulas are made up and placed in the bottles, the caps screwed on loosely, and the bottles placed in a large pot with three inches of water.
• The pot is covered and the water boiled for 25 minutes.
• The bottles, with the nipple rings screwed on tightly, are refrigerated and used within 48 hours.

Method 3:
• The bottles are filled with the required amount of water and sterilized as in Method 2.
• These bottles are stored at room temperature for no more than three days.
• When needed, the correct amount of concentrate or formula is added, shaken in, and fed to the infant.

a living, often on the farm, the needs of the group outweighed the needs of the baby. And it was thought that to indulge babies in their private demands would encourage a kind of self-centeredness that the group could not tolerate easily.

Later, as people moved off the farm to work in industry, thereby breaking the old family patterns, science also came of age, bringing with it new and powerful opinions about proper infant feeding techniques. Schedules were developed, and pediatricians advised parents to follow them. Most parents did, fearing that failure to do so may hurt their baby's development.

After World War II, many families moved to the suburbs, trading the extended families of farm life for the isolation of the nuclear family. Women stayed at home and made rearing the children their entire business. At that time, when and how a child was fed more often reflected the pressures for perfection on the mother than an understanding of the needs of the baby. Because most pediatricians still thought that a fixed schedule was a sign of a "well-brought-up" infant, most mothers arranged their babies' feedings accordingly.

With the new freedoms of the 1960s, the rigidity of many of these schedules finally relaxed. As the individuality of the child was increasingly recognized, more and more mothers began to feed babies according to their own inner schedule, rather than according to the clock.

For most people, feeding babies on demand has become the accepted practice today. Most pediatricians believe that babies know best how much to eat and how frequently they need to eat. Their bodies seem to have a built-in regulator that works with astonishing precision. Breast-fed babies usually feed more often than formula-fed babies. Gradually, over the first two or three months, most babies arrive at a fairly regular schedule.

Many babies want to be fed at bedtime or during the night,

Parents should never give the baby a bottle and go back to bed, allowing the baby to fall asleep with the bottle in his or her mouth. The sugar in milk, lactose, if allowed to stay in a baby's mouth for prolonged periods of time, can cause extensive tooth decay.

which leads to interrupted sleep for parents. If the baby is breast fed then the mother, obviously, has all the feeding responsibilities — day and night. If the baby is bottle fed (formula or expressed breast milk), the father can share these feeding duties.

People who are feeding babies should watch for signs of hunger and satiety and learn to recognize the particular signals of their own baby. Crying, for example, does not always mean a baby is hungry. It is best to consider other possible causes first: change the baby's diapers; play with the baby; check to see whether the baby is warm or cool enough. Only after ruling out these other needs should feeding be tried. In this way babies learn that food is not the remedy for all ills.

The baby will indicate by various signs — turning the head, playing with the nipple, sleeping — when feeding is completed. On some days the baby will eat more; on some days, less; and on some days, more frequently than on others. Forcing the baby to finish a bottle or to conform to the amounts prescribed on some chart is, in most instances, a mistake.

It may relieve new parents to know that by the end of the first year the baby will be eating at the family table, usually on the family schedule. The demand feeding of infancy soon will give way to the needs of the whole family.

SUPPLEMENTS

Although most needs are met by breast milk or formula, certain supplements may be suggested for infants:

Fluoride may be recommended for breast-fed babies (no fluoride is received from the mother) and for babies fed ready-to-feed formulas. If a baby is fed concentrated formulas that are diluted with nonfluoridated water, supplements also may be necessary.

Vitamin D supplements are recommended for breast-fed babies, particularly if they are exposed to little sunlight, as during winter, and if they are dark skinned. Most pediatricians recommend vitamin D supplementation at 3 months.

Vitamin C supplements are needed by only those babies who are fed evaporated milk formulas.

Iron is vitally important during this rapid growth period. Full-term infants, however, are born with enough iron to last six full months. Iron-supplemented formula is the best source of iron for infants. Breast-fed babies are likely to receive enough iron from the mother's milk until about age 6 months, when they begin to eat solids. At that time, iron-fortified cereals should be added.

Multivitamin supplements, however, are *not* needed by most infants and should be introduced only on the pediatrician's recommendation.

INTRODUCING SOLIDS

The age at which to introduce solid foods to infants has changed significantly over the past few decades. While introducing solids at an early age was once considered a mark of the baby's precocity, most pediatricians today recommend that babies not be given solid foods until they are at least 4 months of age. Many doctors recommend that solid foods be delayed until 6 months, especially if the baby is breast fed and is gaining weight well. Babies younger than 4 months are not developmentally ready for solid foods, and the agonies of such early feedings are wasted efforts because little food actually ends up in the baby. Babies, themselves, will provide the best clues as to when they are ready for solid foods. Table 3.8 outlines the various reflexes and developmental patterns that can help parents determine what type of food to provide and at what age to offer these foods.

As Table 3.8 shows, babies younger than 4 to 6 months of age have an inherited tongue-thrusting reflex that causes them to push most solid objects (except fingers, nipples, and other objects that cannot be swallowed) out of their mouths. This reflex, called the extrusion reflex, helps prevent them from choking on foreign objects. Between 4 and 6 months of age, however, the extrusion reflex begins to disappear. Also at this time, the baby begins to lift the head and develops some hand-eye coordination. At this stage, babies are ready for the introduction of solids.

Parents may notice that as the suckle-swallow reflex weakens, the tongue begins to thrust food toward the back of the mouth and the up-and-down, munching-type motion continues to mature. Babies at this age become able to hold up their heads and

Table 3.8
DEVELOPMENT OF FEEDING PATTERNS

Birth

Rooting reflex	Lips, tongue, and head turn toward an object that touches the mouth area, enabling the infant to locate a nipple. The reflex remains until 3 to 5 months of age.
Suckle-swallow reflex	The infant vigorously sucks on an object placed in the mouth. Tongue moves back and forth to express milk from the nipple. The swallowing reflex is automatic if liquid is present while sucking. This reflex remains until 5 to 6 months of age.
Extrusion reflex	The infant pushes solid objects out of the mouth. This reflex remains until 4 to 6 months of age.
Biting reflex	The infant bites down then releases when pressure is applied to the gums. This reflex remains until 6 to 9 months of age.
Gag reflex	Muscles located at the rear of the mouth tighten when pressure is applied to the back of the tongue or the soft part of the roof of the mouth. This reflex remains throughout life.

6 to 10 weeks
Infant recognizes the standard position for feeding and begins to make automatic sucking motions when in this position.

2 to 3 months
Infant's swallowing pattern changes, and tongue no longer moves forward automatically during feedings. Jaw begins to move in a more definite up-and-down motion.

4 months
Drooling begins and steadily increases as teething occurs. Drooling stops by about 1 year of age. Tongue begins to transfer food from front to back of mouth. Infant brings hand up to mouth and sucks on hand and fingers.

5 to 6 months
Infant begins to control hand movements, grasps at objects, and can sit up without much support. Infant sees food, opens mouth to accept it, closes mouth over spoon, and slides food from spoon with lips. Tongue moves up and down to transfer food to back of mouth.

Table 3.8
Continued

6 to 8 months
Infant begins to use index finger and thumb to pick up objects.
  Swallowing is controlled, and infant holds food in mouth longer.
  Tongue moves from side to side, allowing better control over the
  location of food in the mouth. Jaw is able to munch and mash
  foods. Infant can place lips on rim of cup, but most liquid runs
  from corners of mouth. Infant begins to bring food to mouth when
  teething.

9 to 12 months
Infant can hold onto bottle and self-feeds finger foods. Begins self-
  feeding with spoon; however, usually turns over spoon before it
  gets to mouth. Uses cup with some spilling. Biting, chewing, and
  swallowing motions continue to mature.

sit without support. They lean forward with their mouths open to show interest in food, and can lean back or turn away to show disinterest or rejection. Until the baby is able to do these things it is not advisable to begin solid feedings. Again, the baby is best able to regulate when and how much to eat. Parents should pay close attention to these signals and realize that their babies, when healthy, can express their own needs.

There is no strong reason why one group of solids should be started before another group. Most pediatricians, however, recommend beginning with iron-fortified dry cereals because these are easy for the baby to eat and digest. Only one new food should be introduced at a time in order to make identifying any food sensitivities easier. Iron-fortified rice cereal is the least allergenic cereal, and this is usually the first food offered. If this is tolerated, then barley or oatmeal can be tried.

Cereal may be mixed with breast milk or formula for the fats, protein, vitamins, minerals. At first the mixture should be very thin, just slightly thicker than breast milk or formula, and over a few weeks the consistency can gradually become thicker, as the baby becomes more accepting of solid foods. It is best to begin with one to two teaspoons of cereal once a day, and increase this gradually to one-third to one-half a cup total, fed twice a day. A good deal of food will run out of the baby's mouth at first, as the process is new and unfamiliar. If most seems to be lost over several days, it is advisable to stop and try again several weeks later. The baby may not be ready.

Once cereals are well accepted, usually at 5 to 6 months of age, strained fruits, vegetables, and meats gradually can be added to the diet one at a time. Commercially prepared, and home-strained or pureed baby foods are good. (Most commercially prepared infant foods, like homemade baby foods, contain no preservatives and, therefore, should be stored in the refrigerator after opening. Use them within two or three days of opening.) (See Table 10.5 for more information on storing food.) Figure 3.1 outlines the feeding steps and appropriate food textures from the first solids to table textures.

As Figure 3.1 shows, by 6 or 7 months of age, ripe bananas, cooked, soft, fork-mashed, or junior-texture fruits and vegetables will, in most instances, be enjoyed by the baby. If an increase in texture is delayed beyond 6 or 7 months, the infant may resist change.

The transition from strained food to mashed or junior-texture foods is a crucial step.

A baby's foods should not be seasoned with salt or sugar. The addition of these substances is not necessary and often leads to lifelong eating habits that may cause health problems in later years. Recently the major producers of baby food have become sensitive to nutritional issues and consumer pressures. As a result, salt, sugar, modified starch, and other additives have been removed from their products. Too frequently, parents add these seasonings because the baby's food seems bland to the adult palate. But children, who are unaccustomed to extra salt or sugar, will like food without them.

Between 7 and 9 months, minced foods, including meat, enriched breads, toast, potatoes, rice, macaroni, and crackers can be introduced. Teething begins between 6 and 8 months, and hard toast or crackers, as well as cool liquids, often are soothing.

Between 7 and 10 months, babies can begin to sit with the family at mealtime and enjoy pieces of soft finger foods that can

Figure 3.1
INTRODUCTION OF SOLIDS

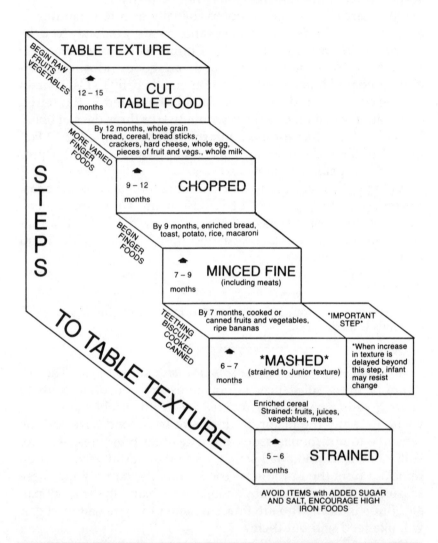

(*Source:* Nutrition Services, Department of Nutrition and Food Service, Children's Hospital, Boston, MA.)

be chewed without molars. By this time, the grasp has developed sufficiently so that babies can manipulate food from table to mouth with increasing accuracy. High-protein foods, such as tender meats (minced), cottage cheese, ricotta cheese, chunks of soft cheese, or egg yolks can be introduced. The iron from egg yolks will not be absorbed unless vitamin C is present in the same meal. In fact, egg yolks will decrease the absorption of iron from other sources if vitamin C is not present.

At this time the baby should be drinking less milk and getting more nourishment from solids. To ensure that the baby does eat enough solids, many find it helpful to offer milk at the end rather than the beginning of the meal. Babies who are 7 to 10 months should be eating three meals plus snacks each day and have moved from a pattern of eating on demand to eating with the family.

Between 8 and 12 months, babies can be weaned from the breast or bottle and moved to the cup. This transition should be approached gradually and in a relaxed manner. Most babies by this time have already begun drinking from a cup. When weaning, the breast or bottle should be eliminated one feeding at a time, over a period of a few weeks. Whole milk should be fed to children until the age of 2 years, when skim, 1-, or 2-percent milk may be introduced. Until then, children need the fats found in whole milk.

By the end of this extraordinarily rapid transition period, at age 10 to 12 months, the child is eating family foods at the family table, and makes hunger pangs clearly known by crawling to the high chair, shaking it, and making noises to get attention. By 12 months, whole-grain breads, cereal, bread sticks, crackers, hard cheese, whole eggs, pieces of fruits and vegetables, and whole milk all should contribute to the child's balanced diet. At this point the Basic Four Food Guide, modified to meet the needs of a small child, can be of value, as shown in Table 3.9.

FOOD AND GROWTH

Babies, like adults, have different frames and different shapes. Parents, therefore, should not worry whether their baby is skinny or a little chubby. Trying to adjust the baby's diet to slim down or fatten up an infant can lead to undernutrition or

Table 3.9
THE BASIC FOUR FOOD GUIDE FOR CHILDREN
(1-year-old child, 900–1,200 calories a day)

Food Group	Recommended Servings Each Day	Average Serving Size
Milk group (or equivalent)	4	
Milk, breast, formula, whole		½ cup
Powdered milk		2 tbsp.
Cheese		¾ oz.
Cottage cheese		½ cup
Yogurt		½ cup
Meat, fish, poultry (or equivalent)	2 or 3	2 tbsp.
Eggs		1 whole
Cooked mashed dried peas or beans		4 tbsp.
Chopped luncheon meat		1 slice
Peanut butter		1 tbsp.
Vegetables and fruits	4 or more	2–3 tbsp.
Citrus fruits (vitamin C source)	1 or more	
Orange or grapefruit juice		¼ cup
Strawberries		¼ cup
Tomatoes or tomato juice		¼ cup
Yellow or green vegetable or fruit (vitamin A source)	1 or more	
Broccoli		2–3 tbsp.
Spinach		2–3 tbsp.
Carrots		2–3 tbsp.
Squash		2–3 tbsp.
Cantaloupe		¼ cup
Apricots		4 halves
Other fruits and vegetables	2 or more	
Fresh, frozen, canned fruits and vegetables		2–3 tbsp.
Potato, turnip, most whole vegetables		¼ veg.
Apple, banana, most whole fruits		¼ fruit
Breads and cereals (whole grain or enriched)	4 or more	
Bread		½ slice
Dry cereal (unsweetened)		½ cup
Cooked cereal, rice, pasta		2–3 tbsp.

Table 3.9
Continued

Food Group	Recommended Servings Each Day	Average Serving Size
Others (to meet calorie needs)	as needed	
Butter, margarine, mayonnaise, oil		1 tbsp.
Desserts		
Pudding		¼ cup
Ice cream or ice milk		¾ cup
Sugar, jelly, jam		2 tbsp.

overnutrition. An excessive focus on slimness or obesity can lead to undernutrition or overnutrition. Healthy babies, left to themselves, usually eat the right amount. They will know when they are hungry and when they are full, and they give signals to the parent.

Doctors and dietitians use height-weight charts to check a baby's development and nutritional status. They show height and weight growth for babies within the whole range of normal development, from infants to children. Generally, in infancy, height and weight advance at about the same rate. When the rates vary dramatically, as when a baby grows in length but not in weight, or makes much more rapid weight gains than height gains, doctors will begin to look for the reason. Most parents will be able to notice any important growth abnormalities and should report any concerns to their pediatrician.

In summary, good nutrition and good eating habits begin before pregnancy. A well-nourished, healthy mother has the best chance of giving birth to a healthy baby. Pregnant women should pay close attention to their increased needs, especially for calcium and iron.

A well-planned diet is essential throughout the baby's first year, as growth and development continue at a rapid pace. The diet for infants up to 6 months of age consists primarily of breast milk or formula, and feeding usually takes place on demand rather than three times a day. Solid foods generally are introduced (one at a time) at 4 to 6 months of age. As infants get closer to their first birthdays, feedings become more routine and consist of foods from the Basic Four Food Groups. They begin to eat three meals and several snacks a day, sit at the family table, and eat adult foods that have been minced to the appropriate texture. The development of healthful lifelong eating habits begins at this early stage.

4

LET'S EAT!
FROM TOTS TO TEENS

"Perhaps" [said the waiter] "you would care to contemplate the sweets." Paddington gave him an odd look. "I'd sooner eat them," he said.

Michael Bond
Paddington Takes the Air

PLANNING A SENSIBLE DIET

Foods that children will eat and foods that they like change constantly. One day a child will eat an entire serving of peas; the next week, that child will stick out his or her tongue, make a face, and say that peas are "yucky." Planning three well-balanced meals and nourishing yet tasty snacks day after day is therefore challenging for parents.

Sometimes a child will ask for the same food for lunch every day for several weeks. Parents may become bored preparing one item over and over, and they may worry about the child's health. Many children refuse to try new foods, and some may refuse to eat almost all varieties of certain kinds of foods, such as green vegetables. It takes creative, patient parents to understand and cope with the capricious eating patterns of children.

Children grow rapidly in their first year of life, but as they enter their toddler years the rate of growth slows down. As a result, their appetites and their need for food also decrease.

Nevertheless, children continue to grow and develop, and they must have nourishing food and a balanced diet.

When planning meals and snacks for toddlers, preschoolers, school-aged children, and adolescents, it is important to know which nutrients children need for normal growth and development, how much of each is needed, and which foods are good sources of these raw materials. Parents can combine this general information with familiarity with the foods their children will eat or are likely to try. Finally, parents should work with their children to foster and nurture sensible eating habits.

The Recommended Dietary Allowances (outlined in Table 2.1) may offer some help planning meals; however, it may be difficult translating the RDA tables into real life. For example, how do parents feed their 2-year-old daughter so that each day she receives 23 grams of protein, 2,000 International Units of vitamin A, and 0.8 milligrams of riboflavin, as well as all the other required nutrients? How do parents remember which foods are rich — and how rich — in iron, calcium, thiamin, and zinc? And then, how should parents put all that into a daily menu that makes sense and is not too complicated or time consuming? The goal, after all, is to feed children in a way that promotes good health and normal growth but also fits naturally into the other patterns of family life.

The most practical way to plan meals for children is to use the Basic Four Food Groups — milk and dairy products; meat or protein equivalent; fruit and vegetables; and bread and cereal (see Table 2.33). These foods should be provided according to the recommendations in the Basic Four Food Guide for Children, which has been broken down by age group in this chapter (see Tables 4.1, 4.2, and 4.3). These guidelines provide for a variety of foods in serving sizes that supply the necessary nutrients for growing children. In general, foods from each of the four groups should be eaten at each meal, and a wide variety of foods from within each group should be chosen.

The Basic Four Food Guide for Children has been adapted from the current set of national standards for an adequate diet, called the Daily Food Guide. The Basic Four Food Guide, however, has been designed to better suit the needs of children and to be more specific in showing parents how to accomplish this.

The original set of national dietary guidelines, known as the Basic Seven, was developed in the early 1940s, soon after the first RDA were published. In the mid-1950s, various government and nutrition committees revised the Basic Seven into the Basic Four. The Daily Food Guide was then published to show how to use the four food groups to eat a well-balanced, nourishing diet.

Over the years the Daily Food Guide has been modified to take into account fat, cholesterol, sodium, and sugar. The food suggestions and portion sizes listed in the guide provide the recommended amounts of protein, vitamin A, riboflavin, ascorbic acid (vitamin C), calcium, and phosphorus, and most of the thiamin and niacin. The Daily Food Guide, however, is low in zinc, supplies only half the iron required by women, and may provide from one-third to one-half the calories recommended (although many will find the caloric intake sufficient).

MEALS AND MEALTIMES

The need for three meals a day remains controversial. Some contend that it is better to eat four or more smaller meals during the day. The three-meals-a-day schedule, however, is the eating pattern that most American families follow. Each meal plays a key role in supplying the daily recommended levels of the essential nutrients.

The Morning Meal

A good breakfast should be a regular part of every morning, especially for children. Unfortunately, it is the meal most often skipped by people of all ages. Breakfast supplies the nourishment and energy necessary to carry children through an active morning. The following example shows what can happen when a child starts the day without breakfast.

A fourth-grade boy had always been a bright, cheerful, attentive student. Toward the middle of the school year, however, his teacher noticed that the boy began to get restless about 10 A.M. He was irritable, and appeared to be tired. He became careless about his schoolwork, and his grades suffered.

After talking with the boy's parents, the teacher learned that until recently, the mother, and sometimes both parents, had eaten breakfast with him. The mother, however, had taken a new job and was going to work before her son left for school. She had been putting breakfast out on the table. Apparently the boy did not like the idea of eating alone, and when confronted he admitted that he threw out the food that was left for him.

This problem was easily solved with a minor change in routine. The parents simply roused the boy earlier in the morning — in time for a nourishing family breakfast.

Comprehensive studies have confirmed what this single example shows: *Breakfast is important.* A study by the University of Iowa Medical College found that children who skipped breakfast had trouble concentrating at school and became inattentive and restless by late morning. Another study of schoolchildren conducted by the Massachusetts Institute of Technology found that problem-solving abilities decreased when no breakfast was eaten. This is because after fasting during the night, the level of blood sugar (the energy that is available for the body to use immediately) usually is low. Skipping breakfast causes it to fall even lower, and when blood sugar is low, fatigue, irritability, and restlessness may set in.

To maintain a consistent level of fuel for the body, the morning meal should contain some foods that provide quick energy, as well as some foods that release energy more slowly. Breakfasts, therefore, should include a protein source, a bread and/or cereal, a fruit or vegetable, a small amount of fat, and milk — foods from each of the Basic Four Food Groups.

The Noontime Meal

In previous generations, lunch often was the main meal of the day because many families worked together on farms, and a hearty midday meal (usually called "dinner") was needed to satisfy the hunger that occurred after a morning of physical work. The meal also provided energy for more work in the afternoon. Over the past century, however, fewer families have relied on the land for income, more people have taken jobs further from the home, and more women have entered the work force. As a result, lunches have become the meal that all family members most often eat outside the home.

School-aged children and adolescents eat most of their lunches at school. During vacations or on weekends children often eat lunches at friends' houses or at fast-food restaurants. Even toddlers and preschoolers may eat lunch regularly at the baby sitter's house or a day-care facility.

Lunch is also an important meal for children. Nourishing foods at lunchtime help children remain attentive and alert through the afternoon, as well as curb their hunger pangs.

The Evening Meal

Dinner, or supper, is the major meal of the day in most households today. Family members are most likely to sit down together and share a meal in the evening. As such, dinner is the logical meal in which parents can help make up for possible deficiencies in their children's diets. In many families, however, dinner at home is eaten in shifts to accommodate jobs, meetings, and recreational activities. It may be eaten on the run or in a restaurant, hot off the stove or rewarmed for the fourth time. And yet, no matter what the situation, dinner can consist of food from the Basic Four Food Groups and be well balanced and nourishing.

MEALS FOR TODDLERS

By 1 year of age most children have tripled their birth weights and increased their lengths (height) by 50 percent. At this point, the growth rate slows to between one-half to one-third of what it was before age 12 months — birth weight is not quadrupled until 2 years of age, or birth length until age 4 years. Developmental growth, mastery of social and motor skills, and the environment occupy the child's interest more. At this point the child will eat less and will eat less voraciously.

Feeding toddlers can be extremely challenging, as most parents can attest. One week a certain food will be a favorite; the next week it will be refused dramatically. Sometimes a toddler will eat the whole meal, sometimes only parts of it. Parents

Table 4.1

BASIC FOUR FOOD GUIDE FOR CHILDREN

Toddlers: Age 1–3 Years Old

(1,000 to 1,300 calories a day)

Food Group	Recommended Servings Each Day	Average Serving Size
Milk (or equivalent)	4	
Milk, whole for children younger than 2 years; whole, low fat, or skim for children older than 2 years.		½–¾ cup
Powdered milk		2–3 tbsp.
Cheese		1 oz.
Cottage cheese		½ cup
Yogurt		½ cup
Meat, fish, poultry (or equivalent)	2 or more	2–3 tbsp.
Eggs		1 whole
Peanut butter		1–2 tbsp.
Cooked dried peas or beans		¼ cup
Luncheon meat		1 slice
Vegetables and fruits	4 or more	2–3 tbsp.
Citrus fruits (vitamin C source)	1 or more	
Orange or grapefruit juice		½ cup
Strawberries		¾ cup
Tomatoes or tomato juice		½ cup
Yellow or green vegetable or fruit (vitamin A source)	1 or more	
Broccoli		4 tbsp.
Spinach		4 tbsp.
Carrots		4 tbsp.
Squash		4 tbsp.
Cantaloupe		¼ fruit
Apricots		5 fruit halves
Other fruits and vegetables	2 or more	
Fresh, frozen, canned fruits and vegetables		2–3 tbsp.
Potato, turnip, most whole vegetables		¼–½ veg.
Apple, banana, most whole fruits		¼–½ fruit
Breads and cereals (whole grain or enriched)	4 or more	
Bread		½–1 slice
Dry cereal (unsweetened)		½–¾ cup
Cooked cereal, rice, pasta		2–4 tbsp.

Table 4.1
Continued

Food Group	Recommended Servings Each Day	Average Serving Size
Others (to meet calorie needs)	as needed	
Butter, margarine, mayonnaise, oil		1 tbsp.
Desserts		
Pudding		½ cup
Ice cream or ice milk		1 cup
Cookies		2–3 medium
Cake		1 oz.
Pie		1½ oz.
Sugar, honey, molasses, jelly, jam		2 tbsp.

should expect and accept this but not be overly concerned about it. While children this age often binge on one food or another for a few days, over time they generally will balance their diets effectively.

Table 4.1 outlines the Basic Four Food Guide for toddlers. Following these guidelines, meat or the equivalent, bread or cereal, fruit or vegetable, and milk or the equivalent should be offered at each meal. *Offered* is the key word here: If a food is not offered, it will not be eaten. At least one food the child likes (if that can be predicted) should be included.

Toddlers eat far less than adults — roughly one-fourth to one-third of adult portions. Therefore, it is a good strategy to feed them *small* servings. The rule of thumb for serving sizes is that children eat a measuring tablespoon (as opposed to a serving spoon) of each food for each year of age or, in the case of foods that do not get served in tablespoon sizes, one-quarter of the adult portion.

Breakfast for toddlers should contain adequate amounts of carbohydrates, fat, and protein to provide energy and nourishment for the morning. Iron-fortified cereal, fruit or fruit juice, and milk is one possibility; a whole, soft-cooked egg, toast with a small amount of butter or margarine, fruit or fruit juice, and milk is another.

Variations on these routine breakfasts, however, help introduce new foods to children and encourage them to learn about differences in taste and texture. Rather than a whole egg, young children may enjoy cheese cut up into cubes or strips. Many toddlers prefer dry, cold cereals to moist, hot cereals. Preferably, these should be unsugared. Cubed, sliced, or sectioned fruits, such as apricots, bananas, peaches, pears, strawberries, and oranges, are good sources of carbohydrate (natural sugar), fiber, vitamins, and minerals.

Allowing toddlers to feed themselves (despite the inevitable mess) makes breakfast more enjoyable for them. And if toddlers enjoy breakfast, they are likely to get into the important habit of starting each day with a good meal.

Lunch for toddlers should provide roughly a third of the RDA for all essential nutrients. Ideally, it should consist of one-half to one ounce of lean meat, poultry, fish, peanut butter, legumes, cheese, or an egg (if the child did not have one at breakfast); four tablespoons of a leafy green or deep yellow cooked vegetable; a slice of whole-grain bread; one-third to one-half cup of fruit; and one-half cup of whole milk for children younger than 2 years old, and three-fourths cup of low-fat or skim milk for children older than 2 years.

Toddlers should have one serving of potatoes, rice, or noodles each day, and this may be given at lunchtime or dinner. Raw vegetables, such as carrots, lettuce, tomatoes, and cabbage, also are desirable each day, and these may be included at lunch or dinner. In fact, they could be offered at breakfast!

The variety of possible combinations allows parents to make lunches for toddlers interesting and fun. Spaghetti and meat sauce, or tuna-noodle casserole, may be a hit. Vegetables or noodle soups made with beef or chicken are good ways to provide several nourishing foods in one hearty dish. Parents, however, should make sure the vegetables are soft and in chunks large enough to be picked out with fingers (again, fun for young toddlers). Creamed soups, split-pea soup, and bean soups also are good lunchtime choices.

Sandwiches are the old reliable standby for a nourishing

lunch, but they should be simple so the child can recognize the items inside. Peanut butter is both a favorite of toddlers and a rich source of protein, making it a staple in most homes with children. Tuna fish, chicken, turkey, and beef that have been minced finely are good choices. Grilled-cheese sandwiches are another easy, economical favorite of toddlers. Raw vegetables can be served along with the sandwich, and a piece of fruit and a cup of milk will round out the meal.

Desserts may be served at lunchtime. Raw or cooked fruits make ideal desserts for toddlers. Young children also enjoy pudding, ice cream, yogurt, and custards. These milk-based, egg-rich desserts are good sources of high-quality protein, calcium, and other minerals and vitamins. They should be made with as little sugar as possible. Cakes, brownies, candy, cookies, and pies should not become dessert mainstays, but can be offered from time to time.

Potato and corn chips, coconut, nuts, popcorn, sunflower or pumpkin seeds, whole kernel corn, or cut-up hot dogs are all dangerous for toddlers. These foods are difficult to chew and swallow, and they can be inhaled into the windpipe, causing the child to choke.

A balanced dinner for toddlers consists of one-half to three-fourths cup of milk (whole milk for children younger than 2 years, and low-fat or skim milk for children older than 2 years) or a milk equivalent; three tablespoons of meat, fish, poultry or other protein source, such as cottage cheese, or cheese; four tablespoons of a yellow or green vegetable; two tablespoons of fruit; and one-half slice of bread or two tablespoons of potato, rice, or pasta. Meals will be more appealing and more fun for parents as well as toddlers if the choices of items from each of the food groups vary from day to day.

Iron deficiency can be a problem among children in this age group. Dinner is an ideal time to include some iron-rich foods. Meats (liver, kidney, red meats, and liverwurst, in particular), fish, poultry, whole-grain breads and cereals, wheat germ, iron-fortified cereals, dark green, leafy vegetables, egg yolks, and cooked dried beans and peas all supply iron. (See Table 2.30 for a list of iron-rich foods.)

MEALS FOR PRESCHOOLERS AND CHILDREN UP TO 10

By the time a child is 3 or 4 years of age, many of the eating problems of toddlerhood have been resolved. Children at this age can feed themselves and no longer approach meals as a contest of dominance and control. Growth during this period is slow but steady, and children gradually increase the amount of food they eat. They enjoy meals both because they are hungry and as social events. Many parents, in fact, have noticed that their children — even fussy eaters — are more willing to eat nourishing foods when the entire family sits down to a meal together.

The Basic Four Food Guide for preschoolers and school-aged children, Table 4.2, should be followed, still with serving sizes equal to one tablespoon for each year of life (four tablespoons = one-fourth cup). This rule need not be followed rigidly, but parents might keep in mind that presenting too much food is worse than presenting too little. It is far better to let the child ask, "May I please have some more?"

Preschool children, 3 to 5 years of age, and school-aged children 6 to 10 years old, need a nourishing breakfast every day. The food choices are greater than for toddlers, primarily because older children have tasted and will eat a wider range of foods. Variety and diversity can work wonders in encouraging children to eat a good breakfast.

The conventional breakfast of eggs, toast, juice, and milk may please some children, but many children will not eat eggs in any recognizable form. Eggs are dependable sources of high-quality protein, iron, fats, and essential vitamins and minerals. If children refuse to eat egg dishes, they may enjoy pancakes, French toast, or waffles, all of which are made with eggs. Another possibility is to add an egg to a blender shake, along with fruit juice, fruit, and milk or yogurt. Children will not notice that the shake contains an egg, and they usually are delighted with the frothy texture. Children also may enjoy less conventional breakfasts

Table 4.2
BASIC FOUR FOOD GUIDE FOR CHILDREN
Preschoolers and School-Aged Children: 4–10 years
(1,700–2,100 calories a day)

Food Group	Recommended Number of Servings	Average Serving Size
Milk (or equivalent)	4	
Milk, preferably low fat or skim		¾–1 cup
Powdered milk		3–4 tbsp.
Cheese		¾–1½ oz.
Cottage cheese		¾–1 cup
Yogurt		¾–1 cup
Meat, fish, poultry (or equivalent)	2 or more	2–3 oz.
Eggs		1 whole
Peanut butter		2–3 tbsp.
Cooked dried peas or beans		½–¾ cup
Luncheon meat		2 slices
Vegetables and fruits	4 or more	
Citrus fruits (vitamin C source)	1 or more	
Orange or grapefruit juice		½–1 cup
Strawberries		1 cup
Tomatoes or tomato juice		½–1 cup
Yellow or green vegetable or fruit (vitamin A source)	1 or more	
Broccoli		¼ cup
Spinach		¼ cup
Carrots		¼ cup
Squash		¼ cup
Cantaloupe		¼–½ fruit
Apricots		5–8 halves
Other fruits and vegetables	2 or more	
Fresh, frozen, canned fruits and vegetables		½ cup
Potato, turnip, most whole vegetables		½–1 veg.
Apple, banana, most whole fruits		½–1 fruit
Breads and cereals (whole grain or enriched)	4 or more	
Bread		1–2 slices
Dry cereal (unsweetened)		1 cup
Cooked cereal, rice, pasta		½ cup

Table 4.2
Continued

Food Group	Recommended Number of Servings	Average Serving Size
Others (to meet calorie needs)	as needed	
Butter, margarine, mayonnaise, oil		1–2 tbsp.
Desserts		
Pudding		½ cup
Ice cream or ice milk		1 cup
Cookies		2–3 medium
Cake		1 oz.
Pie		1½ oz.
Sugar, honey, molasses, jelly, jam		2 tbsp.

such as spaghetti, English muffins or pita bread covered with peanut butter or tomato sauce and cheese, bananas or apples with peanut butter, and toasted cheese sandwiches.

Many preschool and school-aged children insist on highly sugared cereals for breakfast. These cereals appeal to children because they taste sweet, fruity, or chocolatey; are named after, endorsed by, or resemble favorite cartoon characters, television and movie celebrities, or sports stars; or are advertised on children's commercial television programs. On the surface, many of these cereals appear to be a nutritional plus because they have been heavily fortified with vitamins and minerals that are needed by growing children. Most of the benefits, however, are outweighed by the high sugar and salt content of many popular cereals (see Tables 2.13 and 2.28). Excess sugar and salt (as described in Chapter 2) are unnecessary.

Parents can quickly get into the habit of reading the labels of cereals to check the amount of sugar. (See Chapter 10 for more information on reading food labels.)

Ingredients used in a product are listed on the label from most prevalent to least prevalent by weight.

Many commercial cereals are made with whole-grain oats, rice, corn or wheat without added sugar. They are rich in vitamins, minerals, and fiber. Commercial granola is a good source of these valuable raw materials, but many brands are laden with sugar, salt, and saturated fats such as coconut oil. Nourishing granola can be made easily at home without excess amounts of these ingredients.

If parents are trying to break their children from the sugar-coated-cereal-for-breakfast habit, a good idea is to serve an unsugared cereal with a small amount of a sugar-coated cereal sprinkled on top. If that does not work, parents can fill the bowl with half sugared and half unsugared cereal and gradually decrease the amount of sugar-coated cereal until there is none. Strawberries, blueberries, raisins, sliced bananas, and sliced peaches also may make unsugared whole-grain cereals more appealing to children. Adding fruit to the bowl adds natural sweetness as well as a healthy dose of vitamin C and fiber.

A school breakfast program is available in some school districts. For a nominal cost, school cafeterias provide a nourishing, hot breakfast to children before the start of each school day. This can be a help if both parents must go to work early.

Good lunches for children who are 4 to 10 years of age are similar to lunches fed to toddlers. Foods from the four food groups should be included, but portions should be slightly larger. On the average, portions for preschoolers should be anywhere from one-half to two-thirds the amount of a normal adult serving. Portions for school-aged children should be from three-fourths to a standard adult serving.

Sandwiches, especially peanut butter, often become routine lunch fare; many children like them and ask for them day after day. Some children may enjoy combination sandwiches, such as peanut butter with bananas or apples. This is a good way to add fruits to the meal.

For children who are still eating at home, pasta dishes, such as spaghetti, ravioli, ziti, and macaroni with cheese or meat sauce, combine nourishing ingredients from various food groups. Beef or chicken stew served over noodles also is a favorite of some children. It is a good idea to put carrots, peas, and green beans into casseroles or stews because children —

even the youngsters who refuse to eat most vegetables — are more likely to eat them in this form. Some children dislike cooked vegetables, but crisp raw vegetables (carrots, peppers, zucchini, green beans, celery, broccoli, cauliflower), which are full of vitamins, minerals, and fiber, tend to be more tempting.

Preschool children often eat lunches that have been prepared and served by baby sitters, day-care supervisors, relatives, or neighbors. In these situations, parents lose much control over what foods their children eat for lunch. Some children refuse to eat foods that have been prepared by people other than family members, and parents may need to whet their children's noontime appetites by making comments such as, "Mrs. Long sure worked hard to make this lunch. She thinks you are really going to like it." Or, "Dorothy sure is a terrific cook. I wish she would make my lunch." If all else fails, nourishing lunches can be prepared by parents and brought from home. Ideas for meals to be served by baby sitters are outlined in Chapter 6.

School-aged children eat most lunches in the school cafeteria, where they are subject to peer pressures. Even if encouraged not to swap or throw away parts of their lunches, children often can be swayed by their friends' suggestions or criticisms. Food served at school, however, can be satisfying. Lunches provided by the National School Lunch Act (see Chapter 9) are regulated by the Department of Agriculture. They must contain one-third of the child's RDA and must include milk, meat or equivalent, vegetable, fruit, bread or another grain food, and butter or margarine. (Even school lunch programs are required to follow the Basic Four!) School cafeteria meals aim to be nutritious and balanced. If a child does not like what is offered, however, all or part of the meal will land in the trash can.

It is a good idea for parents to try to find out what their children are eating at lunch. If a child usually takes a lunch to school, parents may be able to learn what was eaten by asking questions such as, "How did you like the special treat I put in your lunch today?" Or, "Do you remember what you ate for lunch today? I can't remember what I packed for you, and I don't want to give you the same thing tomorrow." If the child buys lunch in the school cafeteria, parents may ask, "What did you think of the butterscotch sundaes they served in the cafeteria today?" Or, "I heard the food in the cafeteria has been pretty good lately. Do you think so?" Both of these techniques may cause a child to think back on the food he or she ate at lunch and give parents some clue as to how nourishing that noontime meal really was.

The typical well-balanced home-packed school lunch contains a protein-rich sandwich (such as peanut butter, cheese, tuna fish, or luncheon meat), milk, fruit or a vegetable, and sometimes a cookie or other dessert. But even the most carefully planned lunch brought from home may be traded across the table for foods that are low in protein, vitamins, and minerals. Suggestions about ways to make school lunches nourishing, appetizing, and attractive are offered in Chapter 6.

Lunches for school-aged children during school vacations and weekends often consist of something quick and easy — without much thought given to protein, vitamin, and mineral content. Many children, without proper guidance, invariably fill up on soft drinks, cookies, cakes, potato chips, and other high-fat, high-sugar foods if they are available. Better lunches are hearty soups, sandwiches, and salads. Parents may want to gently point out the benefits of eating good, nourishing food, especially the ways it can help sustain energy and improve performance in various activities.

Dinner for preschoolers and school-aged children should include three-fourths to one cup of low-fat or skim milk, or a milk equivalent, such as yogurt, cheese, cottage cheese, or pudding; two to three ounces of meat, poultry, or fish or another source of protein, such as cooked dried beans or peanut butter; one-fourth cup of yellow or green vegetable; and one or two slices of enriched or whole-grain bread, or one-half cup of potato, rice, or pasta. A fruit should be served and an iron-rich food should be included in the meal, especially if no good sources of dietary iron have been eaten in other meals of the day.

MEALS FOR TEENAGERS

Adolescence is a time when a child again enters a period of rapid growth and physical change. Teenagers gain about 20 percent of their adult height and 50 percent of their adult weight during their adolescent years. Although the growth period generally extends over several years, most of it occurs in one 18- to 24-month spurt. A girl's growth spurt usually begins at 10 or 11 years of age and continues to about age 15. A boy's growth spurt occurs a little later, beginning at 12 or 13 years of age and continuing to age 19. There is great variation, however, in the age at which a growth spurt starts and the length of time it takes for the growth to occur. For the most part, children (and parents) should not be concerned if they start earlier or later than their peers or seem to be proceeding at a slower or faster rate.

With this rapid growth comes a dramatic increase in the amount of calories and nutrients needed. While boys need more calories than girls, all adolescents need additional calories, protein, vitamins, and minerals. The average adolescent needs more calories than at any other time in life (between 2,100 and 2,200 calories for teenage girls and 2,700 and 2,800 calories for teenage boys). These calories should be distributed among a variety of foods from the Basic Four Food Groups, and include items that are rich in calcium, phosphorus, vitamin D, iron, and B vitamins.

The most common deficiencies in an adolescent diet are calcium, iron, thiamin, and vitamins A and C. The need for calcium increases greatly at this age, as the weight of the skeleton grows 45 percent during adolescence. Iron requirements are high, as boys build muscle mass, a process that requires additional blood, and girls begin to lose blood through monthly menstruation. B vitamins are needed because of the increased calories eaten, and vitamin D also is needed for growth of bones.

Despite these needs, teenagers are more likely to ignore a balanced diet than any other age group. It is still important to follow the Basic Four Food Guide for adolescents (Table 4.3), while adapting it to the changing tastes of teenagers.

Encouraging teenagers to eat a good breakfast becomes a real challenge at this age. Many teenagers try to grab an extra 20 minutes of sleep in the morning and fight a daily battle with the clock as they rush to get dressed, catch the bus, and get to school before the bell rings. Breakfast gets skipped or turns into anything quick and easy on the run or on the road.

If a quick breakfast consists of a glass of low-fat or skim milk,

Table 4.3
BASIC FOUR FOOD GUIDE FOR ADOLESCENTS
Ages 11–17 Years
(2,100–2,800 calories a day)

Food Group	Recommended Servings Each Day	Average Serving Size
Milk (or equivalent)	4 or more	
Milk, preferably low fat or skim		1 cup
Powdered milk		4 tbsp.
Cheese		1½ oz.
Cottage cheese		1 cup
Yogurt		1 cup
Meat, fish, poultry (or equivalent)	3 or more	3–5 oz.
Eggs		1–2 whole
Peanut butter		3 tbsp.
Cooked dried peas or beans		1–1½ cups
Luncheon meat		2–3 slices
Vegetables and fruits	4 or more	½–1 cup
Citrus fruits (vitamin C source)	1 or more	
Orange or grapefruit juice		1 cup
Strawberries		1½ cups
Tomatoes or tomato juice		1 cup
Yellow or green vegetable or fruit (vitamin A source)	1 or more	
Broccoli		½ cup
Spinach		½ cup
Carrots		½ cup
Squash		½ cup
Cantaloupe		½ fruit
Apricots		8–10 halves
Other fruits and vegetables	2 or more	
Fresh, frozen, canned fruits and vegetables		½ cup
Potato, turnip, most whole vegetables		1 veg.
Apple, banana, most whole fruits		1 fruit
Breads and cereals (whole grain or enriched)	4 or more	
Bread		2 slices
Dry cereal (unsweetened)		1–1½ cups
Cooked cereal, rice, pasta		1 cup or more

Table 4.3
Continued

Food Group	Recommended Servings Each Day	Average Serving Size
Others (to meet calorie needs)	as needed	
Butter, margarine, mayonnaise, oil		2–4 tbsp.
Desserts		
Pudding		½–1 cup
Ice cream or ice milk		1–1½ cups
Cookies		3–4 medium
Cake		1½ oz.
Pie		2 oz.
Sugar, honey, molasses, jelly, jam		2–4 tbsp.

whole-wheat toast with butter or margarine, and an orange, it provides much of what the adolescent needs to get through the morning without feeling tired and hungry. A boxed breakfast "to go" or breakfast on the bus may be a good way to provide a nourishing morning meal. A peanut-butter or cheese sandwich, a piece of fruit, or a container of yogurt is quick, easy, enjoyable, and nutritious. It does not matter that these items are not generally thought of as breakfast foods. If, however, the eat-on-the-run breakfast is a doughnut, a danish, a granola bar, a candy bar, or a handful of cookies, breakfast becomes an unbalanced, high-calorie, low-nutrition meal — especially if the "meal" is washed down with a soft drink.

A bran muffin, yogurt, and a grapefruit half is another quick, nourishing meal that many school-aged children enjoy. Oatmeal, orange juice, and milk; or a poached egg on toast, juice, and milk are other easy morning meals that use standard breakfast foods. If a child will not eat these foods, an acceptable, easy alternative might be a powdered instant breakfast drink, which is mixed with milk. The amount of protein, carbohydrate, vitamins, minerals, and fat in an instant breakfast is comparable to that of the abovementioned meals. Most instant breakfasts, however, contain many additives, so if parents are concerned about additives they should read the labels carefully before buying these products. (See Chapter 11.)

Breakfast may be more enticing to adolescents, as may be the case for younger children, if it is a bit out of the ordinary and fun to eat. Soups made with beef or chicken, vegetables, and noodles, served with bread and cheese or nuts makes a wholesome breakfast. Leftover vegetables, possibly used as a filling for an omelet, also provide a nice break from the traditional breakfast fare. English-muffin or pita-bread pizzas, as mentioned previously, are appetizing, easy, and nutritious, and these can be made up ahead of time, frozen, and reheated when desired.

No matter how much time parents spend preparing nourishing breakfasts, some teenagers simply are not hungry first thing in the morning and will not eat. One way parents can send these children to school with something in their stomachs is to try to wake them earlier in the morning. This may give them a little more time to become hungry. Before leaving the house, they may be willing to eat a bran muffin, a piece of fruit, a bowl of cereal, or drink a shake — a glass of juice blended with milk, egg, and fruit. The boxed breakfast mentioned above is also a solution.

The school breakfast program is another option some teenagers may want to take advantage of. This program, although in jeopardy of government cutbacks, still is available in many public schools. (See Chapter 9.)

Lunch for adolescents may be purchased in school cafeterias or brought from home. Ideally, lunches should contain one-third of the RDA for this age group and should include foods from all four groups. Parents, however, can rarely be sure that the wholesome foods served in the cafeteria or brought from home are the foods that teenagers actually eat for lunch. (Blind faith, hope, and confidence in their children's eating habits will help get most parents through those challenging times.)

Fast-food restaurants are popular lunch hangouts for teenagers. Fast food (hamburgers, milk shakes, french fries, fried chicken, pizza) tends to be very high in fat and salt, and low in fiber, iron, and vitamins A and C. Even at a fast-food restaurant, however, careful choices can result in a fairly nourishing meal.

(Chapter 6 offers suggestions for making the most of fast foods. It may be a good idea to encourage teenagers to read the fast-food section in that chapter.)

A nourishing dinner is a parent's best opportunity to make sure adolescents are well fed. During these years the final growth spurt occurs, and calories, protein, vitamins, and minerals must satisfy all the demands of a rapidly changing body. Many adolescents are too busy or disinterested to eat a balanced meal in the morning. They may eat unbalanced lunches and fill up on low-quality snacks between meals. Dinner, therefore, becomes the key meal.

Dinner for adolescents should consist of one glass of milk or a calcium-rich substitute, such as cheese or yogurt; four to five ounces of meat, poultry, or fish, or other source of high-quality protein, such as chili, an omelet, or vegetable lasagna; one-half cup of a green leafy or yellow vegetable; fruit or fruit juice; and two slices of bread or one cup of rice or pasta. It is a good idea to serve fresh fruit and vegetables and whole-grain or enriched breads at dinner, because these foods tend to be missing from other meals that the adolescent eats away from home.

SNACKS

Snacks are an important and inevitable part of children's diets. Young children and adolescents, in fact, need to eat snacks because it is difficult for them to obtain enough calories in just three meals. Parents should try to provide snacks that will be nourishing as well as enjoyable. If children grow accustomed to eating wholesome snacks at an early age, they will be more likely to continue this habit when the food choice is theirs.

Most children snack throughout the day to curb hunger that sets in between meals. Midmorning, midafternoon (especially after school for older children), and after-dinner snacks become part of the daily eating routine for many children. Eating three meals and several snacks a day is perfectly acceptable if the snacks contain protein, vitamins, minerals, and calories and if the levels of fat, sugar, and salt are kept reasonably low. Table 4.4 offers some ideas for nourishing snacks.

Table 4.4
SENSIBLE SNACKING

Fresh fruits	Apples, apricots, bananas, oranges, grapefruit, grapes, melons, pears, peaches, pineapple chunks, plums
Dried fruits	Apricots, apples, dates, peaches, figs, prunes, raisins
	(*Note:* Dried fruits stick to the teeth and children should brush after eating them.)
Vegetables	Raw broccoli, carrots, cauliflower, celery, cucumbers, green beans, squash, green peppers; cooked artichoke hearts, turnips, sweet potatoes (peeled and eaten like a candy bar)
	(*Note:* Raw and cooked vegetables may be more enjoyable if served with a yogurt-based dip.)
Seeds and nuts	Sunflower seeds, pumpkin seeds, peanuts, cashews, walnuts, pecans, soybeans
	(*Note:* Seeds and nuts are not suitable for children younger than 3 years of age because they may cause choking.)
Meat, cheese, and eggs	Cubed chicken, turkey, or beef, peanut-butter sandwiches, tuna-fish sandwiches, hard-boiled eggs, cheese cubes, cottage cheese, yogurt
Breads and cereals	Whole-wheat or enriched bread or toast spread with cottage cheese or ricotta cheese, graham crackers, popcorn (sprinkled with grated cheese), bagels, wheat or rye crackers
Milk and dairy products	Whole milk for children younger than 2 years of age, low-fat and skim milk for older children and adolescents, cottage cheese, ricotta cheese, other cheeses, yogurt
Beverages	Water, fruit juice, low-fat and skim milk, fruit juice mixed with seltzer water

Many discussions of snacks frequently mention "junk foods" and "empty calories," referring generally to foods high in calories from sugar or fat and limited in protein, vitamins, and minerals. While many foods are needlessly high in sugar and fat, no food by itself can be considered entirely useless. Sugar and fat are necessary. At times of exceptional need (e.g., during physical exercise) extra calories from concentrated sweets and fat may be the most accessible source of energy.

For example, many parents consider a brownie to be junk food. A feverish child, however, often is not hungry but needs extra calories to fight infection. If the sick child would eat a brownie, then this sweet snack becomes an important source of nourishment; it certainly is not junk. Conversely, if a healthy, active child eats two large brownies just before dinner and then refuses spaghetti, meat sauce, and salad, those brownies — generally low in protein, vitamins, and minerals — were a poor snack choice. They made the child lose any appetite for a much more nourishing meal. Again, providing children with a variety of foods is the best way to ensure that they eat a balanced diet.

While parents play a major role in influencing their children's eating patterns, unfortunately, there are many other factors that constantly affect the foods that children want and eat. Television advertising, of course, stimulates children's desires for sweets when it promotes snack foods. Grandparents, friends, and peers may offer candy, cookies, cakes, chips, and soft drinks to children, sometimes making these foods an all-too-common part of the daily diet.

While it is difficult to maintain complete control over children's snacks — and may be unwise to try — parents can and should control the foods that are available under their own roofs. If high-sugar, high-salt, high-fat, low-nutrient foods are not available, a hungry child will be forced to choose a snack that is more nutritious.

Parents who do not want their children to consume potato chips, cookies, cakes, and soft drinks should not keep these foods in the house.

Most parents will be able to find several nourishing snack foods that are pleasing to their children. A snack should not take the place of a meal, but with some forethought it can become a valuable "minimeal" that supplies protein, vitamins, minerals, and calories.

PICKY EATERS

Toddlers, preschoolers, and young school-aged children tend to be picky about food. Interest in mealtime declines as they begin to discover and learn about the world around them; interest in snacking increases as they discover the social uses of food.

All parents should be prepared to deal with refusals to eat certain types of food, refusals to eat anything during a meal, and/or poor eating habits. When these situations arise — and they will — parents should handle them with encouragement rather than by being forceful, demanding, or unyielding.

Forcing a child to eat a certain food often ends up in an uncomfortable confrontation that the parent cannot win. An 8-year-old boy, for example, was told that he could not leave the table until he took at least one bite of beets. After a tearful battle of wills his mother picked up the spoon and forced a beet into the boy's mouth. He sat there with the beet in his cheek for nearly an hour before chewing and swallowing it. That was 15 years ago. Now, as an adult, he cannot bring himself to eat beets, even though he says he would probably enjoy the taste.

Such negative encounters with food are totally unnecessary. Refusing certain foods is normal behavior for children. Children, like adults, have favorite foods as well as foods that they dislike. Parents should respect food preferences, not try to dictate them. There are, however, certain techniques that parents can use to encourage a child to eat foods that are nourishing. There are also ways to make eating good food easier, more enjoyable, and more comfortable.

If a Child Refuses Milk

Some toddlers and preschoolers refuse to drink milk, causing parents to worry about lack of calcium. The reason, however, may be simple. A teething child's mouth, for example, may be sensitive to cold temperatures. Pouring the cup of milk 10 or 15 minutes before it is to be served may solve the problem. (Milk must be stored in the refrigerator to prevent bacteria that could cause food poisoning or spoilage. See Chapter 10 for other guidelines.)

The usual cup of milk served with every meal every day can become tiresome to the child. Putting the milk in a new mug or letting the child pour it from a small pitcher or drink it through a fancy straw may add enough interest to make the milk more enticing. Serving fruit juice or water with a meal and using another source of calcium during the meal, at dessert, or for snacktime may be a welcome break from the milk routine. Ice cream can be blended with milk for milk shakes or frappes, and favorite fruit juices can be mixed with milk for a nourishing drink with interesting flavor.

If children still refuse to drink milk, there are plenty of other ways parents can provide calcium in the diet. Hot cereals, for example, can be cooked with milk, or milk can be poured on top or mixed in before serving them. Cream soups, ice cream, pudding, and custard use milk as a base. Cottage cheese, cheese slices, and yogurt also are rich sources of calcium as well as high-quality protein.

If a Child Refuses Meat

Meats are sometimes unappealing to toddlers and preschoolers. Parents need not worry about this because there are many alternatives to ensure that children get enough high-quality protein. First, parents can try to make eating meat a little easier for their young children, using easy-to-chew meats such as chicken and turkey, or mincing or grinding red meat in a food mill, blender, or food processor for children younger than 1 year, and cutting it into bite-sized pieces for toddlers.

Fish is a good, easy-to-eat protein source for children, but the fish should have a mild flavor and be free of bones. Flounder, halibut, haddock, sole, and tuna are mild-flavored fish that can be offered. Eggs, peanut butter, cooked dried beans, milk, and cheese also are good sources of protein.

If a Child Refuses Bread and Cereal

Children who reject cold cereals may enjoy cooked cereal that is served warm rather than hot. Raisins or fresh fruit may be added to warm or cold cereals to make them more appealing. Some children will eat toast even though they will not eat bread, and toast or bread that is cut into interesting shapes with cookie cutters may be fun for them to eat. In addition, rice, pasta, and potatoes can provide most of the same vitamins and minerals as bread and cereal.

If a Child Refuses Fruits and/or Vegetables

Most toddlers and preschoolers enjoy some types of fruit and fruit juice. If children turn up their noses at fruit, however, they may be willing to eat it if it is added to cereals, Jello, puddings, custard, or ice cream. Chopped fresh fruit, fruit juice, ice, and milk (or any combination of these) can be blended together to form a smooth, frothy blender shake that many young children will enjoy.

The most well-known and prevalent eating problem among children is their refusal to eat vegetables, especially the green varieties. Many children will eat potatoes, and some will like corn, carrots, or peas; but, on the whole, vegetables are the food group most often refused by children. Again, parents should stay calm; there is no reason to be anxious or worried.

Although dark green, leafy vegetables and yellow vegetables are rich sources of vitamins and minerals, these nutrients are usually available in other foods that picky eaters will eat (see Tables 2.20 and 2.21). There are also many ways to "hide" vegetables in foods. Shredded lettuce, for example, may be eaten if it is in a tuna fish sandwich. Chopped celery and carrots can be added to sandwich spreads. Zucchini and pumpkin breads are delicious foods that most children readily eat without realizing they are "good" for them. Tomato sauce can be a good vegetable source, and vegetables can be added to it before it is poured on top of spaghetti, lasagna, ravioli, or other pasta. Soups and stews also are convenient ways to serve vegetables to children.

Many children refuse to eat vegetables that have been boiled until they become soft, mushy, and pale. Crunchy, brightly colored vegetables, which generally contain more vitamins and minerals than cooked vegetables, may be appealing to children. Raw vegetables — carrots, celery, green peppers, broccoli, cauliflower, green beans, cucumbers, and tomatoes — usually are accepted readily if they are coined or cut into easy-to-eat strips. Quickly stir-frying or steaming vegetables are cooking methods that help retain color and crunch.

Other Suggestions

Brightly colored foods often are enjoyed by young children. Strawberries, blueberries, oranges, carrots, raw broccoli, tomatoes, cheeses, corn, and grapes might be eaten because they are pretty. Adding small amounts of colorful foods (not food coloring) to other foods, such as carrot shavings or minced sweet red peppers or green beans or spinach, may tempt young children.

Parents of picky eaters can make the few foods that their children eat more nutritious by adding certain ingredients that may go unnoticed by most children. For example, powdered milk and/or egg whites can be easily added to macaroni and cheese or beef-noodle casseroles to increase the level of calcium, protein, riboflavin, and vitamin A. Powdered milk also can be added to regular, low-fat, or skim milk to increase the already-high food value. Wheat germ can be added to homemade cookies, pancakes, cereal, cakes, and meatloaf to provide a boost of folic acid, vitamin B_6, and zinc.

If, however, children will not try new foods or will not eat certain foods, parents should not feel routinely obligated to provide a substitute. It will not harm a child's health if the vegetable or the meat is left on the plate for a meal or two. Cooking well-liked green beans to replace the untouched broccoli, for example, is asking for trouble. Children may become unwilling to try new foods, expecting that a favorite food always will be available if they reject a new one. Additionally, this practice reinforces the child's behavior and may contribute to poor eating habits in the future.

As mentioned earlier, serving a nutritious, well-balanced diet is likely if parents get into the habit of using a variety of foods from the four groups at each meal. Parents should be concerned about proper nutrition, but they should not panic or fret if a child fails to eat the recommended number of servings from a food group or a particular iron-rich food. If nourishing meals are offered daily, chances are good that over time children will receive everything their bodies need to grow. Food charts and recommendations can offer some help in planning meals; however, variety, flexibility, and a relaxed, happy atmosphere are certainly the best ways to keep a child well fed.

5

THERE'S MORE TO EATING THAN FOOD

They say fingers were made before
forks, and hands before knives.

Jonathan Swift
Polite Conversation

Eating, in theory, is a simple process. There are people, there is hunger, there is food. Hungry people pick up food, put it in their mouths, chew, and swallow. Hunger is quickly satisfied. Simple.

In reality, however, eating is a complicated process that encompasses a vast realm of emotions, needs, and situations. It begins as an instinctive means by which an infant satisfies hunger. The baby soon equates eating with satisfaction, and food becomes a symbol of love, security, and comfort.

Most parents of young children would agree that eating is no simple matter. The mother who has just washed the morning oatmeal from her 1-year-old son's hair and catches him wiping his cottage-cheese-covered fingers on the sofa probably wishes eating were simpler. The father who wears a raincoat to the breakfast table when it is his turn to feed baby might agree.

Despite the messes and spills, eating involves a lot of learning. Through eating, children gradually explore the world and the many differences in taste, color, shape, and texture. Children also learn social interaction, sharing, and manners through eating. To young children, eating and food can mean adventure, excitement, discovery, and challenge. And, of course, what the child eats influences growth, development, and health.

A child's early experiences with food are parent-dependent. It is a parent's responsibility not only to provide nourishing meals and snacks, but also to set a solid foundation for the way a child will eat for a lifetime. Parents must recognize their young children's need to experiment with and experience the foods that they are served. It is natural for the 2-year-old to fingerpaint with ketchup, squish lima beans into a pale green goo, stir chicken soup with one finger, and upset a cup of milk to see the puddle form on the tray. All this exploring — although unacceptable by adult standards — is natural, normal, and desirable.

This chapter discusses ways to teach children good mealtime habits. Suggestions are presented for appropriate times, places, moods, and settings to encourage and nurture sound eating patterns. Also included are some ideas for getting children involved in cooking, an ideal way for them to learn the importance of food and diet.

TEACHING A CHILD GOOD MEALTIME HABITS

Good mealtime habits must be taught directly and indirectly, demonstrated by example, emphasized, and repeated. Happy encounters with food at an early age, as discussed earlier, help establish sensible eating habits for life.

When children begin to eat meals at the family table, they observe and imitate the behavior and manners of others in the family. A young child's world revolves around the immediate family, particularly parents. Table manners and eating patterns are, therefore, modeled on those of family members.

It is important for parents and older brothers and sisters to set a good example at meals for young children to follow.

Toddlers who are included in family meals have the chance to see for themselves how they should behave. For example, they see their parents and siblings using forks, spoons, and knives. They observe family members placing napkins in their laps before eating, and they may hear the words "please," as requests are made for dishes of food, and "thank you," as dishes are received.

Toddlers, unfortunately, may also notice and imitate less mannerly mealtime behavior and the dislikes as well as the likes of those around the table. If father, for example, announces that he hates squash and refuses a helping of zucchini, the toddler may imitate this action and, bingo — zucchini is rejected. As mentioned in Chapter 1, parents' food preferences are reliable predictors of a child's lifelong food preferences. If parents simply practice sensible eating habits themselves they will be more influential than if they criticize, nag, or lay down long lists of "what to eat" and "what not to eat." The do-as-I-say-not-as-I-do approach rarely works with children!

The road to good manners is paved with countless messes and spills. Parents will find it helpful to take any precautions possible to make this stage easier for them and the child. It may help to put newspapers on the floor under the toddler's chair before each meal. Providing child-sized utensils that are easy to grasp, and serving meals on a plate with a rim so food can be pushed against it, also may reduce the number of accidents. Clever parents have lined high chairs with bath towels, spread dropcloths on the carpet, and discovered plastic bibs with little troughs at the bottom to catch stray morsels. One mother even decided it was time to get a faithful family dog to help clean the floor below the high chair!

The precautions, however, should never go as far as excluding the mess-prone toddler from the family dinner table. This will make it impossible for the child to learn how to behave at meals the natural way, *through example.* Young children really want to become part of the family and need as many opportunities as possible to watch and learn how grown-ups eat.

Toddlers are experimenters. They dip bananas into ketchup and marvel at the pretty color contrast. They plop a spoonful of chocolate pudding onto peas, add minced chicken, poke their fingers into the concoction, smear it around the plate, then hungrily eat it (usually to their parents' dismay). Before napkins are used, fingers will be wiped on overalls, furniture, hair, and parents.

Toddlers between 1 and 2 years of age are naturally curious. They have a lot to learn about the world, and experiencing things through their senses is their chief means of grasping concepts. Food and eating affect the senses — taste, touch, sight, and smell — in the most vivid way. Feeling the various textures of foods, for instance, helps young children recognize what they are eating.

There is a difference between experimenting and playing with food, albeit subtle. Allowing toddlers to play with food on the plate is not a good idea. If the food becomes more of a toy and less of a way to satisfy hunger (and curiosity), it is best to remove the plate — without punishing or criticizing the child. Scolding toddlers for playing might make the parent feel better but could lead to future eating problems for the child.

A toddler's desire to experiment picks up momentum during early tries at self-feeding. When the texture and consistency of food become familiar to toddlers, however, they usually are ready to pick up a spoon and attempt to master the art of using utensils. The transition from self-feeding with fingers to self-feeding with utensils occurs naturally, yet gradually. The only way a parent can help a toddler develop self-feeding skills is through good humor, understanding, and faith that all good things happen to those who wait patiently. Toddlers need plenty of time and many opportunities to practice manipulating the spoon or fork under the food and into the mouth. This is no easy task.

At first, most of the food will end up on the child's face, hair, or lap, or on the food tray or floor. After several months of persistence, however, the spoon or fork will reach its destination. As the child grows more efficient, parents will notice — with relief — that fingers play less of a role.

The transition from a bottle to a cup occurs similarly, but more damply. Special spillproof cups may be a useful stepping stone for 1- to 2-year-olds. These plastic cups are covered by a lid with a small spout. Only a few drops of liquid will spill from the cup if dropped or upset. By the age of 2 years, however, the toddler who has been drinking from a spouted cup should be able to drink from a regular cup without too much dripping and spilling. Nevertheless, parents should always be prepared for an occasional waterfall if a child is tired or excited.

The atmosphere and mood at mealtime have a great effect on how a child approaches food. If parents hold expectations of mealtime behavior that are unrealistically high for the child's age and developmental level (see Table 3.8), the youngster may become frustrated, angry, or fearful, especially if scolding and punishment are used.

Children should learn as early as possible to enjoy family meals, not fear or dread them.

Asserting independence becomes one of the most vital struggles for 2-year-olds. Children at this age must be given the opportunity to make choices, refuse foods they do not want, and offer opinions. At the same time it is important that they know and respect limits set by their parents. In other words, children between 2 and 3 years of age need enough freedom to develop and learn, yet enough limits to feel protected and loved.

Parents of toddlers and preschoolers need to be flexible, firm, and tactful as they try to encourage good habits while maintaining a tension-free and enjoyable atmosphere at the table. Children should be reminded gently about slips in their behavior, but they should not be dealt a steady stream of "Put your napkin in your lap," "Get your elbows off of the table," "Clean your plate," or "Don't talk with your mouth full." Children respond best to positive reinforcement. Finding even one thing a child does well at each meal and emphasizing it will lead to willing cooperation. If meals are relaxed times in which all family members, including toddlers and preschoolers, are involved in the conversation, the emphasis will be taken off every little detail of manners. Mealtimes should be full of love and caring. This atmosphere helps a child develop a sensible attitude about food and eating, and it promotes the child's positive self-image.

Most toddlers and preschoolers are unable to sit still for long periods of time. To maintain a relaxed, comfortable atmosphere throughout a meal, young children should be excused from the table when they begin to become restless and irritable, even if it has been only 5 or 10 minutes. Permitting toddlers to leave when they are finished helps prevent upsetting mealtime battles and allows other family members to enjoy the food and each other without making impossible demands on young children.

School-aged children, those who are 6 to 10 years old, continue to need gentle guidance and examples at meals. Children have lots to tell about their activities at this age if parents are willing to listen. If meals are used as parental platforms for lectures, however, children will be glum, restless, and not very interested in eating. Mealtime is not the time to discuss bad grades, inappropriate behavior, or fights with siblings or friends. It is the time for each family member to talk about at least one positive event of the day.

By the time children reach adolescence, their eating habits — good or bad — are firmly established. There is little a parent can do to coax or force teenagers to change their ways. When parents think their teenagers are sloppy or eat the wrong foods at the wrong time in the wrong way, the most effective response usually is to continue providing nourishing meals, offer information, and set a positive example that may influence the teenagers to try some more agreeable behavior.

Many adolescents operate on rigid schedules in which school, social activities, after-school jobs, and sports compete for the limited time in each day. This means that meals often are eaten when the adolescent wants and/or has the time. This pattern may not be conducive to planning family meals on a regular basis. Parents of adolescents should remain flexible and understand the teenagers' needs for independence and involvement in outside activities. Establishing or maintaining an enjoyable, comfortable mealtime atmosphere may encourage the teenager to sit down, relax, and dine with the family.

MAKING FOOD APPEALING

The way food is presented to young children greatly influences both their short- and long-term eating patterns. The amount of food offered, the way it is prepared, the color, smell, shape, and texture of the food may determine whether and how much a child eats.

Too much food on the plate at one time, for example, may not only be impossible for a toddler to eat but may seem overwhelming. Toddlers want to be like the others around the table, and they want to have the foods that others have. But they can eat only a fraction of the normal adult-sized portion.

When serving meals to toddlers, erring on the side of too little is better than heaping too much on the plate.

Child-sized portions on an adult-sized plate may appear meager, and parents may be tempted to fill a regular dinner plate with servings that are too large and too discouraging for toddlers. A child-sized plate or salad plate filled with small portions will be less overwhelming and more appealing. If toddlers are still hungry after the plate is clean, they can ask for seconds.

One of the most difficult challenges facing parents of young children is introducing food. While some toddlers are open-minded about accepting new food, others prefer to eat just a few items that are familiar to them and refuse to taste most unfamiliar foods. One way to deal with this reluctance is to try introducing a very small portion of the new food when the child is the hungriest, along with familiar, well-liked items on the same plate. If the child still refuses to taste the new food, it should be removed and reintroduced at a later time. If children are unwilling to try new food, parents should not pressure, force, or punish them.

Food should not be hard to eat. Toddlers, for example, are unable to slice meat with a knife, cut open a baked potato, or eat peas with a fork. Foods that require too much effort may be frustrating and discouraging to the toddler. There are many ways in which parents can make mealtimes enjoyable and easy for their young children. Meat should be cut into bite-sized pieces before it is served to toddlers. Baked potatoes should be opened, milk or butter should be added, and they should be fork-mashed for easy eating.

It also is important to serve young children food that is at a comfortable temperature. Food that is too hot will not only be rejected immediately, but it can cause totally unnecessary and painful mouth burns.

The temperature of all hot food should be tested before the food is served to young children.

Spoons and forks are needed for food such as macaroni and cheese, soup, and creamed corn, and toddlers may find eating these foods frustrating. Parents might try serving some easy-to-eat finger foods, such as crackers, cubed cheese, or carrot and celery sticks, at the same meal. These familiar finger foods will give the child a needed break from the struggle with the spoon.

At this age, meals should be kept simple. Most young children prefer plain food with no gravy, sauce, or toppings. Gourmet cooking is not appreciated, and if parents insist on preparing dishes that require complicated and lengthy preparation, they may be needlessly disappointed or hurt.

This is not to say that parents cannot use their imaginations. Cutting sandwiches or cheese slices into unusual shapes with cookie cutters is one way to encourage a child to eat good food. Serving several types of finger foods, such as raw vegetables, cut-up fruit, and cheese, and including a small portion of peanut butter or yogurt, may be an enjoyable way for a young child to experiment by dipping and mixing wholesome ingredients.

Many toddlers and young children like their food to be separated on their plates. Some children, in fact, refuse to eat any parts of food that have touched each other, even though they will eat the foods plain. Other children enjoy combining different items, but they want to be the ones to decide what to mix together. If a child has mixed rice with peas at one meal, parents should not assume that the child will always want rice mixed with peas. Perhaps at another meal the child will mix rice with chicken and eat the peas separately. Not surprisingly, children are often unpredictable.

Part of the fun for a child is putting things together to see and taste the result. These experiments change frequently, and parents should not try to pre-empt the experimentation. The parent is responsible for placing a balanced meal on the table. The child is responsible for eating the food in whatever way best suits his or her current moods and preferences. This entire exploring process can be challenging — and exasperating — to parents. If parents expect and accept the constant choosing, mixing, and testing, mealtimes can become an interesting experience for all.

TIMES, PLACES, AND SETTINGS

The mealtime environment — the physical as well as emotional surroundings — has a strong influence on how a child will feel about food. Although it is difficult to set up the ideal situation at every meal, parents should try for a relaxed and warm mood whenever possible.

The precise time at which meals are served is of no major importance, as long as it remains fairly consistent. Most families can establish a routine that takes into consideration jobs, school, and other activities.

Children can adapt to almost any eating schedule. If the family dinner is to be served late one evening, for example, a light snack at the regular dinner time may curb hunger pangs. When work schedules, guests, or other activities delay the dinner hour, parents may decide to feed their children early in the evening. This is all right occasionally; however, in general, children benefit a great deal from participating in family meals, even if they are served earlier or later than usual.

Although activity and play are good ways to stimulate appetite, young children who are playing intently may not realize they are hungry and may refuse to come to the table. Children who are tired also may not want to eat. If a child is either excited or tired before a meal, spending some quiet time reading a story, talking, or letting the youngster help in the kitchen immediately before eating may stimulate interest in food.

If a child announces he or she is not hungry and does not want to come to the table, one possible solution is to explain gently that mealtime is a family time. Even if the child is not hungry, parents might point out that they expect all family members to sit at the table during meals. Usually the youngster will discover that he or she is hungry and eventually will decide to eat something.

If a child still refuses to eat, parents should not apply too much pressure or be overly concerned. It is, however, reasonable to insist that even if the child chooses not to eat the meal, he or she is expected to stay at the table for a while. The amount of time the child remains at the table should not be so long that it seems like punishment, yet it should be long enough to allow the child to calm down and take part in mealtime conversation.

Young children have short attention spans and may not be able to sit still and remain interested during an adult-length meal. As mentioned earlier, when children have finished eating or begin to get restless, they should be allowed to leave the table.

The dessert course, which frequently is higher in calories and lower in vitamins, minerals, and protein than other parts of the meal, often is used as an incentive for children to eat what they do not want or like. Using food or a part of a meal as a bribe, however, such as rewarding a child with ice cream for cleaning his or her plate or offering a cookie or a piece of candy for taking a bite of peas, is setting the stage for later eating problems.

For the same reasons, children should not be denied food or meals as punishment. Sending a naughty youngster to bed without dinner also makes food seem like a reward for good behavior. Nourishing food, like affection, is the natural birthright of a child. Parents who withhold either are endangering their child's development. *Denying food to children can lead to eating problems in later years.*

The physical setting of meals is also important. One or two special places in the home should be reserved for meals, usually the dining room, alcove, or kitchen. During mealtimes, eating should be the main event. Coloring books, dolls, and especially television can distract from the atmosphere. Watching television while eating, for example, leaves little room for conversation. When the meal goes on, the television should go off. If television becomes identified with eating, snacking may increase. Many children — as well as adults — spend hours in front of the television, and the combination of overeating and underactivity can lead to weight problems.

When sitting at the table it is important for children to be comfortable. They should be able to rest their feet on the floor or a footboard. The table should be at a suitable level, which can be accomplished by using high chairs for young children and booster seats for older children. Pillows and telephone books can give the necessary lift when special chairs are not available.

Sometimes it may be fun for the toddler to eat some meals at a special child-sized table with child-sized chairs. When this is allowed, however, the toddler should be served the same meal, in the same room, at the same time that other family members are eating. The child should not be allowed to leave the table and run around until excused (which can be before the rest of the family, as mentioned before).

Bowls, plates, and cups for children should be nonbreakable and heavy enough to resist spilling. Many ingenious items have been invented, such as cups that are weighted at the bottom and plates with suction cups, and these can help make mealtime easier and more enjoyable for both parents and toddler. Utensils should be small enough to fit easily into the child's mouth. Forks and spoons with short, thick handles are easier for the child to manipulate than standard-sized utensils. If a glass is to be used it should have a broad base, and the child should be able to encircle it with two hands.

A helpful strategy for all parents is to keep food out of sight until mealtime or snacktime. Often the sight of the full cookie jar or a bag of potato chips on the kitchen counter will stimulate the appetite, and young children will ask (beg, implore!) for snacks. Keeping these hidden can help reserve eating, whenever possible, for the planned times.

Snacks, like meals, should be offered at fairly regular times each day, and if possible, spaced evenly between meals. Even though it may be difficult to prevent children from accepting snacks from relatives, neighbors, or friends, parents can limit the number of opportunities young children have to obtain snacks. Continuous snacking takes away from the atmosphere of family meals and can lead to undesirable eating habits.

GETTING CHILDREN INVOLVED IN COOKING

Children love to help in the kitchen. To them tasks such as cooking, washing dishes, and setting the table are not work; they are play. Helping parents in the kitchen makes children feel important and useful. It is a chance for children to become part of the adult world, to make the same types of creations that adults make. The kitchen is the ideal setting for children to experiment and be imaginative while developing skills they will need throughout life.

Children learn best when they are directly involved in an activity. An astonishing range of skills and concepts are involved in cooking. Motor skills, science, math, and social skills all come into play during the cooking and cleaning process. Through experiences with food, young children use all their senses and learn about shape, size, amount, color, and texture. This is also an ideal time and way to begin to teach children the basics of a balanced diet. Cooking also allows parents and children to enjoy the satisfaction of constructing something important together.

There are plenty of jobs that children as young as 2 can do in the kitchen. They can pull a chair up to the sink and will wash anything (including themselves and the floor) for long periods of time. Young children love digging into things, so mixing meatloaf, kneading and punching down bread dough, cutting out and decorating cookies, and stirring anything (as long as it is not hot) can be entertaining for them, as well as labor-saving for parents. Typical 3-year-olds can wash vegetables, tear up lettuce, snap beans, shell peas, and husk corn. They can fold napkins, arrange rolls on a cookie sheet, spread peanut butter on bread, pour measured amounts from one container to another, and wipe off the table.

In general, 4-year-olds can pour, mix, break eggs, and do simple measuring. They can use butter knives, graters, and parers with supervision, and many 4-year-olds can set the table correctly. Preschool children will learn that all foods do not come from the grocery store when they participate in such activities as planting seeds, growing bean sprouts, and watching and smelling bread baking. Parents may want to take their young children out to pick apples, peaches, strawberries, or cherries, then let them watch and help use these fruits to make pies and jams.

By the time children turn 5 they should be able to peel carrots and potatoes with a peeling utensil, and wash breakable dishes. Some children at this age also *may* be ready to use the stove and the oven and begin cooking and baking in the presence of and with the assistance of an adult.

Safety is a vitally important issue when cooking with children. Children who are old enough to use knives should be taught how to slice and chop safely. Children younger than 6 years old should be taught to stay away from grills, griddles, blenders, food processors, or hand mixers, as just one accident can be too costly. Parents, however, can show their young children these appliances and explain why they are dangerous if used incorrectly. All adults should remember the importance of keeping the handles of pots and pans turned toward the back of the stove and be sure to teach this to children once they are old enough to reach properly.

Children's first cooking projects should be simple, involving two or maybe three steps. Scrambled eggs, steamed vegetables, applesauce, popcorn, peanut butter, oatmeal cookies, or homemade granola are good foods to try when teaching a child to cook. When the time comes to boil, bake, steam, or fry, parents should *not* let children younger than 6 handle hot pans or stand alone at the stove. Gradually, cooking can involve more steps, complicated procedures, and a bit more independence for the child.

Children may want to test new ways to prepare and combine foods. If a child wants to add broccoli to macaroni and cheese casserole, for example, parents should encourage it. Some good ideas just might come out of these experiments!

Allowing children to help in the kitchen has another advantage: They are more willing to eat food that they helped prepare. Children are curious, and they usually will want to taste their creations, even when made with ingredients that are normally refused.

When children are old enough to read recipes and use the kitchen without constant adult supervision, the result, at first, may be burned casseroles, lumpy gravies, rock-hard muffins, and runny eggs. Children should never be scolded or punished for their mistakes. Rather, they should be praised for their interest in food and cooking. The failures are as important as the successes in cooking. When mistakes do happen, children should be helped to understand why the food did not turn out as planned. Children will be able to see — and taste — firsthand what the result is when they forget to add the egg, leave the casserole in the oven too long, or add too much salt.

Cooking can be the source of great pride and feelings of accomplishment for children of nearly all ages. It provides valuable opportunities to experiment independently and learn a vast array of concepts, skills, and techniques. It helps them discover where food comes from before it is placed on the table. The best part of cooking, however, is the sense of achievement and triumph children have when they finish preparing and cooking and start eating their very own creations.

6

WHEN THERE'S NOT ENOUGH TIME OR MONEY

Its habit of getting up late you'll
  agree
That it carries too far when I say
That it frequently breakfasts at five
  o'clock tea
And dines on the following day.

Lewis Carroll
The Hunting of the Snark

Lack of time and money are two reasons often given to justify poor eating habits. Where children are concerned, however, a well-balanced diet must come before a busy schedule and wholesome food should be a top priority in the family budget. With planning and foresight, nourishing meals and snacks can be offered to children every day, even when time is tight and money is scarce. Except in cases of extreme poverty, it just takes common sense, imagination, and some understanding of nutrition.

Today, more than half of all families have either two working parents or a working single parent. In these households, parents are unable to spend hours planning, shopping, and preparing three wonderful meals a day. Balancing job obligations with family responsibilities is no easy task. Add participation in sports, classes, civic and political activities, and competition for time becomes fierce.

Parents' best intentions for preparing meals that are appetizing and nourishing sometimes do fail for lack of time. Often,
arrangements must be made for others to care for and feed children. Baby sitters, relatives, day-care centers, schools, and the
children themselves may be responsible for meals and snacks.
In all of these situations parents surrender some control over
their children's diets. If parents carefully plan and prepare meals
for other caretakers to serve, however, much of that control can
be retained.

PREPARING MEALS TO BE SERVED BY OTHERS

Parents should tell any person who takes care of their infants
and young children what to serve for meals and snacks as well
as when and how that food should be offered. If children always
have a glass of milk before going to bed, and parents want this
practice to continue, then the caretaker must be informed of this.
Also, all caretakers should know about any food allergies or food
intolerances that children have.

Teenagers and first-time baby sitters usually will require more
specific, detailed instructions about feeding children than regular sitters or relatives, who most likely feel more comfortable
with the child and in the home. For example, all baby sitters
should know what time the child should eat, whether the child
or the sitter should hold the bottle during a baby's feeding, how
often the child should be burped — if at all — and whether an
older child needs assistance cutting meat or opening a baked
potato.

If possible, parents should arrange a time for a new baby sitter
to watch and help them feed infants and toddlers before the sitter tackles this responsibility alone. This will make everyone
more comfortable in the long run — the sitter will have a better
idea of how to feed the child, the parents can see firsthand that
the sitter knows the routine, and the child will have a chance to
get to know a new person in his or her parents' presence. Again,
any food allergies, food-related health problems, or forbidden
foods must be explained in detail.

It is a good idea to make up infant formula and put it in bottles
before the sitter arrives. Baby sitters need to be told how to

warm the bottles and the way to temperature test the formula before feeding. If the baby is eating solid foods, the sitter should know how much of which foods are to be offered. If the baby eats finger food, such as cheese chunks or raw vegetables, parents should tell the sitter exactly what foods are and are not appropriate for the child's age. Foods should be cut to the right size beforehand and stored in labeled containers. Some parents prefer to prepare whole meals for their children and the sitter ahead of time and store them in the freezer or refrigerator on individual plates.

If the baby sitter is expected to prepare all or some parts of the meal, the necessary equipment, utensils, and ingredients, along with detailed instructions for preparation, should be laid out on the table or counter. If possible, an alternative meal plan should be available just in case the original meal does not work out.

In general, it is a good idea to plan meals that are simple, keeping any preparation on the part of the sitter to a minimum. Sandwiches, pizza, casseroles, soups, hamburgers, and macaroni and cheese are favorites of both teenagers and young children. Best of all, these nourishing meals are easy to prepare.

Baby sitters should spend time with the children, not with the stove.

Complicated dishes that require a lot of adding, stirring, mixing, measuring, pouring, and cooking should be avoided. If parents want their children to have meals that require a lot of preparation time, these dishes should be prepared in advance so the sitter will need only to heat and serve them.

Parents who are trying to limit the amount of sugar, salt, fat, fast food, cholesterol, or calories in their children's diets should be sure that all off-limit foods are unavailable to their children — and, preferably, are not in the house. Baby sitters must be told about foods in the house that neither they nor the children should eat.

Many baby sitters bring treats for their little charges, and frequently these treats are high in sugar. If parents do not want their children to eat these sweets they should diplomatically let the sitter know this ahead of time. A few suitable snacks should be on hand and reviewed with the sitter.

When close relatives, such as grandparents, are caring for young children, parents may feel more comfortable leaving meal decisions up to them. Grandparents often have favorite recipes that they enjoy preparing and serving to their grandchildren. Some grandparents, however, appreciate it when all or most of the food preparation has been done for them. Unless arrangements have been worked out ahead of time, it is the parents' responsibility to do the shopping and meal planning. If parents expect grandparents to bake the chicken breasts and steam the broccoli flowerets, these foods should be in the refrigerator, thawed and ready for use.

Grandparents and other relatives also may bring cookies, candy, baked goods, and other sugary foods to children as treats. Parents who do not want these snacks offered to their children should gently inform well-intentioned relatives of this before they begin to baby sit and provide them with suggestions for treats that are more acceptable.

If parents want to retain control over their children's diets then it usually is a better idea to have grandparents or the baby sitter come into the child's home. If the child goes to someone's home, then that person usually plans and prepares the meal. Parents who are strict about their children's diets may object to some of the foods offered by others. If parents, however, explain their personal ideas about food and diet to all baby sitters, the result usually will be meals that are acceptable to all, even if the child goes to another home.

In day-care centers or cooperative groups there is less a parent can do to maintain control over what is served and when and how it is served — unless, of course, parents send food with their children. Some day-care centers provide hot meals, which usually are included in the cost of the service. The best way to make sure meals are acceptable is for parents to visit the center and check the type and quality of food before choosing that center for their child.

The directors, teachers, and supervisors at the center should be informed of any food restrictions a child may have. If parents do not approve of a meal that is being served at the center, they can pack a lunch for the child. Parents, however, will need to be in touch with day-care supervisors to make sure they will serve the child a lunch brought from home.

When other parents or neighbors take care of children through cooperative arrangements, meal plans can be discussed in advance. Co-op members usually can agree on nourishing meals and snacks that parents and children both will find acceptable.

While it is important for parents to be concerned and interested in their children's diets, they should avoid taking their concerns to unnecessary extremes. Rather, parents should relax and not try to control everything their children eat. No matter how much effort is put into keeping sweets out of a child's diet, friends will bring cookies, relatives will offer soft drinks, and bank tellers will send lollipops out to the car through the drive-in window tray. Parents will be fighting a running battle if they forbid these foods. They can, however, make sure their children do not consume too many sweets and treats. Little damage results if children eat foods high in sugar, fats, or salt every now and then. The problems occur when children acquire such a strong desire for these high-calorie, low-nutrient foods that they continuously ask (or beg) for them and eat them to the exclusion of other more nourishing foods. If parents and other caretakers serve hearty meals and keep most commercial snack food out of the house, children will consume the raw materials they need to grow and develop.

SCHOOL LUNCHES — BRINGING AND BUYING

Teaching sensible, healthful eating habits to young children is crucial because once they troop off to school with lunch pail in hand or lunch money jingling in their pockets, parents have little say about what and how their children eat in the school cafeteria.

A carefully home-packed lunch of orange sections and peanut-butter-filled celery stalks may be traded across the table for a prepackaged fruit pie or a bag of potato chips. A well-bal-

anced hot lunch bought in the school cafeteria will remain untouched if a child does not like the way it looks, no matter how
nourishing it is. Observers have seen, and studies have confirmed, that much cafeteria food — with the possible exception
of the dessert — is wasted.

The best way to encourage children to eat well is to find good
foods that they like. For example, if a child likes peanut butter
slathered on white bread but refuses to eat it on whole-wheat
bread, sending peanut butter on whole wheat usually means the
sandwich will be traded or discarded. Although some whole-
wheat bread contains more fiber and vitamins than white bread,
peanut butter on white bread — especially enriched white bread
— provides many essential nutrients. In addition, most children
like cookies, and almost all kinds (even chocolate chip) can be
homemade with bran, wheat germ, or whole-wheat flour. These
fiber-rich treats will be gobbled up at lunch, rather than traded
or thrown away.

Acceptance is crucial for many school-aged children. They
want to be like their peers, and this extends to the foods they
eat. If a child is sensitive about fitting in, packing unusual food
in the lunch bag could lead to unnecessary social problems. At
certain schools, a tofu and alfalfa-sprout sandwich, for example,
could make a child very self-conscious and fearful that the other
children at the lunch table will laugh and make fun. All that
well-intentioned nourishment could end up in the garbage can.
In other school environments, however, unusual or innovative
lunches attract positive attention, and tasty, nourishing food is
the rule rather than the exception.

When packing lunches, it is a good idea for parents to consider the child's food preferences, his or her peer group, and the
school environment. Within those guidelines, a balanced lunch
should include a protein-rich food, a fresh fruit or vegetable, a
food containing cereal or grains, a special treat, and a beverage
or milk money. Lunch does not have to be the traditional sandwich, apple, cookies, and milk. Instead, the source of protein
could be chunks of leftover roasted chicken, a slice of meatloaf,
nuts, cheese cubes, or a hard-boiled egg. Slices of green pepper,
cherry tomatoes, pineapple chunks, or carrot coins are good

lunch-bag items. Graham crackers, cocktail bread spread with peanut butter, or a rice cake could be included instead of the usual two slices of white bread.

A pita pocket stuffed with an assortment of vegetables is another lunch idea that older children may find appealing. Small plastic bags of chopped carrots, celery, green peppers, tomatoes, and lettuce can be placed in the lunch bag, and these vegetables can be added to the pita bread in the cafeteria. Chunks of roast beef, chicken, turkey, meatloaf, or canned tuna (preferably packed in water) also can be included in a separate container for a protein boost.

Sandwiches made with mayonnaise or mayonnaise-based spreads — chicken salad, tuna salad, or egg salad — may not hold up well if the lunch bag is kept in a warm room for too many hours. Unrefrigerated mayonnaise, especially the homemade kind, is an ideal growth medium for bacteria that can cause food poisoning. Mayonnaise in the lunch box, therefore, is best avoided.

Some types of sandwiches (peanut butter or meatloaf, for example), banana, cranberry, and zucchini bread, and cookies freeze well. These items can be individually wrapped and placed into the lunch bag directly from the freezer. By lunchtime they should be completely thawed but still cool and appealing.

Cutting sandwich bread into stars, circles, triangles, or other shapes may add a little excitement to the usual brown-bag fare for young children. One giant oatmeal cookie or a cookie shaped like a person, an animal, or another familiar object may be more fun to eat than several little round ones. Including a holiday or fancy napkin is another way to make lunchtime at school a little special. Also, putting a little note, a drawing, or a photograph into the bag makes the lunch more exciting. If the lunch seems fun and personal, children may be more eager to eat the nourishing foods contained in it.

Whenever possible, children should be involved in planning and preparing their lunches. They frequently have interesting, inventive ideas about what can go into a lunch box. Often they are more willing to eat nourishing food if they have had some say in the daily "what-to-pack-for-lunch" decisions.

Buying a hot meal in the school cafeteria is another school-lunch option. The appeal and quality of the food served varies greatly from state to state, district to district, and even school to school, despite the fact that the lunch program operates under federal guidelines.

The National School Lunch Program is administered by the United States Department of Agriculture. The meals, planned by qualified personnel, are intended to provide one-third of the daily Recommended Dietary Allowances for children, and consist of a protein source, vegetable, fruit, bread or grain source, butter or margarine, and milk.

Parents may provide lunch money, thinking that their children will receive a hot nourishing meal. The children may be *served* a nutritious meal, but if they do not like what is offered they may pass over the vegetable and meat and point their forks straight toward the cake or pie.

It seems that no matter what is served or how appetizing it is, school children feel it is their duty to complain about cafeteria food — all the kids do it. It is fun, after all, to think up new names for foods. According to students, school cafeterias offer such temptations as "mystery meat" (usually breaded veal or meatloaf), "greenie weenies" (hot dogs), "lice" (rice), "FBI Jello" (thumbprint embedded in the dessert), "mud" (gravy), "blood and guts" (ketchup and mustard), and "bug juice" (red fruit punch).

It is not only the students, however, who do the complaining. Many parents have criticized school lunches, expressing concern about the high starch and fat content of many of the meals. Parent groups also have found fault with portion size, which often is standard even though the appetites of children vary. Also, in most schools, especially in the lower grades, all the food items are placed on the plate or tray even if the child does not like some or any of them. This adds up to a whopping amount of wasted food each year.

In the past few years, however, some school districts have cut down on waste by allowing students to take only what they want and by offering flexible portion sizes. Also, many school cafeterias have worked to improve their image by offering a varied menu, a brighter lunchroom atmosphere, and special meals in conjunction with holidays and festivals. Some cafeterias have reduced the amount of sugar, fat, and salt in the most popular items (hamburgers, french fries, and pizza), and a few offer whole-wheat bread and brown rice. Many parents, teachers, and students have become actively involved in planning menus. As a result, in some districts salad bars have become an option, fresh whole fruit is now available, and students are given the opportunity to regularly evaluate the lunch program.

In addition, many schools distribute weekly or monthly calendars outlining meals. Some local newspapers publish weekly school menus so parents *and* children can decide whether to buy or bring lunch. (Occasionally, the actual menu varies from the schedule.) One thing is certain: If children do not like what is served on a given day, they will not eat it! On these days, sending children to school with a home-packed lunch may be one way to help them get some nourishment in the middle of the day.

WHEN CHILDREN ARE IN CHARGE

Few parents today can afford to make full-time careers of caring for their homes and children. When the school day ends, therefore, more and more children go to empty homes. The term latch-key has evolved to describe children who carry their own house keys to let themselves in before their parents come home.

Many children spend anywhere from a few minutes to six or seven hours in the house without parental supervision. The majority of latch-key children spend about two or three hours alone — from 3:00 or 3:30 P.M. to 5:00 or 6:00 P.M. These hours, of course, are prime snacking times for children.

Working parents should be sure that after-school snacks are easy to find, easy to prepare, and easy to eat. The snacks must be enjoyable to the child and should be nutritionally acceptable to parents. It also is a good idea to limit the number of snacks available. If parents, for example, have left carrot sticks in the refrigerator as an after-school snack, but there is a bag of chocolate-chip cookies in the cupboard, most children would reject the carrots for the cookies.

Parents who do not want their children to eat ice cream, brownies, potato chips, or candy after school should not keep these tempting items around the house.

Children enjoy coming home to unusual and fun snacks. A plastic container can become the snack box, which is stored in a special place in the refrigerator. Parents can place different kinds of after-school treats in the box.

Most children enjoy whole fresh fruit, such as apples, oranges, plums, peaches, grapes, and pears as snacks. Cut-up raw vegetables also make satisfying after-school fare. Sliced green peppers, carrot and celery sticks, cherry tomatoes, broccoli and cauliflower, and radishes are crunchy and nourishing. Some children may enjoy raw vegetables more when they are served with a tasty yogurt-based dip. Cooked artichoke is another interesting and well-liked vegetable snack, and it can be served with French dressing or yogurt-lemon dip.

Cookies, coffee cakes, and cakes may be acceptable treats every so often, especially if homemade. Baking at home enables parents to better regulate the amount of sugar and salt in food and add some extra protein or fiber. Some types of cookies and cakes are more nutritious than others. Oatmeal-raisin cookies, for example, provide more fiber, vitamins, and minerals than most kinds of chocolate-chip cookies. Any type of cookie, however, can become more nourishing by adding bran or wheat germ. Angel food cake, although high in sugar, has less cholesterol than pound cake and most iced cakes.

Granola (preferably homemade with a minimum of added sugar or honey), cereal and skim milk, popcorn, ice pops made with unsweetened fruit juice, frozen bananas, and sherbet made with real fruit are enjoyable treats that can be served as after-school snacks. Slices of homemade banana, carrot, zucchini, cranberry, and pumpkin breads are favorites of many children. Sandwiches made with peanut butter, tuna fish, cheese, or meat slices may curb predinner hunger pangs.

Parents who allow their older children to use the stove, oven, toaster, or microwave oven can put more variety in snack planning. English-muffin or pita-bread pizzas (half an English muffin or pita bread covered with tomato sauce and cheese) can be made in advance, frozen, and heated in the oven. Cheese slices melted on toast or crackers also are nourishing snacks. Cups of homemade soup are tasty and warming, especially in the winter.

A word of caution, however, is advised before allowing older children to use the stove while they are alone in the house. Parents should make sure that their children know what to do if something catches on fire. A *working* fire extinguisher should be located near the stove, and older children should be shown how to use it. Parents should emphasize, however, that it is important for children not to try to fight a fire for longer than a minute, especially if it spreads. Children should be told to leave the house and call the fire department from a neighbor's house or get an adult to help put out the fire. All children should know several neighbors who will be available if emergencies occur.

After a long day at school, children often enjoy something cold and refreshing to drink. It is a good idea to keep plenty of nourishing drinks on hand. Unsweetened fruit juice (apple, orange, grapefruit, pineapple, and grape) and skim milk are good thirst quenchers. Iced water, though often overlooked, is an inexpensive, excellent option. (It may be more appealing if served with a twist of lemon rind.)

Whatever the after-school snack, children will enjoy it more when parents leave a note, clipping, cartoon, or photograph in a prominent place. After all, children should smile and feel happy to be back at home. A loving memento from parents somehow makes the house seem a little less empty in those after-school hours.

FAST FOOD

No matter how valiant an effort parents make in teaching their children the fundamentals of good nutrition, when adolescence sets in, fast food often becomes irresistible. Fast-food restaurants, to begin with, offer teenagers a convenient place to congregate. They serve foods that top the list of teenage favorites — burgers, pizza, fries, fried chicken, tacos, milk shakes, soft drinks.

Parents often worry whether their teenagers are getting ade-

Table 6.1
WHAT'S IN THAT FAST-FOOD MEAL?
(Cheeseburger, french fries, milk shake)

Fast Food	Food Group
Hamburger	Meat or equivalent
Cheese	Milk and dairy products
Hamburger bun	Bread or cereal
Lettuce, tomato (if included)	Vegetable and fruit
French fries	Bread or cereal (starch)
Milk shake	Milk and dairy products

quate nourishment from fast foods. After all a cheeseburger, side of fries, and chocolate shake may not be considered a well-balanced, nourishing meal. But before parents get too worried, they should take a closer look at what their children are actually getting when they consume fast food.

When this cheeseburger, fries, and shake — the typical fast-food meal — are eaten, three of the Basic Four Food Groups are represented, as Table 6.1 shows. If the cheeseburger is served with lettuce and tomato, the fourth group — fruit and vegetables — would also be provided, albeit in limited amounts.

This popular trio of fast foods *does* provide protein, carbohydrate, fat, vitamin A, the B vitamins, calcium, and other essential nutrients. Lacking, however, are vitamin C, folic acid, and fiber — nutrients that are abundant in many green vegetables and fruits. Fiber is also limited because most fast-food restaurants have not, yet, added whole-grain breads to their fare, and many customers do not ask for lettuce and tomato on their burgers, or opt for a side salad (if a salad bar is available) instead of french fries.

The main problem with fast foods is not what they lack, but rather what they provide. As Table 6.2 shows, fast foods generally are *extremely* high in fat (mostly saturated fat), sodium, and calories. Shakes, soft drinks, and desserts are especially high in sugar. Fast-food burgers, fried chicken, chicken sandwiches, fish sandwiches, and french fries are generally very high in fat and salt. Eating too much of any of these over time can potentially lead to a variety of health problems, including heart disease, high blood pressure, and/or obesity.

The key to maintaining a balanced diet among the members of the fast-food generation is to try to promote sensible fast-food eating habits. Parents can encourage adolescents to make wise food choices. As explained by the earlier example, meals that are fairly well balanced and nutritious are available at most fast-food restaurants. In pizzerias — popular hangouts among teenagers — pizza and many of the pasta dishes served in these types of restaurants contain nourishing ingredients, although they, too, may be very high in fat and salt.

When teenagers gather at a hamburger stand, they face a variety of choices. Coleslaw, if available, is more nourishing than french fries or onion rings. (Granted, few teenagers can be persuaded to swap french fries for coleslaw, but a few diet-conscious adolescents might, and it is worth a try!) Also, many fast-food places now provide salad bars. Salad bars offer weight-conscious and nutrition-conscious people the chance to eat a nourishing, high-fiber meal with limited calories — especially when the creamy dressings are bypassed in favor of low-cal choices. But the problem remains: How can teenagers be enticed to the salad bar? There may be no simple answer, but if a child learns to eat salad from an early age, there is a chance that the salad bar will not be totally shunned.

If the local teen hangout is a fried-chicken place, parents might encourage their children to select larger pieces of white-meat chicken, such as the breast. Likewise, when ordering fast-food seafood, adolescents can be encouraged to order larger pieces of fish. More salty, fatty batter covers small pieces, such as chicken nuggets, fried clams, and fried shrimp, and more fat is absorbed into each piece.

Shakes add calcium, vitamin A, and some B vitamins to the diet, but they tend to be high in saturated fat, salt, sugar, and additives if prepared from special mixes. A better choice is low-fat milk, which often is available in fast-food restaurants. Fruit juice (as opposed to sugar-laden fruit drinks) has become widely available in fast-food restaurants, especially those that have a breakfast menu. Plain water, however boring, may be the best drink bet — and the least costly.

Table 6.2
NUTRITIONAL ANALYSES OF FAST FOODS

	Calories	Protein (gm)	Carbohydrate (gm)	Fat (gm)	Cholesterol (mg)	Sodium (mg)**
ARBY'S						
Roast Beef	350	22	32	15	45	880
Beef and Cheese	450	27	36	22	55	1220
Super Roast Beef	620	30	61	28	85	1420
Junior Roast Beef	220	12	21	9	35	530
Ham and Cheese	380	23	33	17	60	1350
Turkey Deluxe	510	28	46	24	70	1220
Club Sandwich	560	30	43	30	100	1610

(*Source:* Consumer Affairs, Arby's Inc., Atlanta, GA. Nutritional analysis by Technological Resources, Camden, NJ.)

	Calories	Protein (gm)	Carbohydrate (gm)	Fat (gm)	Cholesterol (mg)	Sodium (mg)**
BURGER CHEF						
Hamburger	244	11	29	9	27	480
Cheeseburger	290	14	29	13	39	641
Double Cheeseburger	420	24	30	22	77	835
Fish Filet	547	21	46	31	43	—
Super Shef Sandwich	563	29	44	30	105	1088
Big Shef Sandwich	569	23	38	36	81	840
Funmeal Feast	545	15	55	30	27	513
Rancher Platter	640	32	33	42	106	444
Mariner Platter	734	29	78	34	35	882
French Fries, small	250	2	20	19	0	33
Vanilla Shake	380	13	60	10	40	325

(*Source:* Burger Chef Systems, Inc., Indianapolis, IN. Nutritional analysis from *Handbook No. 8*, US Dept. of Agriculture.)

DAIRY QUEEN

DQ Cone, regular size	230	6	35	7	20	80
DQ Dip Cone, regular size	300	7	40	13	20	100
DQ Sundae, regular size	290	6	51	7	20	120
DQ Malt, regular size	600	15	89	20	50	260
DQ Float	330	6	59	8	20	85
DQ Banana Split	540	10	91	15	30	150
DQ Parfait	460	10	81	11	30	140
DQ Freeze	520	11	89	13	35	180
Mr. Misty Freeze	500	10	87	12	35	140
Mr. Misty Float	440	6	85	8	20	95
Dilly Bar	240	4	22	15	10	50
DQ Sandwich	140	3	24	4	10	40
Mr. Misty Kiss	70	0	17	0	0	tr
Brazier Chili Dog	330	13	25	20	—	939
Brazier Dog	273	11	23	15	—	868
Fish Sandwich	400	20	41	17	—	875
Super Brazier Dog	518	20	41	30	—	1552
Super Brazier Dog, with cheese	593	26	43	36	—	1986
Brazier Fries, small	200	2	25	10	—	115
Brazier Onion Rings	300	6	33	17	—	140

(*Source:* International Dairy Queen, Inc., Minneapolis, MN. Nutritional analysis by Raltech Scientific Services, Inc. Madison, WI. Nutritional analysis not applicable in Texas.)

Table 6.2
Continued

	Calories	Protein (gm)	Carbohydrate (gm)	Fat (gm)	Cholesterol (mg)	Sodium (mg)**
JACK IN THE BOX						
Hamburger	263	13	29	11	26	566
Cheeseburger	310	16	28	15	32	877
Jumbo Jack Burger	551	28	45	29	80	1134
Super Taco	285	12	20	17	37	968
Moby Jack Sandwich	455	17	38	26	56	837
Breakfast Jack	301	18	28	13	182	1037
Apple Turnover	411	4	45	24	17	352
Vanilla Shake	342	10	54	9	36	263
Ham & Cheese Omelet	425	21	32	23	355	975
Ranchero Omelet	414	20	33	23	343	1098
French Toast	537	15	54	29	115	1130
Pancakes	626	16	79	27	87	1670
Scrambled Eggs	719	26	55	44	259	1110

(*Source:* Jack-in-the-Box, Foodmaker, Inc., San Diego, CA. Nutritional analysis by Raltech Scientific Services, Inc., Madison, WI.)

KENTUCKY FRIED CHICKEN

Original Recipe Dinner*						
Wing & Rib	603	30	48	32	133	1528
Wing & Thigh	661	33	48	38	172	1536
Drumstick & Thigh	643	35	46	35	180	1441
Extra Crispy Dinner*						
Wing & Rib	755	33	60	43	132	1544
Wing & Thigh	812	36	58	48	176	1529
Drumstick & Thigh	765	38	55	44	183	1480
Mashed Potatoes	64	2	12	1	0	268
Gravy	23	0	1	2	0	57
Roll	61	2	11	1	1	118
Corn (5.5″ ear)	169	5	31	3	X	11

*Two pieces chicken, mashed potato, gravy, cole slaw, roll.

(*Source:* Kentucky Fried Chicken, Inc., Louisville, KY. Nutritional analysis by Raltech Scientific Services, Inc., Madison, WI.)

Table 6.2
Continued

	Calories	Protein (gm)	Carbohydrate (gm)	Fat (gm)	Cholesterol (mg)	Sodium (mg)**
McDONALD'S						
Egg McMuffin	327	19	31	15	229	885
English Muffin, butter	186	5	30	5	13	318
Hotcakes, butter, syrup	500	8	94	10	47	1070
Sausage (pork)	206	9	tr	19	43	615
Scrambled Eggs	180	13	3	13	349	205
Hashbrowns	125	2	14	7	7	325
Big Mac	563	26	41	33	86	1010
Cheeseburger	307	15	30	14	37	767
Hamburger	255	12	30	10	25	520
Quarter Pounder	424	24	33	22	67	735
Quarter Pounder, with cheese	524	30	32	31	96	1236
Filet-O-Fish	432	14	37	25	47	781
French Fries, regular size	220	3	26	12	9	109
Apple Pie	253	2	29	14	12	398
Cherry Pie	260	2	32	14	13	427
McDonaldland Cookies	308	4	49	11	10	358
Vanilla Shake	352	9	60	8	31	201
Hot Fudge Sundae	310	7	46	11	18	175
Caramel Sundae	328	7	53	10	26	195
Strawberry Sundae	289	7	46	9	20	96

(*Source:* McDonald's Corporation, Oak Brook, IL. Nutritional analysis by Raltech Scientific Services, Inc., Madison, WI.)

TACO BELL

Bean Burrito	343	11	48	12	—	272
Beef Burrito	466	30	37	21	—	327
Beefy Tostada	291	19	21	15	—	138
Bellbeefer	221	15	23	7	—	231
Burrito Supreme	457	21	43	22	—	367
Combination Burrito	404	21	43	16	—	300
Enchirito	454	25	42	21	—	1175
Pintos 'N Cheese	168	11	21	5	—	102
Taco	186	15	14	8	—	79
Tostada	179	9	25	6	—	101

(*Sources:* (1) *Menu Item Portions*, San Antonio, Texas; Taco Bell Co., July 1976. (2) Adams, C. F.: "Nutritive Value of American Foods in Common Units," in *Handbook No. 456*. Washington, D.C.: USDA Agricultural Research Service, November 1975. (3) Church, E. F., Church, H. N. (eds.), *Food Values of Portions Commonly Used*, Twelfth Edition. Philadelphia: J. B. Lippincott Co., 1975. (4) Valley Baptist Medical Center, Food Service Department: *Descriptions of Mexican-American Foods*. Fort Atkinson, WI: NASCO.)

Table 6.2
Continued

	Calories	Protein (gm)	Carbohydrate (gm)	Fat (gm)	Cholesterol (mg)	Sodium (mg)**
WENDY'S						
Double Hamburger	670	44	34	40	125	980
Double with cheese	800	50	41	48	155	1414
Chili	230	19	21	8	25	1065
French Fries	330	5	42	16	45	112
Frosty	390	9	54	16	45	247

(*Source:* Wendy's International, Inc., Dublin, OH. Nutritional analysis by Medallion Laboratories, Minneapolis, MN.)

Beverages

Coffee +	2	tr	tr	tr	—	2
Tea +	2	tr	—	tr	—	—
Orange Juice	82	1	20	tr	—	2
Chocolate Milk	213	9	28	9	—	118
Skim Milk	88	9	13	tr	—	127
Whole Milk	159	9	12	9	27	122
Coca-Cola	96	0	24	0	—	20 + +
Fanta Ginger Ale	84	0	21	0	—	30 + +
Fanta Grape	114	0	29	0	—	21 + +
Fanta Orange	117	0	30	0	—	21 + +
Fanta Root Beer	103	0	27	0	—	23 + +
Mr. Pibb	95	0	25	0	—	23 + +
Mr. Pibb w/o sugar	1	0	tr	0	—	37 + +
Sprite	95	0	24	0	—	42 + +
Sprite w/o sugar	3	0	0	0	—	42 + +
Tab	tr	0	tr	0	—	30 + +
Fresca	2	0	0	0	—	38

Note: + = a 6 oz. serving; all other data are for 8-oz. servings.

+ + = value when bottling water with average sodium content (12 mg/8 oz.) is used.

(*Sources:* 1. Adams, CF, *Nutritive Value of American Foods in Common Units, Handbook No. 456,* Washington, D.C., USDA Agricultural Research Service, November 1975; 2. The Coca-Cola Company, Atlanta, Georgia, January 1977; 3. *American Hospital Formulary Service,* Washington, D.C., American Society of Hospital Pharmacists, Section 28:20, March 1978.)

(*Source:* Young, E. A., "Perspectives on Fast Food," *Public Health Currents,* Vol. 21, No. 3, Ross Laboratories, Columbus, OH, 1981.)

Note: Some of the information on this table may be outdated. Since 1981, many fast-food restaurants have altered their recipes and ingredients in response to consumer demands.

** = Salt information adapted from *Salt: The Brand Name Guide to Sodium Content.* New York: Center for Science in the Public Interest/Workman Publishing, 1983. Also: *Guide to Salt Content of Your Foods* by R. L. Berko. South Orange, NJ: Consumer Education Research Center, 1983.

X = less than 2% USRDA; tr = trace; — = no data available.

As consumers have become more aware of the importance of a sensible diet, fast-food restaurants have become more responsive to their demands. As mentioned above, salad bars have caught on in many fast-food chains and franchises. In addition, a few restaurants have added fish that has been baked or broiled or chicken that has been roasted instead of fried. Whole-grain buns are available in at least one fast-food chain, and baked potatoes have appeared on some menus; however, some of the toppings (cheese, sour cream, bacon, chili) may raise the fat and salt levels of these potatoes, putting them on par with bacon cheeseburgers and fried-chicken sandwiches.

Despite the recent headway made toward creating a better fast-food meal, there still is *plenty* of room for improvement. Concerned parents can make an impact by talking to restaurant managers and writing to the fast-food company, asking for information on ingredients, and expressing interest in seeing a greater number of low-salt, low-fat foods on the menu. Consumer pressure can work! Many fast-food chains continue to add large quantities of salt to their food and use saturated fat (usually a blend of mostly beef fat with some vegetable oil) for frying. The reason: "Our customers like the way our food tastes."

While burgers, fries, pizza, chicken, and shakes cannot be recommended as a steady diet, it is unrealistic for parents to prohibit children from eating fast food and expect them to willingly comply. Fast food is not all bad. The important thing for parents to remember is that they should compensate for the shortcomings of fast food by serving well-balanced meals and snacks at home. If most of a teenager's meals are nutritionally sound, some fast-food meals and snacks are not a problem.

MEALS WHILE TRAVELING

To many people, eating on the road means making quickie stops at fast-food restaurants or buying peanut-butter cheese crackers and soda pop from gas-station vending machines. Traveling and a poor diet, however, need not go hand in hand. Satisfying meals and snacks can be packed at home and eaten in the car, or on the train, plane, or bus.

Roadside picnics are a great way to make meals on the road a lot of fun. While in transit, snacking on easy-to-carry, easy-to-serve, and easy-to-eat treats will save time and money, and help make a happier, healthier family outing.

The best on-the-road snacks are finger foods, and the best finger foods for travel are the ones that are not too crumbly, drippy, or sticky. Cubes or slices of cheese, chunks of roasted chicken, and hard-boiled eggs are convenient and nourishing protein-rich snacks that are easy to eat in a moving vehicle. Tiny sandwiches made on cocktail bread also are ideal for snacking. Peanut butter, sliced meat, plain tuna, and cheese are the best sandwich choices because these are less likely to spoil than mayonnaise-based sandwich spreads. Mayonnaise, however, can be used on sandwiches that will be refrigerated in a cooler or eaten soon after they are made.

Fruits and vegetables are refreshing and convenient foods to eat on the road. The most popular choices — carrot and celery sticks, radishes, cherry tomatoes, and slices of green pepper — are good for munching and low in calories. Apples, pears, and bananas make good snacks, and orange and grapefruit sections and pineapple chunks, though sticky, also are sweet, delectable treats. Seedless grapes, raisins, and dried apricots, peaches, pears, and apples are good snacks small enough to be popped right into the mouth. Plastic garbage bags are a must for cores, seeds, and peels, and premoistened towelettes are great for wiping sticky fingers.

Other snacks that travel well include popcorn, pretzels, cookies, dry cereal, and bagels. Crackers, especially the kind made with whole grains and low salt, also make good on-the-road snacks, as long as parents can live with the crumbs for a while.

Children often are more thirsty than hungry when traveling long distances. Water is by far the best drink choice. Not only does it quench the thirst, but if it is spilled it does not stain, stick, or attract unwanted flies. It also can be used to wipe sticky little hands and faces. Fruit juices are available in little cans and single-serving boxes, which can be frozen beforehand and enjoyed while they are cold.

Canned soft drinks are all right for traveling, but they are loaded with sugar. A better "fizzy" choice is to mix fruit juice with seltzer water in resealable plastic bottles and pack these in a cooler. When traveling, milk can be a poor drink choice, especially for children prone to motion sickness, because it can upset the stomach.

Meals on the road present more of a challenge than snacks. Serving meals on a flimsy paper plate while riding in a car is no treat, especially for parents, who bear most of the clean-up burden. Fortunately there are plenty of rest areas, picnic areas, parks, and roadside tables on most roads. When the weather is good, stopping at these outside areas is a welcomed, much needed break for everyone.

Picnic areas and parks usually provide charcoal grills for hungry travelers to use. Hamburgers are picnic favorites if a barbecue is possible. Chicken, precooked or barbecued, may be a better choice than hamburger for roadside picnics. (Precooking or parboiling chicken before it is placed on the grill reduces barbecue time, which otherwise is about an hour.) Leftover chicken can be taken off the bone, stored in plastic bags, and distributed later as an on-the-road snack. Hard-boiled eggs and grilled-cheese sandwiches are good alternatives to hamburgers, and some fish, such as swordfish and bluefish, grill well.

During long trips it may be a good idea to make several stops at grocery stores along the way rather than try to bring enough food for many meals. Grocery-store deli counters often offer a wide variety of fresh potato salad, macaroni salad, and coleslaw, as well as meat and cheese for sandwiches. Prepared salads, however, do not travel well, and leftovers always should be discarded unless they can be adequately refrigerated. Take-out salad bars also have sprung up in supermarkets in many parts of the country. They provide a wonderful alternative when eating while traveling.

MICROWAVE COOKING

Microwave ovens have shortened the long process of thawing, preparing, and cooking. Baked potatoes, which take at least an hour to cook in a standard oven, can be popped into the microwave oven a mere five minutes before they are brought to the table. Frozen hamburger, which takes roughly 12 hours to thaw in the refrigerator, can be thawed in a microwave oven in eight minutes.

Microwave ovens use special radar waves that either pass directly through objects (such as paper or glass), reflect off objects (such as metals), or penetrate into the cells of objects (such as foods). Radar waves cause food molecules to move rapidly, creating friction, thereby building up heat. This heat cooks the food as it spreads through the molecules.

Microwave ovens are especially helpful when cooking single dishes, small meals, or snacks. The more food that is placed into a microwave oven, the longer the cooking time will be. In large families, when many busy schedules do not allow one big family dinner, meals can be cooked and easily reheated in the microwave oven as needed.

Microwaves also are helpful in warming and softening bread for sandwiches, softening or melting butter or margarine for cooking, clarifying honey, softening brown sugar, and semi-cooking meats before they are placed on a grill to barbecue. Vegetables can be cooked in a microwave without adding water, which helps retain more of the vitamins and minerals. Cooking food in a microwave also helps ensure that the food is heated sufficiently to destroy harmful bacteria.

One major problem with microwave ovens is that overheating and uneven distribution of heat is fairly common. The liquid or food inside the container (dish, jar, or bottle) may become dangerously hot — even though the outside of the container feels cool. Parents should always stir or shake the food or liquid after it has been heated in the microwave oven, then test the temperature before feeding it to infants or young children.

Because microwave ovens are becoming more affordable, are easy to use, and save considerable time, they are finding their way into a great many homes. (An estimated 25 percent of the homes in the United States currently have microwave ovens.) As a result, more and more parents of infants are regularly taking bottles of formula or expressed breast milk from the refrigerator, placing the bottle in the microwave oven, and heating the formula. While this heating method is quick and easy it is not without potential problems.

Baby bottles, especially those with disposable plastic liners or those that are tightly covered, can — and do — explode because steam and pressure build up inside the closed container. Severe burns have occurred as a result of this practice. Extreme caution is advised because heating *tightly closed* baby bottles in a microwave oven can be dangerous. If a microwave is used, the nipple and cap should be removed before the bottle is placed in the oven, or the formula should be heated in a clean dish and then poured into the bottle.

Additionally, although less dramatic or dangerous, overheating formula or expressed breast milk destroys certain vitamins and may inactivate some elements of the mother's natural immunities found in breast milk.

Alternative methods to heating baby bottles in microwave ovens can be found in Table 3.6.

As infants move out of the formula phase and into solid foods, microwave ovens can be a time and labor saver for parents. Cereals are easily heated in the microwave oven. Homemade baby foods can be pureed or mashed ahead of time, frozen in ice-cube trays, and heated in the microwave oven (for approximately one minute) as needed. Commercial baby food can also be heated easily by removing the cap and placing the jar in the microwave oven for 20 to 30 seconds. *Again, all food must be temperature tested before it is served to young children.*

As mentioned earlier, microwave ovens are useful in providing quick and nourishing after-school snacks, such as melted cheese on bread or crackers, soups, and hot sandwiches. The federal government has established safety standards for microwave ovens; for example, the oven must turn off automatically as soon as the door is opened. Because they are safe and easy, children can become skillful in using microwave ovens. There is less of a chance for burned fingers because the dishes in which the foods are cooked stay relatively cool. *Nonetheless, microwave ovens always must be used carefully by children as well as adults.*

Table 6.3 offers tips for safe use of the microwave oven.

GOOD FOOD ON A LIMITED BUDGET

Providing a sound, balanced diet is enough of a challenge when money is plentiful. When there is not enough money, however, the job of meeting the body's need for food is more

Table 6.3
MICROWAVE OVEN SAFETY TIPS

• The food temperature (not the temperature of the bottle, jar, or container) should *always* be tested before food is served, especially for infants and young children.

• Containers that are to be placed in a microwave oven should be open or have some openings to allow steam to escape. Steam can build up inside closed containers, causing them to explode.

• Parents should *never* hold babies when removing food from a microwave oven.

• The microwave oven instruction booklet should be kept handy, and the directions should be followed carefully.

• If food labels offer instructions for microwave cooking, these should be followed *exactly*.

---

challenging. The best way to ensure a sound diet while cutting costs is to buy only foods that are nourishing and filling. Many foods that are high in sugar, fat, and salt — potato chips, candy, cakes, and soft drinks, for example — contain few nutrients and, therefore, are a poor value for the money. Food money instead should be spent on fruits and vegetables, milk, eggs, whole-grain and enriched breads and cereals, dried beans, meat, and/or cheese.

Meat, a major source of protein for many people, usually is the highest priced item in most food baskets. One way to cut costs, therefore, is to reduce the amount of meat purchased. Most people in developed countries eat much more protein than they need. Cutting back and choosing among the many other less expensive sources of protein is an economical move. Dairy products — milk, cheese, yogurt, cottage cheese, and eggs — are excellent sources of high-quality protein and are less expensive than meat. Milk is an extremely important protein source for most children. When budgets are tight, powdered milk and evaporated milk (both requiring dilution with water) cost less and provide most of the vitamins and minerals found in whole, low-fat, or skim milk.

Learning ways to use other nonmeat protein sources and how to combine them to obtain high-quality protein is important to families on a restricted budget. Combining beans with rice or cornmeal, for example, provides high-quality protein at a low cost. Lentils, chickpeas, black beans, pinto beans, and kidney beans can be combined with other vegetables to make inexpensive, colorful, and appealing meals. (Methods for combining nonmeat sources to improve protein quality are found in Chapter 7.) Several vegetarian cookbooks (many of which are available in most libraries) are listed in the Useful Reading section at the end of this book. These titles supply a range of recipe ideas for families with all sorts of tastes and life-styles.

Vegetables and other foods can be purchased less expensively at food cooperatives, which are growing in number and popularity. Lower prices and the high quality of fruit, vegetables, and processed food make joining a food co-op highly attractive for many families.

Buying in bulk is another way to cut costs. Sometimes neighbors and friends can get together to buy large quantities of food at a lower cost per unit. In some areas there are discount food warehouses that sell food, in large quantities, at lower prices. Sharing the cost of transportation to a food warehouse or co-op can result in additional savings.

Costs also can be reduced by buying food that requires cooking, baking, or preparation at home. Ready-to-serve or partially prepared foods tend to be more expensive than their raw ingredients. For example, instant hot cereals are more expensive than hot cereals that demand a longer cooking time; fully prepared spaghetti sauce is more expensive than homemade sauce; cornbread bought in the bakery or prepared from a boxed mix is more expensive than the homemade kind; frozen french fries are more expensive than a baked potato.

Depending on the time of year, some canned fruits and vegetables may be less expensive than their fresh or frozen counterparts. In addition, buying fruits and vegetables in season and freezing them for later use can save money — if there is adequate freezer space available.

The U.S. Department of Agriculture (USDA) has prepared food plans for four economic levels. The Thrifty Food Plan is used as a basis for food-stamp allotments; the Low-Cost Plan, Moderate-Cost Plan, and the Liberal Plan also may prove helpful to people on limited budgets. These food plans suggest appropriate amounts of different foods for a family to buy each week or each month to meet most of the nutritional requirements at a cost that fits its budget. Booklets that include menu plans and recipes for nutritious, low-cost meals are also available from the USDA. (See the Resources section for the address of the U.S. Department of Agriculture offices.)

Besides the National School Lunch Program and the School Breakfast Program, the federal government runs the Supplemental Food Program for Women, Infants, and Children, known as the WIC program. This program provides selected staple foods to a limited number of pregnant and lactating women and children up to 5 years of age who are at nutritional risk. It also provides nutrition education and health services for mothers and their children who qualify.

The Food Stamp Program, established in 1964, supplements the food-buying power of individuals or families who meet the strict financial requirements. In this program, eligible participants buy food stamps, which allow them to buy food at reduced cost.

All these programs are important; they help fulfill basic food needs and are a means of combating the health problems often associated with poverty. Not all low-income families in the United States, however, benefit from these federal subsidies. In addition, most of the existing programs are in danger of reduction or elimination because of government budget cutbacks. The 1985 *Hunger in America* report asserts that, "Today we have a public health crisis which threatens a significant segment of our population." Expanding these programs, the report states, could eliminate hunger in the United States within six months.

Parents who care about the future of these programs should write to their representatives and senators and ask that funding for these vital programs be increased. After all, no child should be deprived of the right to grow up to be a strong and healthy adult.

In conclusion, providing nourishing meals and snacks to children need not involve a lot of time or money. The wide range of foods and the assortment of preparation methods allows a variety of wholesome foods to be prepared quickly and economically. The subsidized programs and assistance available in many communities provide some means by which low-income families can obtain necessary funding and information to buy nourishing food.

All children must eat nourishing food in order to grow and develop into healthy adults. It is a parent's responsibility to make sure all the necessary raw materials are present in their children's diets. This task is challenging, but it is not impossible — even when time and money are limited.

7

ALTERNATIVE DIETS: THE GOOD, THE BAD, AND THE UGLY

First he ate some lettuces
and some French beans;
and then he ate some radishes;
and then, feeling rather sick,
he went to look for some parsley.

Beatrix Potter
The Tale of Peter Rabbit

Countless books, articles, and advertisements describe diets that claim to melt pounds away, promote good health, cure cancer, or increase intelligence. According to these enthusiastic reports, eating certain foods at the right times in the prescribed amounts can lead to nearly anything — calm children, thin thighs, long life, self-satisfaction, or unity with the universe. Among these magic diet schemes are mounds of carrots and celery, half a grapefruit before each meal, no meat, just meat, massive quantities of water, just rice, and enormous doses of various vitamins.

Some alternative diets are sensible and balanced; others are dangerous and can lead to temporary or permanent health problems — even death. Fortunately, most of the dangerous food fads are short-lived. People try them, and sometimes lose weight or feel better. In most cases, however, the menus are too restrictive, impractical, expensive, or boring to follow, and people either discover that the claims are false, or lose interest.

A few diets, once thought of as faddish, however, have met the tests of time and scientific scrutiny and have become accepted as sensible, healthful ways to eat. The vegetarian diet is the best example of a diet that many people have claimed was just a fad. Millions of people throughout the world, however, are vegetarians, and the diet continues to grow in popularity in developed countries. The case that follows shows that vegetarian diets, when carefully planned, can suit the needs of growing children.

VEGETARIAN DIETS

A mother of three who had recently moved to the Boston area brought her children — aged 10 years, 4 years, and 6 months — to her new pediatrician for a well-child examination. During this first visit, the mother made it clear that she and her husband were vegans. (They ate no meat, poultry, fish, dairy products, or eggs.) She had read extensively about nutrition, however, and was careful when planning meals during her pregnancies and for her children.

During all three pregnancies and while breast feeding, this mother had supplemented her diet with milk, cheese, and eggs (in addition to her prenatal vitamins) to make sure she got enough calories, calcium, protein, vitamins D and B_{12}, riboflavin, iron, and zinc. She also understood that growing children had different requirements from adults. As a result, she included milk and eggs in her children's diets, though she did not give them meat, poultry, or fish.

The mother explained that she understood some vegetables (especially beans) contained substances called phytates and oxylates, which might interfere with absorption of iron and calcium. Iron deficiency could lead to fatigue and learning difficulties, and she wanted to make sure her children were getting enough of this mineral. Finally, the mother said that most of the foods she normally used were low in calories, so she never restricted snacks, although she did not let the children have candy, cakes, or cookies except as rare treats.

The pediatrician, feeling as though she had just received a crash course in nutrition, examined the children and found them to be "bright, active, and engaging." They were all at the 75th percentile for weight and height, except the baby, who was at the 90th percentile for weight. All three children had rosy cheeks, shiny hair, and were well proportioned.

After the examination, the pediatrician suggested that the mother continue this diet because all the children were thriving on it. She then asked if the mother were planning to phase out milk and eggs from her children's diets. The mother explained that she knew her children needed these foods, at least until they stopped growing, and by that time she would not have much say about what they ate.

A vegetarian diet, as this example shows, can be a nutritious way to eat, but it must be planned carefully to meet all the body's needs for vitamins, minerals, and protein. For centuries, people have survived — and thrived — on vegetarian diets. Vegetarianism has economic, geographic, and religious roots. Buddhists, for example, have followed strict vegetarian diets as far back as 483 B.C., when Gautama Buddha founded their religion. Orthodox Hindus, who believe that all living things possess a part of the divine spirit, also follow vegetarian diets. Seventh-Day Adventists, who supplement their diets with milk and eggs, and Trappist Monks, who use dairy products but no eggs, also are examples of healthy groups that use vegetarian-type diets. In the Himalayas of Pakistan, the Hunza tribe has practiced vegetarianism for years, with an emphasis on grains, vegetables, dairy products, and apricots. The Hunza are renowned for their health and longevity, and have been the subject of many books, articles, and documentaries.

In early America, vegetarian diets were considered strange by the meat-eating masses. But in 1838, participants at an American Health Convention learned about a study concluding that a vegetarian diet was a sensible way to eat. The message spread quickly, and vegetarianism became widely accepted.

People adopt vegetarian diets for a variety of reasons — religious beliefs, health concerns, environmental considerations, humane views, economic pressures, social status, and political

Table 7.1
TYPES OF VEGETARIAN DIETS

Partial vegetarian	Diet includes dairy products, eggs, seafood, and usually poultry. Diet excludes meat, and sometimes poultry.
Lacto-ovo-vegetarian	Diet includes dairy products and eggs in addition to vegetables, fruits, cereals, grains, nuts, and seeds. Diet excludes meat, seafood, poultry.
Lacto-vegetarian	Diet includes dairy products in addition to vegetables, fruits, cereals, grains, nuts, and seeds. Diet excludes eggs, meat, seafood, poultry.
Vegan (total vegetarian)	Diet includes vegetables, fruits, cereals, grains, nuts, and seeds. Diet excludes all foods from animal sources — meat, eggs, seafood, poultry, dairy products.
Fruitarian	Diet includes raw or dried fruits, seeds, and nuts. Diet excludes vegetables, grains, and all foods from animal sources — meat, eggs, seafood, poultry, dairy products.

beliefs. Today, vegetarians in the United States number more than 3 million. This figure is on the rise as a health-conscious society is drawn more and more to fresh vegetables, fruits, and whole grains, rather than red meat.

There are several types of vegetarian diets, ranging from partial vegetarianism, which includes poultry, seafood, eggs, milk, and dairy products, to fruitarian, which includes only fruits, seeds, and nuts. Table 7.1 outlines the most common forms of vegetarian diets.

Many types of vegetarian diets are nourishing and balanced. Partial-vegetarian, lacto-ovo-vegetarian and lacto-vegetarian diets, for example, can provide all the raw materials that children need to grow and thrive. Vegan diets, which omit all sources of animal protein, however, are not suitable and, in fact, are dangerous for growing children. Children on vegan diets tend to weigh less than their peers.

A fruitarian diet also lacks too many of the nutrients that children need to grow — especially protein. A severe protein deficiency can lead to problems with both mental and physical development.

Fruitarian diets are dangerous for children — and adults.

Meat, poultry, or seafood are the primary sources of protein for people in developed countries. They all contain high-quality protein (protein in which all essential amino acids are present in the right proportions — see Chapter 2). Milk, dairy products, and eggs also contain high-quality protein. So when these foods are included in the diet there is no problem getting enough high-quality protein.

Protein from all nonanimal sources is considered low quality because it lacks sufficient amounts of one or more essential amino acids. If the amino acids are not present in the right proportions, then the body cannot use the other amino acids in the food. Different foods, however, lack different amino acids. The key to a sensible vegetarian diet, therefore, is to combine foods to form high-quality protein.

There are four groups of nonanimal proteins:

1. *Grains* (rice, wheat, corn, oats, barley, buckwheat, rye, millet, bulgur, pasta, bread, flour)

2. *Legumes* (pinto, kidney, navy, black, mung, lima, broad, and white beans; black-eyed peas; lentils; soybeans, soy grits, tofu; chickpeas; dried peas)

3. *Seeds and Nuts* (sesame, sunflower, pumpkin seeds; almonds, Brazil nuts, cashews, peanuts, pecans, pistachio, walnuts, filberts, macadamias)

4. *Vegetables* (asparagus, broccoli, cauliflower, potatoes, Brussels sprouts, spinach, kale, greens, green peas, mushrooms)

In addition, milk, dairy products, and eggs can be mixed in or eaten along with any food from these four groups to enhance the protein in the vegetable source. Combining milk and eggs with grains, nuts, and seeds is especially good, because the amino acid lysine is abundant in milk and eggs, and deficient in grains, nuts, and seeds. Table 7.2 provides guidelines for combining foods to achieve high-quality protein.

A vegan diet is hazardous to a child's health because it lacks sufficient amounts of vitamin B_{12} (found only in animal proteins), calcium, zinc, iron, riboflavin, and possibly vitamin D, all of which are necessary for proper growth and development.

Using the guidelines outlined in Table 7.2, many tasty, appealing vegetarian meals can be easily prepared and enjoyed. Table 7.3 offers some suggestions for dishes that use nonmeat foods to form high-quality protein. Recipes for these dishes can be found in most of the vegetarian cookbooks listed in the Useful Reading section of this book, as well as in the excellent books by Frances Moore Lappé, a pioneer in this field.

Parents' religious convictions often dictate the type of family diet. As mentioned earlier, Zen Buddhists, Hindus, and Seventh-Day Adventists eat various types of vegetarian diets. Parents should understand the needs of their children and the nutrients provided by or lacking in the diet they follow. They should make sure that their dietary beliefs do not endanger their children's health. If the guidelines raise questions, registered dietitians or physicians can discuss ways to meet children's needs while following various vegetarian diets.

MACROBIOTIC DIETS

The parents of a 1-year-old boy noticed that their son was not growing well or gaining much weight, so they brought him to Boston Children's Hospital. Doctors there found the boy to be thin, frail, and irritable. His crying was very weak and his temperature was below normal. He was underweight — in fact, his

Table 7.2
FORMING HIGH-QUALITY PROTEIN

Food Group	Some High-quality Combinations
Grains (all)	Grains and milk and dairy products Grains and eggs
Rice	Rice and legumes Rice and soybeans and wheat Rice and sesame seeds Rice and peanuts and soybeans and wheat Rice and spinach and cauliflower
Wheat	Wheat and legumes Wheat and soybeans and rice Wheat and soybeans and sesame seeds Wheat and soybeans and peanuts Wheat and spinach and broccoli
Corn	Corn and legumes Corn and cauliflower and potatoes Corn and soybeans and sesame seeds
Legumes	Legumes and milk and dairy products Legumes and eggs Legumes and rice Legumes and barley Legumes and oats Legumes and millet Beans and wheat Beans and corn Soybeans and rice and wheat Soybeans and wheat and sesame seeds Soybeans and peanuts and sesame seeds Peas and sesame seeds and Brazil nuts
Vegetables*	Vegetables and milk and dairy products Vegetables and eggs Vegetables and sesame seeds Vegetables and pumpkin seeds Broccoli and mushrooms and lima beans Cauliflower and spinach and cashews
Seeds and nuts	Nuts and milk and dairy products Nuts and eggs Seeds and milk and dairy products Seeds and eggs

Table 7.2
Continued

Food Group	Some High-quality Combinations
Seeds and nuts *continued*	Seeds and legumes Sesame seeds, peanuts, and soybeans Sesame seeds, soybeans, and wheat Peanuts and sunflower seeds Sesame seeds and rice

*Vegetables, in general, are low in protein.

Table 7.3
HIGH-QUALITY VEGETARIAN DISHES

Vegetarian chili with rice
Pea soup with corn bread
Black-eyed peas and rice
Broccoli-noodle casserole
Vegetable lasagna
Frittata (an open omelet with onions and vegetables)
French toast
Pizza
Lentil pot pie
Vegetable stroganoff
Bean tostadas
Baked zucchini, tomato, and rice casserole
Broccoli-cheese baked potato
Macaroni and cheese
Hummus (chickpea and sesame paste) and pita bread
Egg foo yung
Green peppers stuffed with rice and tomato

weight compared to that of a normal 4-month-old baby. In addition, he had reached only the 6- to 8-month developmental level.

The boy had been breast fed for 6 months and then he was introduced to solid food. This solid food, however, consisted mainly of kohkoh — a pureed mixture of soybeans, kombu beans, seaweed, aduki beans, whole oats, sweet rice, brown rice, and spring water. Sometimes millet, bulgur, mugwort, or sesame seeds were added to the mixture. On a few occasions, the boy was given radish tops, carrots, broccoli, kale, mustard greens, green beans, kali beans, onions, miso soup, barley malt, yini syrup, and whole oat cream.

To many people some of these ingredients sound strange, but they are familiar items to people on macrobiotic diets, the diet followed by this boy's parents.

The boy was admitted to the hospital, and tests showed he was anemic and deficient in iron, vitamin B_{12}, calcium, magnesium, and phosphorus. He also had severe diarrhea and an upper respiratory infection. His parents, convinced that their macrobiotic lifestyle was the key to a happy, healthy life, were reluctant to feed the boy differently. Eventually, however, they agreed to let doctors change his diet. He was immediately started on cow's milk, and soon after this, fruits, vegetables, and meat were added. He also was given vitamin and mineral supplements.

During his hospital stay, the boy grew and thrived on his new diet. His weight climbed dramatically, his appetite was voracious, and he became more active. One of the most noticeable improvements, however, was in the boy's personality. He changed from an apathetic, irritable boy into a warm and loving child who smiled brightly at the nurses when they came into his room.

The child left the hospital nearly a month later. His parents, convinced that their macrobiotic diet was not suitable for their son, began feeding him a balanced diet by adapting the Basic Four Food Groups. When he came back for a routine check-up six months later, his weight, height, and developmental level were normal for an 18-month-old child.

This example clearly shows the strong link between diet and health and the importance of providing children with everything they need to grow and develop normally. Certain types of macrobiotic diets may be suitable for adults, but macrobiotic and many other alternative diets can be harmful for children.

Asian cultures have followed Zen Buddhist macrobiotic diets for centuries, but in Western civilization the diet has become popular only during the past 10 to 15 years. The premise behind the macrobiotic diet is that good health and happiness depend upon a delicate balance of yin and yang, the two primary forces that exist in the universe. These forces are opposites, and they complement each other to maintain harmony.

The yin is thought of as an outward-moving, expansive force, while the yang is seen as pulling together and consolidating all the forces in nature. Foods are classified as either yin or yang, and macrobiotic diets seek to balance the intake of these two categories of foods.

Followers of macrobiotic diets progress through ten stages of dietary restraint. The lowest level is a diet containing 30 percent vegetables, 30 percent animal products (usually fish), 15 percent salads and fruits, 10 percent soups, 10 percent cereals, and 5 percent desserts. These percentages change gradually until the person has reached a diet that consists of 100 percent cereals and grains (usually brown rice) and herbal tea. The idea is to reduce food intake to the bare minimum necessary for continued activity and survival, which is said to enhance consciousness.

Children, however, must do more than survive. They must grow, develop, and thrive. A macrobiotic diet, especially at the highest levels, *eliminates* most of the vital proteins, fats, minerals, vitamins, and calories that help nurture a child through to a healthy adulthood.

Most levels of the Zen macrobiotic diet are unsuitable for children.

Fortunately, most people who follow macrobiotic plans stick to the low levels of the diet, which contain most of the essential nutrients. Low levels may lack enough calcium and calories for a child's proper development, but these deficiencies can be corrected easily with a few additions, such as cow's milk. High macrobiotic levels are deficient in protein, calories, riboflavin, vitamin C, iron, calcium, vitamin B_{12}, and vitamin D. Diseases such as rickets, scurvy, anemia, malnutrition, failure to thrive, and stunted physical and mental growth are likely among children who follow strict macrobiotic diets, as seen in the above example. Several deaths have even occurred because people have stayed on high levels of the diet for long periods of time.

Some parents who do not themselves follow a macrobiotic lifestyle may become concerned if their teenage child decides to adopt such a diet. Adolescence is a natural time for experimentation, and some teenagers turn to exotic eating patterns as a way to assert independence.

Parents can maintain an open mind and try to discuss ways of keeping the diet nutritious. Perhaps the teenager would be willing to talk to an informed adult, such as a physician, registered dietitian, biology teacher, or coach, to design a macrobiotic diet that is balanced, nourishing, and acceptable. The low levels of a macrobiotic diet, for example, contain cereals, vegetables, fruits, fish, and desserts, and this plan can be nutritionally sound. If adolescents remain at these levels, their development and growth will not be hampered. Parents might also keep on hand supplies of simple, nourishing foods, such as nuts, seeds, rice, vegetables, or local fruit, that are acceptable to macrobiotic devotees.

If the teenager insists on progressing to the more restrictive levels of the diet, however, parents should calmly help the child understand the dangers. Information and compromise usually are more successful than attempts to steer a determined teenager from a particular course of action.

HIGH-FIBER DIETS

In the past century, the emphasis on fiber in the American diet has come full circle. In the early 1900s, fiber (also called roughage) was a mainstay of each meal. People consumed large quantities of whole-grain breads, porridge, and plain vegetables such as potatoes, turnips, and cabbage. As the general standard of living rose and technology led to more types of processed foods, people in developed countries, in general, switched from grains and vegetables to refined foods, well-marbled meats, and sweets.

This increased consumption of fatty meats and highly processed and refined foods has been associated with a rise in the incidence of health problems, such as cardiovascular disease, diverticulosis (creation of small pockets in the intestinal lining), colon and rectal cancer, and constipation.

In 1970, two British physicians, Dr. Denis Burkitt and Dr. Hugh Trowell, published *Diseases of Civilization*, a study showing a relationship between the rise in intestinal diseases in Western civilization and the increased use of processed foods. They concluded that removing much of the undigestible fiber from common plant sources of carbohydrates had affected human health. These findings were highly publicized and, as a result, consumption of fiber-rich foods began to increase. High-fiber diets became the new American nutrition rage.

Studies continue to confirm the benefits of increased fiber in the diet. Today, diets in which fiber is plentiful are no longer considered faddish. Fiber-rich diets are, in fact, beneficial and encouraged.

Fiber is a complex carbohydrate found in the walls of plant cells. It is the tough, structural part of the plant, for example, the stringy part of celery and the bran (the outer shell) of wheat. The best sources of fiber include whole-grain breads and cereals, dried beans, nuts, fresh fruits, and fresh vegetables.

In the digestive tract, fiber is not broken down by enzymes. It remains virtually intact, acting like a sponge in the intestine, absorbing many times its weight in water. The result is a bulkier, softer stool, which is easy to pass. People who consume a lot cf fiber also get rid of wastes sooner after eating than persons who consume little fiber. This is known as a shorter gut-transit time.

In developed countries, the average person consumes anywhere from 15 to 25 grams of dietary fiber a day, even though 35 to 45 grams a day is considered the ideal amount. It is difficult, however, to determine exactly how much dietary fiber people eat. There are many types of fiber — cellulose, hemicellulose, gums, pectin, lignin, and mucilage. Most methods used to measure fiber content are inexact. The fiber content listed on a product often represents the crude fiber, which is what remains after the food has been treated with chemicals. These chemicals destroy many types of valuable fiber, leaving only a portion of the lignin, cellulose, and hemicellulose to measure. New testing methods, which try to simulate human digestion, can more accurately assess the dietary fiber content of foods. These methods, however, continue to have drawbacks, making dietary fiber figures still somewhat imprecise, but more reliable than crude-fiber figures.

High-fiber diets contain anywhere from 30 to 70 grams of dietary fiber a day. These diet plans are prescribed frequently to relieve the symptoms associated with constipation, hemorrhoids, and diverticulosis. Increasing fiber may prevent the onset of these conditions. Additionally, some diabetic *adults* placed on high-fiber diets have been able to reduce significantly or eliminate the amount of insulin they require. Fiber slows down the process by which carbohydrates are converted into blood sugar, or glucose. When less sugar is absorbed into the bloodstream, less insulin is needed to regulate the glucose level (see Chapter 8). To date, this has not been well documented in diabetes among children.

There is some speculation that a high-fiber diet can help prevent cancers of the colon and rectum. The ability of fiber to move wastes quickly through the body means that possible toxins and carcinogens are eliminated quickly as well.

High-fiber diets can be effective means of weight loss and control. Fibrous foods, especially fruits and vegetables, tend to have fewer calories than low-fiber foods. Also, fiber expands in the digestive tract as it absorbs water, so the feeling of fullness comes sooner, and a person tends to eat less. Because fiber passes through the body quickly, it may carry with it small amounts of fats and proteins that have not yet been absorbed into the system.

If levels of fiber are increased *gradually*, the digestive system generally adjusts quite well.

Adding fibrous foods to the average diet is generally a good idea. Too much fiber, however, can cause problems, especially if a person's digestive system is not accustomed to high levels. The most common problems associated with overconsumption of fiber are diarrhea, increased gas, bloating, and stomach cramps. Most of these symptoms, however, are temporary. They usually stem from adding too much fiber too fast.

Another possible problem with high-fiber diets involves the ability of some forms of fiber to interfere with the absorption of iron, calcium, zinc, copper, magnesium, phosphorus, and vitamin B_{12}. When fiber binds with these essential minerals, it carries them out of the body as waste.

Most people, however, consume more of these minerals than they need, so high-fiber diets present few mineral deficiency problems. The body regulates the balance of most of these minerals, so after a few weeks on a high-fiber diet the minerals that are available usually are absorbed more effectively.

Calcium, however, may be the exception. Researchers have estimated that high-fiber diets may interfere with the absorption of sufficient amounts of calcium. Short-term studies have shown that a significant increase of fiber may lead to a need for more calcium in the diet.

Very-high-fiber diets, therefore, may not be suitable for children, adolescents, elderly people who suffer from osteoporosis (degeneration and weakening of bone), or people who are poorly nourished. These groups need higher levels of calcium and other minerals. Robbing even small amounts of these minerals from the body could lead to nutritional problems. Parents should remember the need for milk and other sources of calcium and add fiber to meals in *moderation*.

Parents should not place their children on a high-fiber diet without the advice and guidance of a physician or registered dietitian.

MEGAVITAMINS

As society became more health conscious in the mid-1970s, many people focused on the importance of vitamins. Studies linked several health problems to vitamin deficiencies, which led to the belief that supplementing diets with vitamins would alleviate symptoms. Vitamin supplements were touted as a means to counter the dangers of a poor diet.

From that belief grew the philosophy that if a little of a certain vitamin was good, then more was better. Thus, megavitamins, or taking high concentrations of vitamins in doses ranging from 10 to 2,000 times the RDA, became a fad. Consuming vitamins in excess, however, has not proven to be the cure-all for which many people hoped. In fact, this practice can be dangerous, as the following example shows.

A worried mother brought her 4-year-old daughter to Boston Children's Hospital after the child failed to gain weight for three months. Usually bright, warm, and enthusiastic, the child lately had been irritable, temperamental, and cross. At night she had trouble falling asleep and woke up often. She complained of a sore head, blurred vision, stomachaches, leg pains, and had little appetite. At nursery school, the child lacked interest in almost all activities.

Doctors discovered an itchy rash on the child's body. Her hair was thin and coarse — she appeared to be going bald. There were cuts at the corners of her mouth, and her tongue and gums were cracking and bleeding. Her liver was larger than normal, and there were tender, swollen areas on some of her bones and joints.

The source of the problem became clear when, in passing, her mother noted how peculiar it was for the child to become sick right after the family had started to take an interest in health and fitness. Sure enough, part of the family's fitness plan included megadoses of vitamin A.

When the supplements were stopped, the child slowly regained her appetite, began to gain weight, and slept well. Her hair, skin, mouth, liver, and bones improved significantly. Soon her enthusiasm, warmth, and vigor for life returned to normal.

When high levels of vitamins are ingested they can act like drugs in the body. High concentrations of the fat-soluble vitamins, such as vitamins A and D, are particularly harmful, as the above example shows. In the case of water-soluble vitamins such as vitamin C, most of the excess is excreted in the urine. This, however, does not mean that massive doses of vitamin C and other water-soluble vitamins are harmless.

A brief review of the potentially harmful side effects of megavitamins follows.

Vitamin A

Although it is not common, vitamin A toxicity *does* occur. The adult body needs no more than 5,000 International Units (IUs) of vitamin A a day, while infants and children require approximately 2,500 IUs. This amount is easily obtained through food such as liver, eggs, cheese, fortified milk, and yellow, orange, or dark-green fruits and vegetables (see Table 2.20).

Vitamin A toxicity is unlikely if people stick to food sources for this vitamin. Incidences of toxicity, however, have been reported in adults who have taken megadoses of 50,000 IUs over a period of several months. In infants and young children, toxicity may occur when 20,000 IUs are taken daily for as little as one month.

Approximately 95 percent of the body's vitamin A supply is stored in the liver. Because of this, excess amounts of vitamin A can impede liver function and cause damage. High concentrations of this vitamin also can cause fluid buildup inside the brain, which may lead to headaches, blurred vision, fatigue, insomnia, lack of concentration, depression, and irritability. Other symptoms of vitamin A toxicity are loss of appetite, weight loss, joint pain, menstrual problems, rash, abnormal bone growth, nausea, and cracked lips.

When large amounts of the type of vitamin A found in plants (called beta carotene) are eaten, the result may be a yellowing of the skin. This condition, known as carotenemia, is not harmful and it usually subsides when people reduce the amount of beta carotene in their diet.

Vitamin D

The RDA of vitamin D is 400 IUs a day for infants and children, and 200 IUs for adults. This level can be attained easily from the diet. Vitamin D is contained in fortified milk, egg yolk, liver, and tuna, and it is manufactured on the skin with the aid of the ultraviolet rays of sunlight (see Table 2.20).

Doses of 3,000 to 4,000 IUs daily over a period of several months can lead to the formation of calcium deposits in the kidney, intestinal tract, and bloodstream. Continuous doses as high as 10,000 IUs can lead to kidney stones, kidney failure, bone degeneration, heart damage, and reduced mental function.

Symptoms of vitamin D toxicity include weakness, weight loss, nausea, diarrhea, cramps, deafness, appetite loss, and high blood pressure.

Vitamin E

Although vitamin E, also known as alpha-tocopherol, is fat soluble, the effects of massive doses do not appear to be as severe as those associated with taking megadoses of vitamins A and D. The RDA for vitamin E is 3 to 4 milligrams (approximately 10 IUs) of alpha-tocopherol units for infants, 5 to 8 milligrams (15 to 20 IUs) for children and adolescents, and 8 to 10 milligrams (30 IUs) for adults.

Supplementary doses of vitamin E are unnecessary because this vitamin is plentiful in food that is consumed every day by most people. Good vitamin E sources include vegetable oils, margarine, wheat germ, cereals, green leafy vegetables, liver, seeds, dried beans, egg yolks, and nuts. Despite the plentiful food sources, many people have taken daily supplements ranging anywhere from 200 to 8,000 IUs of vitamin E (see Table 2.20).

Taking megadoses of vitamin E became quite fashionable after limited laboratory experiments suggested that the vitamin could delay the aging process by decreasing deterioration of cells. The popularity of vitamin E also grew when it was mentioned as a possible aid in increasing sexual responsiveness and fertility. Further research has not confirmed the sexual or youth-restorative powers of the vitamin. As a result, megadoses of vitamin E have decreased in popularity.

To date, massive doses of vitamin E have not proved to be dangerous. Some evidence exists, however, that high vitamin E levels are linked with decreased function of vitamin K, which is necessary for proper blood clotting. People who have taken high concentrations of vitamin E also have reported vision problems, fatigue, weakness, headache, high blood pressure, and reduced function of the thyroid hormone, thyroxine.

Vitamin C

The RDA for vitamin C (also called ascorbic acid) for infants is 35 milligrams, 45 milligrams for children, and 60 milligrams for adults. This amount is easily obtained from fruit and fruit juices (especially citrus fruits) and some vegetables, such as broccoli, green peppers, and greens (see Table 2.20).

Vitamin C is water soluble, so it is not stored in the body. Body tissues can accommodate no more than approximately 150 milligrams of vitamin C a day, and most of the additional vitamin C is excreted in the urine.

The use of megadoses of vitamin C became popular in the early 1970s, soon after Nobel Laureate Dr. Linus Pauling noted that vitamin C helped reduce many of the uncomfortable symptoms associated with the common cold and helped prevent the onset of this annoying malady. Shortly after Pauling's report, many people began to swallow megadoses of vitamin C in strengths ranging from 500 to 10,000 milligrams a day. Recent studies, however, have shown that high doses of vitamin C do little more than turn urine bright yellow. Megadoses will not prevent the common cold, but for some people vitamin C may reduce the severity of some of the symptoms.

In the late 1970s and early 1980s there was speculation that megadoses of vitamin C (10,000 milligrams a day) could help protect against the development and spread of some types of cancer. But new research indicates that vitamin C has no effect as an anticancer agent, and the vitamin does not improve chances for survival among cancer patients.

Megadoses of vitamin C have not been found to cause major toxic effects in the body, but some problems have been linked with continuous high concentrations of the vitamin. Massive doses taken over a long period of time may result in permanent dependency on supplements because the body will lose its ability to use smaller amounts of the vitamin. *If pregnant women take large doses of vitamin C, permanent dependency on high levels of the vitamin may carry over to the fetus.*

Other problems associated with vitamin C megadoses include kidney stones, diarrhea, abnormal absorption of vitamin B_{12}, and overclotting of blood.

The B Vitamins

The vitamins in the B group — B_1, or thiamin; B_2, or riboflavin; B_3, or niacin; B_6, or pyridoxine; folic acid; pantothenic acid; biotin; and B_{12}, or cobalamin — are water soluble and are not stored in the body. Excess amounts of most B vitamins are excreted. Folic acid, however, is absorbed and stored in the liver (see Table 2.21).

To date, few toxic effects have been shown when B-complex vitamins are taken in megadoses. Recently, however, very high levels of vitamin B_6, pyridoxine, have been linked to neurologic abnormalities such as unstable gait, difficulty in walking (especially at night), numbness in feet and hands, and clumsiness when handling objects. These abnormalities usually disappear when the vitamin is stopped. Massive doses of niacin have been blamed for such side effects as tingling sensations, flushing of the skin, abnormal liver function, high blood sugar, digestion problems, and throbbing in the head.

Megavitamin therapy can be dangerous.

BRAIN-FOOD DIETS

The idea that eating certain "brain foods" such as fish and eggs could make a person smarter has been in existence for centuries. Unlike most miracle-food rumors, these claims have some basis in fact.

Fish, for example, especially salt-water fish, is a good source of iodine. Before iodine was routinely added to salt, many people who lived inland lacked this mineral in their diets. This often caused a condition called goiter, where the thyroid gland enlarges and production of the thyroid hormone, thyroxine, decreases. Thyroxine is necessary for proper mental function. When a person who suffered from iodine deficiency ate fish, the thyroid was stimulated into producing more of the essential hormone. The person usually became alert and able to think clearly.

The idea that eating eggs will make a person smarter also may have slight merit. Egg yolks, as well as liver and legumes, are rich sources of a substance known as lecithin. In the body, lecithin is broken down into its components, one of which is choline. Choline aids in the production of acetylcholine, which helps transport nerve impulses to the brain.

Although foods such as fish and egg yolks may have a slight influence on brain function, no single food has the power to increase intelligence or improve mental capacity. In short, *there are no brain foods.*

Brain-food diets, however, have become more sophisticated and complicated than merely fish and eggs. Today, several intricate diet plans outline exact amounts of specific foods at particular times of the day, claiming that this eating pattern will increase a child's IQ by 15 or more points.

The basic principle behind some of these diets is sound. Good nutrition during pregnancy and in the first few years of life will provide a better chance for intelligence in later life. Poor nutrition, after all, can affect all the body's organs and systems, including the brain and the nervous system. In the fetus, the brain grows as the cells in the brain continually divide and increase in number. After the infant is born, brain growth occurs as the cells increase in size as well as numbers. When the infant is approximately 18 months of age, the number of cells in the brain stops increasing, but the existing cells continue to grow in size. Brain-cell growth continues until the child is approximately 5 years old.

Severe malnutrition at any time in this developmental process can stunt brain growth. If the fetus and the newborn are not properly nourished, the result may be fewer brain cells. If the child is malnourished between the ages of 18 months and 5 years, the permanent size of the cells in the brain may be smaller than normal. Both of these conditions could result in reduced mental capacity. Good nutrition during pregnancy and the early years is thus vital.

Proponents of brain-food diets prescribe food plans that are rich in egg yolks, fish, peanut butter, cheese, yogurt, meat, dried beans, and other vegetables. Most of these diets are relatively high in fats — up to 50 percent. (Fat is thought to be vital for proper formation of the brain cells and for construction of the protective shields around these cells.) Brain-food diets often prescribe nutrients in roughly the same concentrations that would be found in human breast milk. Besides the 50 percent fats, these diets usually consist of anywhere from 35 to 45 percent complex carbohydrates, and 5 to 15 percent protein. This proportion of fat in the diet of a child older than 6 months can cause later problems with weight and heart disease.

Parents should evaluate these diets the way they would any other food plan. If the specific brain-food menu concentrates too heavily on any particular food or food group, chances are that it is not a suitable program for a growing, developing child. If the diet is flexible, balanced, and provides essential nutrients from each of the Basic Four Food Groups, it is no different from the recommendations elsewhere in this book.

It should be made clear, however, that there is no evidence to support the claim that adhering faithfully to a brain-food diet while pregnant or placing a child on a brain-food regimen will produce a genius. Mental capacity, after all, is determined by more than diet.

FEINGOLD DIET

In 1973, San Francisco allergist Benjamin Feingold, M.D., reported that approximately half of the hyperactive children he treated improved significantly when they were placed on a special elimination diet. The late Dr. Feingold published his findings in a book entitled *Why Your Child is Hyperactive*, which caught the attention of parents of hyperactive children across the country. Enthusiastic groups of Feingold Associations were formed nationwide to advocate the diet, and these groups remain active today.

The Feingold plan calls for eliminating two groups of foods. Group I is foods that contain artificial colors, artificial flavors, and three antioxidant preservatives — butylated hydroxyanisole (BHA); butylated hydroxytoluene (BHT); and monotertiary butylhydroxlquinone (TBHQ). Group II consists of foods that contain natural salicylates (aspirinlike compounds) — almonds, apples, apricots, berries, cherries, cloves, tea, coffee, cucumbers and pickles, currants, grapes and raisins, green peppers, tomatoes, nectarines, oranges, peaches, plums and prunes, and tangerines. Aspirin itself and medication containing aspirin also are eliminated.

The second stage of the diet, which begins four to six weeks after both groups of foods have been omitted, calls for the foods from Group II to be reintroduced gradually. These salicylate foods are added one at a time in order to identify any sensitivities that may be linked with behavior problems.

Soon after Feingold's results were published, other researchers launched controlled studies attempting to verify his conclusions. Some of these studies showed slight improvement among hyperactive children, especially preschoolers, on the Feingold diet, but no follow-up study produced a dramatic relationship between additives and hyperactivity.

One of the groups that studied the diet was a panel from the National Institutes of Health. The report issued by this panel stated that the Feingold program may have a positive effect on a *small* number of children. The panel members concluded that the diet may be considered as an initial treatment in the management of hyperactivity, but only if the physician and family agree.

Many physicians and registered dietitians, however, have expressed concern about the nutritional adequacy of the Feingold plan. The diet makes it difficult for children to receive sufficient amounts of some vitamins and minerals, especially vitamin C, because it omits many common fruits. But other physicians and nutritionists have concluded that as long as parents are careful and plan their children's diets to make sure that they receive everything needed for normal growth and development, the Feingold diet may be useful. In fact, eliminating foods with synthetic colors and flavors usually means relying less on sugar- and fat-laden foods and relying more on whole grains, lean meats, and fresh vegetables.

ORGANIC FOODS, NATURAL FOODS, AND HEALTH FOODS

The late 1960s and 1970s brought with it a renewed emphasis on back-to-basics nutrition. Dietary buzzwords became "natural," "organically grown," "no additives," "no artificial ingredients," and "no preservatives." Many people rejected offerings at the typical grocery store, calling them too processed, too commercial, or too far from the producer. Instead, many people started shopping in health-food or natural-food stores.

Health foods, organic foods, and natural foods became big business. They were so big, in fact, that some food manufacturers began using these reassuring words (often inaccurately) on their packages to tempt health-conscious shoppers. Supermarkets began stocking their shelves with herbal teas, whole-grain breads, and products that were natural, additive-free, and organic.

"Organic," "natural," and "health food" are words with rather vague definitions. They also overlap a good deal. Parents need a certain amount of common sense and practicality in evaluating food with these words on the label.

Organic Foods

In the dictionary sense, "organic" simply means the presence of carbon in a molecule, and all plants and animals contain carbon; therefore, all food is organic. The term organically grown food, however, was adopted to mean plants that are grown without the use of synthetic fertilizers, insecticides, fungicides, or herbicides.

The soil in which organic food is grown supposedly contains only naturally occurring organic materials. The farmer who grows organic food enriches the soil with animal manures, humus, compost, or extracts and residues from other organically grown foods.

Most people buy organically grown food to avoid the risks of pesticides and fertilizer residues. Studies on products sold as "organic," however, have turned up levels of pesticides, some that are even higher than levels in commercial foods. There are two reasons for this. First, pesticide residues have found their way into nearly all parts of the environment, and it is difficult to avoid them. Most pesticides break down slowly. If pesticides or synthetic fertilizers ever have been used on the land, it can take several decades before the soil is free of residues. Also, in some areas of the country, residues from neighboring farms, industries, or runoff may contaminate the soil.

The second reason is that the increase in popularity of organic food led to a rise in the number of fraudulent organic-food manufacturers. Some producers and distributors have taken commercially grown foods, slapped "organically grown" labels on them, and hiked up the price of the food to premium levels. This type of activity is difficult to police because by 1985 only three states — California, Maine, and Oregon — and the Federal Trade Commission had legal definitions of what constituted an organic food.

Buying food produced on organic farms in areas where pesticides are not prevalent *may* be a way to reduce exposure to toxic residues; however, there are no guarantees. In many instances, pesticides and other potentially harmful residues have found their way into the soil through the years. People who buy organic foods should check the reputation of the dealer, manufacturer, or farm, if possible.

Some people believe that organic food is more nutritious than commercially grown food. This is not always so. Organic farms use natural substances to introduce nutrients into the soil and to improve soil texture. Most commercial farms use synthetic fertilizers to enrich the soil with nutrients. If the soil in which an organic potato is grown has the same nutrient content as the soil in which a commercial potato is grown, then there will be little difference in the food value of these two potatoes. To most people, the potatoes taste identical.

Natural Foods

The term "natural" is applied to foods that have undergone little or no processing and contain no added flavors, colors, or artificial preservatives. Many of the foods recommended in this book — fresh fruits and vegetables, whole-grain breads and cereals — are examples of natural foods. But, as with organic foods, there is confusion about what the word "natural" actually means.

A large number of highly processed foods have been branded with the words "natural" or "no artificial ingredients." Food manufacturers have found these terms to be psychologically appealing and reassuring to consumers. Many natural foods are nutritionally superior to highly processed products, but other foods that are touted as natural are less nutritious. Labels of many of the natural foods show that these products can be high in sugar, fat, calories, cholesterol, and salt. Some granolas, for example, thought by many to be a nourishing, natural cereal, are loaded with honey (a sugar), brown sugar, or coconut oil (a saturated fat). Although granola is a good source of fiber, vitamins, minerals, and protein, other "non-natural" cereals also provide these nutrients without a high sugar content.

Health Foods

Buying and eating organic or natural foods may have a few advantages; the only problem associated with them is damage to the pocketbook. Using certain so-called health foods, however, is a different story. This practice can lead to some serious health problems.

Health foods are thought to have some therapeutic value. They often serve as home remedies for treating illness, pain, and disease. Many health foods are used with the idea that they will promote wellness and prevent disease.

Common health foods include sea salt, kelp, nutritional yeast, royal jelly, bee pollen, bran, ginseng, fertile eggs, desiccated liver, tiger's milk, and blackstrap molasses. Vitamins and minerals, some taken in megadoses, also fill the shelves of health-food stores. Hundreds of herbs and spices also are sold in health-food stores and are used for a variety of medicinal purposes.

Many of these herbs are used to make herbal teas. While herbal teas have increased in popularity in recent years as a caffeine-free alternative to coffee and regular tea, some of the ingredients used in these drinks can cause a wide range of health problems. Table 7.4 describes problems reported to be associated with some of the herbs used in teas.

When buying herbal teas it is important to read labels to determine whether any ingredients that cause problems are used. If ingredients are not listed on the package it is best to avoid the product. Also, if the label states that the tea can be used to relieve pain, cure disease, reduce stress, or give an energy boost, it may contain an herb that is more like a potent drug than a soothing hot drink. These teas should be avoided as well.

While some health foods, such as rose hips, yeast, and wheatgerm, are rich sources of essential nutrients, most of the claims

Table 7.4
HERBAL TEAS: WHAT CAN THEY DO?

Aloe leaves	Can cause severe diarrhea
Apple (seeds, bark, leaves)	Large amounts can be converted into poisonous cyanide in the body
Apricot (pits, bark, leaves)	Large amounts can be converted into poisonous cyanide in the body
Bayberry	Large amounts can cause vomiting
Bitter almond (bark, leaves)	Large amounts can be converted into poisonous cyanide in the body
Buchu	Increases urine flow
Buckthorn bark	Can cause severe diarrhea
Burdock root	Can cause blurred vision, dry mouth, abnormal behavior, slurred speech, hallucinations, difficulty eliminating body waste
Chamomile	Can cause severe reactions in people who have hayfever or are allergic to goldenrod, ragweed, marigold, yarrow, asters, or chrysanthemums
Cassava bean	Large amounts can be converted into poisonous cyanide in the body
Catnip	Can cause hallucinations, euphoria
Cherry (wild or choke) (pits, bark, leaves)	Large amounts can be converted into poisonous cyanide in the body
Chinese or green tea	Increases urine flow
Dandelion	Increases urine flow
Devil's claw root	Can cause miscarriage or abortion
Dock root	Can cause severe diarrhea
Ginseng	Contains the hormone estrogen; large amounts can cause high blood pressure, insomnia, nervousness, painful breasts
Hydrangea	Can cause hallucinations, delusions
Indian tobacco	Can irritate the digestive tract, large amounts can be fatal

Table 7.4
Continued

Jimson weed	Can cause hallucinations
Juniper berries	Increase urine flow, can irritate digestive tract, cause hallucinations
Licorice root	Large amounts can cause swelling, high blood pressure, cardiac arrest
Lobelia	Can cause hallucinations
Melilot	Can cause blood-clotting problems
Mistletoe (leaves, berries)	Contains toxins that can cause fatal reactions
Nutmeg	Can cause hallucinations
Peach (leaves, pits, bark)	Large amounts can be converted into poisonous cyanide in the body
Pear (leaves, seeds, bark)	Large amounts can be converted into poisonous cyanide in the body
Pennyroyal	Can cause miscarriage
Peppermint	Can cause insomnia
Plum (leaves, pits, bark)	Large amounts can be converted into poisonous cyanide in the body
Poke (pokeweed, inkberry)	Can cause stomach and intestinal problems; large amounts can be fatal
Quack grass	Increases urine flow
St. John's wort	Can cause extreme sensitivity to sunlight and allergic reactions
Sassafras	Contains safrole (a carcinogen)
Senna (leaves, bark, flowers)	Can cause severe diarrhea, cramps, stomach pain
Shave grass (horsetail)	Greatly increases urine flow, toxic
Tonka beans	Can cause blood-clotting problems
Woodruff	Can cause blood-clotting problems
Wormwood	Can cause hallucinations, convulsions, brain deterioration

made about the healing powers of these substances have been proved false. Nonetheless, people are constantly looking for a panacea. They continually search for the magic key to a longer, happier, healthier life.

No evidence has been found linking health foods with extraordinary medicinal capabilities. Those cases in which people have used health foods and been "cured" of a disease usually can be attributed to the placebo effects of the treatment.

Health foods most often are used as dietary supplements. Some of the health foods are substances that also are part of sensible conventional diets, such as bran, sprouts, and wheat germ. These items generally are sold in grocery stores at lower prices than in health-food stores. Other health foods, however, are unusual and difficult to find except in specialty stores.

There are several major problems with health-food diets. The most serious is that some people put too much faith in the healing powers of health foods, and they may delay or forego conventional forms of medical attention. Simple health problems may become severe health risks. Sometimes serious diseases that could be alleviated with proper treatment result in death when people rely extensively on health-food cures.

Another problem with health foods is that some of them produce druglike effects, especially when large amounts of exotic ones are consumed. Some of these medicinal substances can be quite harmful when used incorrectly. Proper medical supervision for these various health-food diets is virtually nonexistent. People too often turn to clerks in health-food stores or door-to-door health-food salespeople for information on how to use various substances. These "experts" may have a strong belief in the powers of health foods, but usually they are not qualified to offer advice and have little knowledge about nutrition and health other than what they have read in brochures and pamphlets that come from their health-food suppliers.

Many people who use health foods also follow unconventional diets, and this combination often leads to dangerous deficiencies or excesses. For example, a person who adheres to an advanced, highly restrictive stage of a macrobiotic diet may supplement the diet with one or more health foods. This combination usually results in severe dietary imbalances.

FADDISH WEIGHT-LOSS PLANS

Thinness is an obsession for many people. To some, thin means beautiful, sexy, happy, and popular. Magazine articles, books, pamphlets, and over-the-counter pills claim to offer the foolproof way to a slim figure. And some people are willing to try just about anything to lose pounds and inches.

Fad weight-loss schemes, however, are neither balanced nor practical. Most of them are low-carbohydrate plans that claim to help dieters shed pounds quickly. The weight reduction that soon shows up on the bathroom scale usually can be attributed to water loss. These liquid pounds will be regained as soon as the dieter replaces the water. Dr. Jean Mayer, former chairman of the White House Conference on Food, Nutrition, and Health, calls this loss–gain pattern common among dieters "the rhythm method of girth control."

Despite warnings about the fad weight-loss diets, many people take their chances and try diets that prove dangerous. Children living in a family with dieting parents may find themselves following a similar eating pattern, usually by default. But fad weight-loss diets are not suitable for growing children, and following these diets can result in serious health problems. (See Chapter 8 for information on effective, sensible ways to feed an overweight child.)

Parents should never place their children on any weight-loss plan without consulting a physician or registered dietitian.

Below are brief descriptions of some of the most popular weight-loss diets and the health risks associated with them.

Atkins Diet

This low-carbohydrate diet permits unlimited quantities of fats and proteins (except cheese), and limits fruits, vegetables, breads, and milk. The diet lacks calcium, vitamins A, D, and C, thiamin, riboflavin, and niacin. It has high levels of saturated fats and cholesterol. It may present serious problems for people with gout, diabetes, kidney disease, or heart problems.

Stillman Diet

This diet, also called the water diet, is similar to the Atkins diet in that it is low in carbohydrates and high in protein and fat. It consists of lean meat, fish, poultry, eggs, low-fat cheeses, and eight glasses of water a day. No fruits, vegetables, breads, or milk are permitted. The diet lacks sufficient levels of vitamins A and C, thiamin, calcium, and iron.

Scarsdale Diet

This diet, while not as restrictive as most low-carbohydrate diets, places the dieter on a two-week eating plan that includes large quantities of protein, limited fat, and some fruits, vegetables, and breads. The diet contains too little vitamin A, calcium, and riboflavin.

Mayo Diet

This diet (which has no relationship to the reputable Mayo Clinic) promotes quick weight loss with high-protein meals consisting of meats and eggs. Grapefruit, and some vegetables, also are included. The diet is extremely high in cholesterol and could present severe problems for people with heart or kidney disease.

Grapefruit Diets

These diets usually call for eating a half of a grapefruit or drinking unsweetened grapefruit juice before every meal. The idea is that grapefruit burns up calories from other foods. There is no evidence to support this theory. Some of the grapefruit diets are low-carbohydrate, and the weight loss is just water. Other grapefruit diets have the dieter eating only low-calorie fruits and vegetables, and these plans lack protein, calcium, iron, and other essential vitamins and minerals.

Beverly Hills Diet

This expensive diet relies heavily on fruit as the way to shed unwanted pounds. Pineapple, in particular, is touted as having special enzymes that burn up fats. Dieters eat nothing but fruit for 10 days, and then breads, vegetables, and some meats are introduced sporadically into the diet. This unbalanced diet is low in protein, calcium, iron, and other vitamins and minerals.

And it may cause serious problems, especially for people with ulcers, diabetes, or gastrointestinal disorders.

Cambridge Diet

This is one of the many very low-calorie diets that came into vogue in the late 1970s and early 1980s (shortly after the once-popular liquid-protein diets were banned because they were linked to 60 deaths). The Cambridge plan consists of powdered formulas that are mixed with water to make a thick drink. Nothing but these drinks are consumed for several weeks. The mixes, while fortified with 100 percent of the RDA for vitamins and minerals, lack fat, are low in carbohydrates, and provide only 330 calories a day. Registered dietitians and physicians, however, say that fewer than 800 calories a day may be harmful.

Herbalife

Another fad weight-loss diet is Herbalife, an assortment of pills and powders that rely on herbs to cleanse and nourish the body to slimness and good health. Herbalife followers make shakes out of special powdered formulas. They take fistfuls of various herbs several times a day. Only one regular meal, usually dinner, is consumed each day. Herbalife products neither cleanse the body nor improve health. Some dieters have experienced diarrhea, nausea, vomiting, dizziness, and indigestion after using the products.

A fad diet is not a wise solution to the problem of being overweight. The only practical way to take off fat is for the body to use more calories than it takes in. The safest way to do this is to increase physical activity while maintaining a balanced, though limited, diet. Children, as mentioned before, should *never* be placed on a weight-loss diet without consulting a physician or registered dietitian.

Eating smaller portions, using less sugar and fat, increasing exercise, and relying on the Basic Four Food Groups are the keys to a slim figure and good health. Sensible eating habits should be followed for a lifetime, not just a few weeks or a few months. It takes time to shed unwanted pounds this way, but the result will be a leaner — and healthier — body.

8

FROM ALLERGIES TO OBESITY: SOME SPECIAL CHALLENGES OF FEEDING CHILDREN

'How long does
getting thin take?'
Pooh asked anxiously.

A. A. Milne
Winnie the Pooh

The "average" child in the "average" family does not exist. There are many kinds of children — some are fat, some are thin, some have allergies, some are athletic, some have colds, some are diabetic, some are active, some are quiet, some get cavities, some have acne. All of them need to eat, and all of them need to eat good food.

Social, medical, athletic, emotional, and economic factors, however, can, indeed, influence a child's appetite and need for certain kinds of food. Parents must be flexible enough to deviate from mealtime routines and plan a short- or long-term diet that will better suit a child's needs.

Should parents feed their children more when they have colds and less when they have fevers? Should the active Little Leaguer continue to eat the recommended 2,400 calories a day? Should teenagers with acne problems be allowed to eat candy bars and potato chips? How does the child who is allergic to milk get enough calcium?

These are only a few of the issues that parents may face. Some of the more common situations calling for changes in diet are outlined in this chapter, along with suggestions for how to handle them.

FOOD ALLERGIES

Food allergies are common disorders among children, especially those younger than 3 years of age. Symptoms are varied, can be mild or severe, and can occur in almost any part of the body, although they usually affect the gastrointestinal tract (vomiting, diarrhea, abdominal cramps), respiratory tract (swelling of the throat, nasal stuffiness, wheezing), and skin (hives, rash, swelling).

Sensitivity to cow's-milk protein is the most common food allergy among infants and young children. Other foods that cause allergic reactions for many children are eggs, wheat, chocolate, nuts, fish and shellfish, corn, soy, peas, tomatoes, citrus fruit, legumes, and strawberries. Almost any food substance can trigger a reaction in a sensitive individual.

Identifying food allergies is important. Delays in growth, resulting from poor absorption of vital nutrients and stress on the body, can be associated with allergies that go untreated. Therefore, children with food allergies should be evaluated and monitored by a physician. Also, early diagnosis of food sensitivities means that parents will not mistakenly withhold foods needed by the child.

Several methods are used to diagnose food allergies. The most common is the elimination diet, in which a suspicious food is omitted and any disappearance or reduction of symptoms is noted. The food being tested is reintroduced a few weeks later to see if symptoms recur. Another diagnostic tool for determining allergies is the scratch or prick test, where a small nick is made on the skin and a drop of the suspected substance, or antigen, is applied to see if a reaction occurs. A diary of all foods and medications taken up to 72 hours before the onset of reaction is another method sometimes used to identify food allergies. A family history of food allergies also may provide clues.

After food allergies are identified, treatment usually involves partially or totally eliminating the offending food, products containing it, and its derivatives. This may not be a problem when children have only one or two food sensitivities. Children who are allergic to many foods, however, require careful menu planning to make sure that they get enough of all the necessary nutrients.

Three common food allergies — milk, eggs, and wheat — are among the most challenging because these ingredients are contained in many processed and prepared foods. Parents of children with any of these sensitivities should take extra care to read labels and recognize ingredients that are byproducts of the offending food. For example, lactose, caseinate, casein, curds, and whey are all derived from milk byproducts. Egg byproducts may be listed as albumin, vitellin, livetin, or globulin. Gluten, bran, food starch, vegetable starch, and vegetable gum can indicate the presence of wheat.

Cow's-Milk-Protein Allergies

Allergy to cow's-milk protein is estimated to affect as many as 12 percent of infants and young children. Because cow's milk is one of the principal sources of calcium, protein, riboflavin, and vitamins A and D, parents of children who are allergic to cow's milk must be sure that adequate levels of these important nutrients are eaten in other foods.

Infants rarely have sensitivities to breast milk, so breast feeding is a good way to avoid the potential problem of milk allergies that may stem from cow's-milk-derived formula. Human milk is available from milk banks in some areas of the country for mothers who are unable or choose not to breast feed their infants.

Cow's-milk-sensitive infants normally grow and develop well when they are given soy-based formulas, which are available in pharmacies and many supermarkets. Some infants, however, also have allergies to soybean milk. These infants generally are fed an elemental diet, or partially digested formula, in which the protein is broken down into amino acids or small groups of amino acids.

Older children with allergies to cow's milk may be able to drink goat's milk without a reaction. Goat's milk, however, is deficient in folic acid, and children fed goat's milk must be given folic-acid supplements. Other milk-sensitive children can tolerate milk that has been heated, and this allows puddings, cakes, soups, and custards to be added to the diet.

Levels of sensitivity may vary from child to child. One child may be unable to tolerate cow's milk but may be able to eat other dairy products in small amounts with no reaction. Another child may be extremely sensitive to cow's milk and all food products derived from it. In this instance, cheeses, butter, cream, ice cream, milk sherbet, cakes, puddings, margarine made with milk solids, milk chocolate, hot breads made with milk (such as pancakes, waffles, biscuits, and muffins), and hot dogs containing milk solids should be avoided.

When cooking and baking for a child with milk allergies, parents can substitute soybean milk for cow's milk. Fruit juices also can replace cow's milk in some recipes. Pancakes, waffles, muffins, and French toast can be made without milk.

Although milk or milk byproducts often are present in breads, cakes, cookies, pastries, soups, and other processed foods, milk-free versions of some of these products are widely available. French and rye bread, for example, usually are made without milk. Graham crackers, saltines, soda crackers, pretzels, most cereals (served with fruit juice or milk substitutes), meats, vegetables (without cream sauces or butter), fruits, potatoes, and pasta also are suitable for children on milk-free diets.

Fortunately, the majority of children with milk-protein allergy outgrow it by the time they are 12 to 24 months of age and are able to drink milk and eat milk byproducts with no reaction.

Egg Allergies

Eggs are another common cause of food sensitivity among infants and young children. Frequently, reactions to eggs are severe, occurring within minutes of eating them. The albumin, or the white part of the egg, usually causes the reaction, but some children are sensitive to yolks as well.

Eggs are rich sources of high-quality protein, fats, and essential vitamins and minerals, but these can also be obtained from meats, fish, and poultry. Unfortunately, eggs are used in most cakes, pastries, and cookies, and some breads, sauces, and glazes. Eggs are used to thicken and bind together ingredients in cooking and baking, and as a result they may be hidden in foods.

Egg-free cooking at home has been simplified with the introduction of egg substitutes — both powder and liquid — which are available in most supermarkets. These egg-free replacements mimic the flavor and color of real eggs and can be used for many egg dishes. (Several of the egg substitutes, however, are designed for people who are trying to lower the cholesterol level in their diets. As a result, some do contain egg whites, and these are not appropriate for children with sensitivities to egg. Careful scrutiny of the label is extremely important.)

Most egg-free substitutes will not duplicate the thickening and binding properties of real eggs that are necessary when baking. To achieve the binding effect, mashed bananas can be substituted for eggs when blending together powdered ingredients of cakes, cookies, or breads, for example. In recipes where eggs are needed to thicken liquid ingredients, an alternative is to combine two tablespoons of whole wheat flour, one-half teaspoon oil, one-half teaspoon baking powder, and two tablespoons milk, water, or fruit juice to replace each egg.

When baking egg-free muffins or other pastries, an additional one-half teaspoon of baking powder may help compensate for the decrease in volume. When eggs are needed to add body to cream sauces and casseroles, extra amounts of flour or cornstarch may produce the right consistency.

Children who are allergic to eggs can eat most commercial and homemade breads (white, whole wheat, pumpernickel, rye, French), saltine and soda crackers, graham crackers, and cereals. Potatoes, rice, and pasta (except egg noodles or pasta made with egg) also are safe for egg-sensitive children. Meats, fish, and poultry are fine unless coated with egg batter before cooking. Cheese, fruit, sherbet, frozen yogurt, pies, and puddings made without eggs are all safe desserts. Better-quality ice cream often is made with egg yolks, so parents should check the labels.

Egg-sensitive children should avoid hot breads such as muffins, pancakes, French toast, and pastries unless they are made without eggs or with egg substitutes. Also, cakes, cookies, frostings, meringues, custards, and creams usually are made with eggs. Salad dressings made with eggs and soups containing egg noodles should be avoided. Hot dogs, sausage, and meat loaf may contain eggs. Again, reading labels is always very important.

Wheat Allergies

Wheat allergy is not as common as milk and egg allergies, but it presents more of a challenge to parents because most baked foods — commercial and homemade — use wheat flour as the primary ingredient. In addition, because most wheat flour is enriched and serves as a good source of iron, thiamin, niacin, and riboflavin, other sources of these vitamins and minerals must be found.

Fortunately, a number of wheat-flour substitutes are available. In most recipes, one cup of wheat flour can be replaced by three-fourths cup of rice flour, one cup of corn flour, three-fourths cup of coarse cornmeal, one cup of fine cornmeal, or five-eighths cup of potato flour. One cup of soy flour also may be a suitable substitute, but one-fourth of it should be replaced by another flour (usually potato flour) to help prevent an unmistakable soybean taste.

Longer, slower baking usually is necessary when flours other than wheat are used. Cornmeal and rice flour tend to have grainier textures, but when they are boiled in the liquid that is used in the recipe they achieve a smoother texture. When this method is used, the mixture should be cooled before the other ingredients are added. Nonwheat flours do not react well with yeast; therefore, other leavening methods must be used to achieve a lighter density, especially with the coarse flours such as cornmeal and rice flour. Adding 2½ teaspoons of baking powder for each cup of coarse flour, beating the egg whites before they are added to the dough, or using sour milk plus baking soda are some possibilities for creating a better texture.

Children with wheat allergy can eat breads made with 100 percent cornmeal, potato flour, and rice flour, and some can tolerate bread made with rye flour and oats. Parents must read labels of commercial breads, however, because most are made with flour mixtures that contain wheat. Corn, oat, or rice cereals usually cause no trouble for children who are allergic to wheat. Meats, fish, and poultry should be prepared without bread-crumbs and without flour-thickened gravy. Gravy and sauces can be thickened with cornstarch or tapioca starch.

Foods to avoid on a wheat-free diet obviously include cakes, pies, cookies, and doughnuts, but also canned soups, salad dressings, pasta, hot dogs, processed cheese, and malted drinks.

Allergy to a component of wheat — gluten (also found in rye, oats, and barley) — is called celiac disease, or gluten enteropa-thy. In this condition, gliadin, an extract of gluten, causes dam-age to the gastrointestinal tract when sensitive children eat it. The damage results in an inability to absorb needed nutrients. Diarrhea and growth failure often occur. Although age and symptoms may vary, most children with celiac disease develop diarrhea between 6 and 24 months of age. When gluten is re-moved from the diet, children with this allergy recover com-pletely and thrive. They must remain on a gluten-free diet for life.

Sensitivities to foods other than milk, eggs, and wheat tend to be easier to manage because most of the offending foods can be avoided with few problems. Fortunately, most food allergies subside as a child gets older; allergies to fish, shellfish, and nuts, however, often last through adulthood. A variety of cookbooks are available with suggestions for preparing foods for people with allergies. Some of these are listed in the Other Reading sec-tion at the end of this book.

As mentioned earlier, parents should work with a physician or a registered dietitian when their children have food allergies.

LACTOSE INTOLERANCE

Intolerance to lactose, the main carbohydrate in cow's milk and breast milk, is a condition that requires special care and planning, especially for infants. This condition is different from milk allergy.

Lactose is composed of two sugars, glucose and galactose. Normally, lactase, an enzyme located on the cells lining the digestive tract, breaks down lactose into its component sugars. Lactose cannot be absorbed unless it is broken down. If it is not digested, it stays in the intestine where bacteria turn it to hydrogen gas and acid. The gas causes bloating and sometimes cramps. The acid irritates the bowel and causes watery stools.

There are three forms of lactose intolerance: congenital (present at birth or hereditary), or primary; secondary (related to another underlying physical disorder); and physiologic, or age related. Congenital lactose intolerance is rare, but it is a permanent condition. Lactase deficiency causes the newborn to have profuse, watery diarrhea. Infants cannot survive on a formula containing lactose, but they do well when fed a lactose-free formula, such as a soybean derivative.

Secondary lactose intolerance can happen after an episode of infectious diarrhea or other gastrointestinal disease. The lactose intolerance develops because most of the enzyme that breaks lactose into its component sugars is located in the mature cells of the gastrointestinal tract. Any process that disrupts normal maturing of cells lining the bowel or injures the gastrointestinal tract can lower levels of lactase and make it hard to digest lactose. This lactose intolerance is not permanent, but the time it takes for lactase to regain normal function varies, depending on what caused the problem and the recuperative powers of the individual.

Finally, a large proportion of the world's population — especially blacks and Orientals — loses the ability to digest lactose with age. The age when this occurs and the degree of lactose intolerance varies. Most people naturally change their eating habits to avoid the uncomfortable symptoms of lactose intolerance. Age-related lactose intolerance does not develop before 3 years of age in black children or 5 years of age in white children.

People with lactase deficiencies are placed on lactose-free or lactose-reduced diets. These diets limit all types of untreated milk (whole, low fat, skim, buttermilk, powdered, evaporated, and condensed). Lactose-free milk, which has been pretreated with lactase, is widely available in supermarkets. Several lactase enzyme preparations, which are added to milk to break down most of the lactose, can be used by people with limited tolerance to lactose. In addition, enzyme capsules, which are taken with meals to process lactose in the body, are available.

Lactose-free diets also avoid milk byproducts such as yogurt, cheese, ice cream, and some kinds of sherbet. Foods containing milk or milk solids — prepared mixes such as muffins, waffles, pancakes, biscuits; some dried cereals and most instant hot cereals; commercial cakes, cookies, and pie crusts; margarine and salad dressings made with milk or milk solids; creamed vegetables; hot dogs made with milk solids; and creamed soups and chowders — also are eliminated. (See also the discussion of milk allergies, earlier in this chapter.) Other lactose-containing foods that may be excluded from the diet are chewing gum, chocolate, peppermint, butterscotch, and many artificial sweeteners. Labels, once again, should be read carefully.

When all products containing milk are eliminated, calcium supplements are necessary. However, parents should consult a physician before giving any supplements to a child. The child's pediatrician, who is most likely familiar with the condition, will be able to recommend the proper supplement.

PREMATURE INFANTS

Premature infants — babies born before 38 weeks of pregnancy — generally weigh less than full-term babies. Their immature digestive systems, poorly coordinated sucking and swallowing motions (especially among infants born before the 34th week), and increased need for many nutrients make overseeing the premature infant's diet a particularly challenging job. This task is best guided by registered dietitians, doctors, and nurses in a hospital setting, where the infant's progress can be monitored, and deficiencies and imbalances can be corrected immediately.

Premature babies have extraordinarily high needs for water, calcium and other minerals, vitamins, protein, and energy (calories) immediately after birth. These needs must be carefully assessed because they will vary according to the developmental stage of the infant, the extent of the infant's medical problems, and the level of adaptation to a new environment.

The main sources of nutrition for premature infants are breast milk and special premature formulas. Both breast milk and formulas, however, usually must be supplemented with some nutrients to more closely meet the preterm infant's additional needs.

Human breast milk, which satisfies the needs of the full-term infant, may not be enough for premature infants. Breast milk provides less than half of the protein needed for maximum growth of premature babies, three-fourths of the sodium, and one-fourth of the calcium and phosphorus requirements. Premature babies on breast milk alone grow more slowly than the rate at which development occurs in the uterus, but studies have shown that these infants tend to catch up over several months. Special supplements, which are added to expressed breast milk, are available to enrich human milk intended for premature infants.

The advantages of feeding breast milk to premature infants appear to outweigh the disadvantages. The fats and proteins in breast milk are more easily digested than the fats and proteins in premature formula. Breast milk also is more appropriate for the infant's immature gastrointestinal tract. The carbohydrate content of breast milk is acceptable for premature infants, and natural immunities against infection and disease are passed from the mother to the infant through breast milk. Although human breast milk does not satisfy the calcium and phosphorus needs of the premature infant, these minerals can be supplemented.

There also are psychological advantages for mothers who provide breast milk for their premature infants. Offering breast milk helps the mother feel involved. Even if the premature infant is too weak to suck from the breast or a bottle, the mother can participate in her baby's care by providing expressed breast milk, which often is fed to the baby through a tube that leads directly into the stomach.

Babies who are born less than 34 weeks into a pregnancy most likely will be fed through a feeding tube and/or intravenously for the first few days or weeks of life. At 34 weeks, sucking and swallowing motions become coordinated enough to attempt nipple feeding.

If a mother cannot or chooses not to provide breast milk, premature infant formulas, which are available only to hospitals and medical professionals, may be used to feed the preterm baby. These formulas are designed to encourage the rate of growth that would occur in the uterus.

Protein levels in premature formulas are greater than in standard infant formulas because protein is essential for the body to build muscles, lay down tissues, and promote growth of red blood cells. Fat is necessary for energy and helps growth and the absorption of vitamins and minerals. The fat content of premature formulas is similar to that of regular infant formulas; however, the type of fat used in most premature formulas is medium-chain-triglyceride (MCT) oil, which is composed of small molecules that are more easily digested. Carbohydrates also are important energy sources for the preterm infant. Premature formulas contain slightly higher carbohydrate levels but less lactose than standard formulas.

Premature formulas have high levels of calcium, phosphorus, and vitamin D for bone development. Premature infants have high needs for vitamin E, iron, folic acid, and sodium. Premature formulas contain sufficient levels of vitamin E; however, supplements of iron, folic acid, and sodium may be necessary.

Premature infants generally are cared for in a hospital — usually in an incubator — until they reach term or weigh more than 5½ pounds. Most hospitals recognize the importance of parental involvement in the care and feeding of premature infants, and more parents are becoming actively involved.

DIABETES

Parents of diabetic children have an unusual and important challenge when it comes to planning meals and snacks. Because diet is such an important part of the care of diabetes, a specific food plan and schedule, prescribed by a physician and planned by a registered dietitian, always is tailored to each diabetic child's needs.

Diabetes is a disorder of the pancreas, the organ responsible for producing insulin. Insulin, a hormone, is needed to regulate blood sugar. When insufficient insulin is produced, blood sugar (glucose) cannot be delivered properly to the tissues of the body. When this occurs, the blood glucose level rises.

Some cases of adult-onset diabetes can be controlled with careful dietary planning. But in children, diabetes must be controlled using insulin injections and diet. Food plans for diabetic children are designed to control both the long- and short-term effects and complications of the disease, while filling needs for normal growth and development. The big hurdle confronted by parents of diabetic children is limiting refined sugar (concentrated sweets). (See Table 2.12.)

Menus for diabetic children generally provide 50 to 60 percent of the calories from carbohydrates (mostly from starches, but also from lactose in milk and fructose in fruits), 25 to 35 percent from fat (mostly polyunsaturated vegetable fats), and 15 to 20 percent from protein. The appropriate number of calories allowed each day varies according to the child's age, weight, height, sex, and level of activity.

Diabetic diets also should contain a high level of fiber — as much as 65 grams a day. Experiments have shown that some adult diabetics on high-fiber, high-carbohydrate diets can substantially reduce the amount of insulin they inject daily because of fiber's ability to make body tissues more sensitive to insulin. The benefits of high-fiber, high-carbohydrate diets for diabetic children, however, have not yet been established. Low-cholesterol and low-saturated-fat diets may also be prescribed.

Although special foods made without refined sugar are available in pharmacies, catalogs, and some supermarkets, these tend to be expensive and offer few advantages other than convenience. The needs of diabetic children can be met with common foods available in supermarkets.

Most food plans for children with diabetes call for three meals and two or three snacks a day. Five or six small meals help prevent the occurrence of wide swings between high and low sugar concentrations in the body. Insulin injections are given at the same times each day, and the child with diabetes should eat regular meals and snacks during the time when the insulin is most active.

Young children and their parents usually can get into a routine that matches eating with insulin injections. Teenagers, however, who experience social pressure to eat foods that are high in sugar, may find the limitations of the diabetic diet too restrictive. Parents should show patience and understanding toward the hardships faced by the adolescent with diabetes; however, the importance of maintaining a sensible diet should be emphasized.

It is a good idea for parents to allow their diabetic children to help plan their diets. This will make them more aware of the types of foods they should eat and the acceptable quantities. Diabetic children who understand their restrictions and the consequences of eating inappropriate foods will be better able to deal with the disease when they are away from home.

WEIGHT PROBLEMS

Children and adolescents with weight problems need a great deal of help and support from their parents. The most common weight problem is obesity. Overeating or improper eating habits and insufficient exercise are two causes of obesity. At the other extreme, undernutrition, which often results because of eating disorders (anorexia nervosa or bulimia), also can be a problem, especially among adolescent girls.

Obesity

The most commonly used criteria to gauge fatness are weight-for-age and weight-for-height standards. Most physicians use growth charts for plotting these figures. If weight is greater than the 90th percentile (i.e., less than 10 percent of the population is heavier), individuals are generally classified as obese. Obesity also often is defined as 10 to 20 percent above the ideal weight for height.

A small percentage of obese children and adolescents carry too much weight because of a physical disorder. Research indicates that heredity may play a role in a child's tendency toward obesity. Most obese children, however, put on excess weight through a combination of overeating and underexercising.

Obesity in childhood is a serious problem. In fact, obesity has been called the major nutritional problem among children in many developed countries. It is not unusual for obese children to become obese adolescents, nor for obese adolescents to become obese adults, although obese infants and children are not automatically destined to obesity in later life. If parents give obese

---

Table 8.1
WHY DO PEOPLE GAIN WEIGHT?

It takes 3,500 calories *above* the number of calories required for basic activity to form one pound of fat. For example:

If a person consumed: 2,000 calories
    and expended: − 1,500 calories in a day;

  he or she consumed: 500 extra calories that day

If 500 extra calories are eaten every day for a week, then:

$$500 \text{ extra calories a day}$$
$$\underline{\times \ 7 \text{ days}}$$
$$3,500 \text{ extra calories for the week}$$

3,500 extra calories = 1 pound fat

The result would be a one pound weight gain for the week.

---

children a good start toward sensible eating and living patterns, they have a good chance to overcome obesity.

Prevention of obesity is much easier than treatment. The best preventive measures are obvious: a balanced, moderate, and nourishing diet and sufficient exercise. During childhood, the body lays down the majority of fat cells that will remain in the body throughout life. Overfeeding and/or underexercising, therefore, could result in the formation of too many fat cells.

After the creation of fat cells stops, continued overconsumption and insufficient activity cause more fat to accumulate inside cells, increasing their size. Too many fat cells, or cells that are too large, can both cause obesity. Together, the combination of too many fat cells that are too large leads to extreme obesity — and health risks.

When people eat more calories than their bodies can use, the extra calories are stored as fat. If extra energy is needed, the body can draw it from these fat cells. As mentioned earlier, each gram of fat supplies nine calories (see Chapter 2). Each pound of body fat can supply 3,500 calories. Table 8.1 shows what happens as the body stores more and more calories.

Poor attitudes toward food during childhood may lead to unhealthful eating habits and obesity. Too often, foods take on an emotional meaning. Some foods — especially sweets — are associated with pleasure, love, and rewards, while lack of food ("Go to bed without your supper") is associated with punishment. Parents should avoid charging food with powerful emotions, as this may set up bad eating habits.

Breast-fed babies may tend to be leaner than formula-fed babies because breast feeding allows babies to adjust the amount of milk they drink to match their hunger. With formulas, parents sometimes encourage an infant to finish the entire bottle, even if the baby does not want it. This can be the first step toward a pattern of eating because food is offered or available rather than eating because of hunger.

Keeping the amount of sugar-laden treats and desserts offered to babies and children to a minimum also may help keep weight problems from developing. Infants need not be exposed to the temptations of sweets, such as cookies, ice cream, cake, candy, and brownies. The longer a child's desire for snacks of low nutritional value can be delayed, the better.

Cutting back on the level of fats in foods also is a way to maintain a child's desirable weight. Adding butter or margarine to potatoes and vegetables during cooking and then putting a pat or two on them before serving is unnecessary. Instead, parents can try to reduce or eliminate the butter or margarine. *Some fat, however, is necessary in the diet.*

Children older than about 2 years of age do not need as much fat as infants. Switching from whole milk to low-fat or skim milk after the second year can be a good way to cut back on fats and calories.

With toddlers and young children, parents may be able to substitute some lower calorie, nutritious foods for high-calorie, low-nutrient snacks. Unsweetened applesauce, yogurt, raisins, or fresh fruit, for example, can be offered instead of ice cream, cakes, or pies. Also, unsweetened fruit juice or skim milk may be just as appealing to the child as soft drinks or sugary fruit drinks.

Children should be served reasonable portions of food, and if they ask for seconds, parents should give them small helpings. For children who have weight problems, parents can eliminate second helpings.

Preventing weight problems, as mentioned, is the best course of action; however, many children are already overweight, and treatment is the immediate concern of their parents. Treatment is essential because the psychological and social impact of childhood obesity can be enormous. Obese children often are rejected and teased by their peers. This may lead to isolation and depression in the short term as well as lifelong problems with self-confidence and self-image.

When dealing with childhood obesity, the parents' first step should be to consult the child's pediatrician. Parents should *never* attempt to put an obese child on a weight-reducing diet without the advice of a physician or registered dietitian because this may lead to a dangerous reduction in some nutrients needed for proper growth and development.

Most often, the goal for young children is not to lose weight, but rather to maintain the current weight while height increases. This can be done gradually — so gradually, in fact, that changes in food selection, preparation, and eating patterns may go unnoticed by the child. Substituting lower-calorie foods for high-calorie foods and preparing meals with less sugar and fat, while maintaining a well-balanced, nourishing diet, are usually the best ways to keep down weight gain.

Meals and snacks for the dieting child should be the same as those served to other members of the family. Serving the child a small piece of broiled fish with some cottage cheese while others at the table eat lasagna and garlic bread could call unnecessary attention to the child's weight problem. For children, dieting alone often results in resentment rather than loss of excess fat. It is important, therefore, for family members to be supportive. Some behavior modification program may be necessary, possibly for the whole family, to redirect the focus from food and eating to other subjects and activities.

Many children put on excess weight because of underactivity. Exercise is essential to help children burn excess energy (calories) and for proper growth and development of the body. Parents should encourage their children to become involved in activities — walking, jogging, bicycling, swimming, and team sports. Many overweight children shun sports, especially team sports, because they are embarrassed about their abilities. Parents may be able to suggest individual sports such as running, swimming, bicycling, skiing, or hiking. If the whole family participates, the child may enjoy these sports more.

Infants and toddlers also need to exercise to expend energy and develop muscles and coordination. Young children, especially overweight children, should not spend the entire day in a crib or a playpen. They should move and crawl. Parents should encourage their toddlers to play actively — pulling toy trains, throwing or rolling balls, riding a tricycle, walking, and running.

Dealing with an obese teenager presents a much more difficult challenge. Issues of control are complex. Adolescence is a time in life when young people struggle to find their own identities, and they may rebel against parents who are overly insistent about eating habits. This is also a period when fat cells are forming quickly, preparing the body for maturation and adulthood, so weight gain at this time of life often is substantial.

"Social snacking" is common among adolescents, and it often goes on in fast-food restaurants, in friends' homes, and at school. Many of the snacks that are offered are laden with calories from sugar and fat. The best way parents can deal with snacking among overweight adolescents is to suggest lower calorie snacks and to set an example. Drinking water, fruit juice, unsweetened iced tea, or diet soft drinks instead of milk shakes saves calories. Eating a few pretzels rather than handfuls of potato chips also is a way to cut back on calories. At parties, eating a few crackers with cheese or raw vegetables and fruits rather than cookies and cakes allows for social snacking without excess calories. If parents can keep high-calorie snacks out of the house, and provide plenty of low calorie ones as well as activities such as games, sports, and music, which do not involve eating, their overweight adolescent may not equate socializing with heavy eating.

Some overweight adolescents, especially girls, try to lose weight during their teen years because they feel social pressure to be thinner. If their weight-reduction plan involves careful food selection and increased exercise, they usually can do well on it. Some teenagers, however, try to lose weight quickly through fad diets, skipped meals, or fasting. Fad diets generally do not work because people tend to regain any lost weight as soon as the diet is stopped (see Chapter 7). Skipping meals and fasting usually result in excessive hunger, often causing the ravenous teenager to snack on large quantities of foods that are high in calories.

Some adolescents who begin to put on weight believe they are socially unacceptable to their peers, and they may console themselves with even more food. Obese adolescents need a great deal of support and help from families and friends. The reasons for the obesity should be identified, and the whole family may need to change its attitudes toward food to promote healthful patterns of eating. Role models of slim, athletic adults — professional sports stars, family members, athletic peers, school coaches, or camp counselors — also can help.

Adolescents who are obese need professional help. A physician should be consulted to prescribe an appropriate eating plan and to monitor the results. Because adolescence is a time of change and self-consciousness, counseling may be useful to help teenagers modify feelings and adopt eating styles that promote health, weight loss, and self-esteem.

Anorexia Nervosa

While obesity is, by far, the greatest weight problem associated with childhood and adolescence, a growing number of teenagers (usually girls) suffer from disorders that involve undereating — specifically, anorexia nervosa and bulimia.

Anorexia nervosa, which affects approximately one in 150 to 200 teenage girls and a very small number of boys, is a condition in which people have a distorted body image, seeing themselves as overweight although they are not. As a result, they restrict their food intake, plan menus meticulously, cut foods into small pieces, and take hours to eat each small meal. In addition, a daily routine of rigorous exercise may be followed.

Although the cause of anorexia nervosa is unknown, it is thought to be a result of the intense society and peer pressure to be as thin as a fashion model. A teenager, equating a slim figure with attractiveness, acceptance, and popularity, decides to lose a few pounds. Dieting, however, becomes an obsession, and the teenager begins to develop strange eating habits such as making odd food choices, insisting on eating alone, or refusing to eat when others are watching.

At first, a person with anorexia nervosa will use enormous willpower to keep from eating, even when extremely hungry. Parents may notice the rapid weight loss and express concern, encouraging — even begging — the teenager to eat. The teenager may comply to please parents, but often will induce vomiting soon after the meal. As more and more pounds come off, the teenager may try to hide this loss from worried parents and friends by wearing baggy clothes, hiding weights under clothes, or dressing and undressing alone.

Most adolescents with anorexia nervosa are from middle- or upper-class, white, close families. Their parents, while usually loving, are often overprotective and controlling. As a result, the teenager may be submissive, dependent, indecisive, and afraid to grow up. Teenagers with anorexia usually are obedient, kind, eager to please others, and appreciative of favors. Many, however, are immature, lack self-confidence, and often criticize themselves for being unattractive, unintelligent, and unpopular.

The physical tolls of anorexia include extreme weight loss, malnutrition, curtailment of growth, and delay of maturation or suspension of menstruation. If uninterrupted, anorexia can lead to death.

Teenagers with anorexia nervosa need medical help. Parents who suspect that their teenager has anorexia nervosa should seek the help of a physician, psychologist, or psychiatrist. Each anorexic person is slightly different, and the course of treatment varies significantly. Physical as well as psychological treatment is necessary because all underlying causes must be identified in order to keep the disorder from recurring. The earlier the treatment can begin, the better the chance for a complete recovery.

Bulimia

Bulimia, which also is a problem among adolescent girls, is an uncontrollable craving for large amounts of food coupled with self-induced vomiting. People with bulimia have frequent secret binges in which they gorge themselves with massive quantities of foods — usually high-calorie foods that are easily swallowed, such as ice cream, cookies, and cakes. Soon after these binges, guilt and shame overwhelm the adolescents, and they force themselves to vomit.

Many cases of bulimia go unsuspected by parents because weight loss with bulimia may not be as severe as with anorexia nervosa. In fact, bulimics may even be slightly overweight. Bulimics usually are discreet about their binges, often taking great pains to avoid being caught while eating. Behavioral changes and refusals of food at family mealtimes may be clues of bulimia. Parents may notice that their adolescent's cheeks appear puffy because of swollen salivary glands. Another sign of bulimia is scratches or abrasions on the back of the hand caused by teeth scraping the skin when fingers are placed far back into the mouth to induce vomiting.

Most teenagers with bulimia recognize that their binging-vomiting episodes are abnormal. Many, however, because of shame and guilt, avoid admitting their problems to anyone. Parents who suspect that their teenager is bulimic should be as supportive and understanding as possible. They should encourage the child to seek professional help, although this suggestion may be rejected at first because of an unwillingness to admit there is a problem. In this case, parents themselves should discuss the problem with a physician.

WHEN CHILDREN ARE SICK

Colds

The most prevalent childhood illness is the common cold, which usually is not very serious and runs its course in one or two weeks. During this time, however, children's appetites may decrease. At the same time they need adequate nourishment to help them fight infection and maintain their strength. Getting the child to eat full meals during a bout with a cold may be unnecessary and impossible. In these cases, parents should take a temporary break from the child's regular eating patterns and work with requests and desires for food and drinks.

Children with colds often want to eat only light soothing foods, such as ice cream, sherbet, puddings, soft drinks, and fruit juices. Parents may want to encourage soothing but wholesome foods such as frozen yogurt, applesauce, soup, or fruit juice. Mixing nutritious ingredients, such as dried non-fat milk or wheat germ, into foods that the child will accept (possibly hot or cold cereals, cookies, milk shakes, soup, or pudding) is another way to give a child some extra nourishment during a bout with the common cold.

Cutting foods into interesting shapes and sizes may entice a sick child. Using different plates, cups, or utensils also may make foods more tempting. Variations on the old favorites (such as chicken alphabet soup rather than chicken noodle soup) may be more readily accepted by children with colds.

Children with colds should be encouraged to drink as much fluid as they want. Water usually is the best choice, closely followed by fruit juice. Milk is acceptable if the child prefers it, and soft drinks also can be offered, but parents should try to limit the amount of these. Fluids are especially important if the child refuses food. Parents should make sure fluids are available; they should not, however, force their child to drink.

It is never a good idea for parents to urge, coax, or force a child to eat a lot during a cold because the child usually is in bed or on a sofa, and activity level is low. Few calories are being used (unless fever is present), so fewer calories are needed. Also, if parents are overly demanding about what is eaten during an illness, the child may develop negative attitudes about a particular food or foods.

Fever

When fever is present, the metabolic rate increases and the body needs extra calories to fight the illness. It may be difficult to encourage children to eat because with a high fever (above 102 degrees Fahrenheit) children generally will lose their appetites. Most feverish children, however, will want to drink liquids. Liquids, especially water, sugar water, or fruit juices are the best choices. These fluids should be offered at least every half hour. Infants are likely to want milk.

Parents should not force the feverish child to eat solid foods for the first day or two. It is, however, necessary to encourage the child to eat or drink more than the recommended number of calories for age (see the chart in Chapter 2, Table 2.19) because breathing rate, heartbeat, and the body's conversion of food to sugars and fats speeds up. The general rule for fevers is that there is a 7 percent increase in the number of calories needed for each degree above normal (usually 98.6 degrees F). In other words, if an average 6-year-old child, who usually needs 1,700 calories a day, has a fever three degrees above normal, he or she would need approximately 360 additional calories, or a total of 2,060 calories.

It may be difficult for parents to encourage the sick child to drink or eat these extra calories. It is important, therefore, to make foods and drinks appealing by arranging them in an interesting, colorful way or serving them in a new cup or with a straw. Ice cream, custards, puddings, milkshakes, and fruit slushes (made in a blender with fruit, fruit juice, an egg, ice, and water or milk) are good choices because these foods are rich in calories and are made with nourishing ingredients. When the child becomes hungry, bland foods such as toast, crackers, cereal, soups and broths, gelatin, and applesauce can be offered. Children with high fevers probably will not be able to digest or keep down vegetables or meats until they feel better.

Parents should call the pediatrician for a fever higher than 100 degrees F in an infant younger than 6 months; higher than 102 degrees F in children between 6 months and 3 years of age; and higher than 103 degrees for all children. A pediatrician also should be notified if the fever persists for more than three days or if the child is unusually drowsy or behaves strangely.

Sore Throats and Coughs

Sore throats and coughs may increase the child's desire for drinks or foods that are hot or very cold. Soups and broths may be soothing to a child's raw throat. If mucus is not present, creamed soups or hot cocoa may appeal to the child. Hot apple juice with cinnamon also may taste and feel good to a child with an irritated throat.

If the child would rather soothe a sore throat with cold foods, fruit slushes (fruit juice, fresh fruit, with crushed ice) and milk shakes can be made in the blender. Frozen yogurt, ice pops, ice cream, sherbet, and ice chips also help alleviate some of the soreness.

A physician should be consulted for sore throats lasting more than 24 to 48 hours, especially if fever also is present.

For coughs, two parts honey mixed with one part lemon juice may provide temporary relief. Parents, however, should not give this homemade cough formula to children younger than 1 year of age because of the link between infant botulism and honey (see Chapter 10).

Vomiting

Vomiting is a common symptom of many childhood illnesses. After vomiting, a child should not eat or drink anything for an hour or two. After this time the child should be given a few sips of clear (transparent) liquids. Simple, clear fluids, such as water, plain fruit-flavored gelatin, diluted broth, and flat soda (preferably caffeine-free varieties) usually are the best choices because they replace the water, salts, and some calories lost. When small amounts of liquid do not upset the stomach, more fluid can be offered gradually during the next few hours.

Dehydration is one of the most serious complications associated with severe vomiting, especially among infants and young children. Forcing fluids, however, is not advised because this may produce more vomiting, which will lead to a greater loss of fluid. If the child refuses liquids repeatedly, parents should consult a physician.

If the child keeps fluids down for several hours, parents should offer dry, bland foods such as dry toast, crackers, or arrowroot cookies. As appetite increases, easily digested foods such as soup may be added. If the child vomits again, however, all foods and drinks should be stopped for several hours, and the same procedure of gradually introducing fluids should be repeated. If vomiting persists, the child's pediatrician should be notified.

Diarrhea

Careful control of food and liquid is the key to effective treatment of diarrhea, with prevention of dehydration as the goal.

Dehydration is the most serious complication associated with diarrhea. Younger children are at greater risk of dehydration because their bodies require more fluid per pound of body weight than older children or adults.

Most cases of diarrhea are mild and can be treated at home. A physician should be consulted, however, if diarrhea persists, especially if stools become excessively watery and large in quantity. Parents should also notify a physician if the stool is red, rust-colored, black, or contains blood.

When a child has frequent loose bowel movements, clear liquids are usually recommended to replace water and electrolytes. Fluids containing fats, such as soups and whole milk, should be avoided. For infants with diarrhea, small amounts of diluted formula or breast milk may be given.

It is better to give small amounts of liquids frequently than large amounts of liquids occasionally. The ill child may not be able to tolerate large quantities at once, and vomiting is likely. Vomiting with diarrhea raises the risk of dehydration.

The severity and frequency of the diarrhea and the age of the child should dictate the diet. The child who has episodes of diarrhea more often than once every three hours should remain on a clear-liquids-only diet. No milk should be offered. Infants should be given an average of two ounces of fluid every hour, or about a cup and a half over the span of six hours. Preschool children need approximately four ounces of fluid every hour, or three cups over the span of six hours. Children who are school aged should be given approximately five ounces of fluid every hour, or four cups during a six-hour period. *Parents should not keep their children on a clear-liquid diet for more than 24 to 48 hours without consulting a physician.*

The diet for children who have diarrheal stools every four to six hours should include plenty of clear liquids. Parents can add soft, bland foods such as mashed bananas, rice cereal, applesauce, dry toast, crackers, and sherbet. Children who have no more than two diarrheal bowel movements within 24 hours usually do well on a simple balanced diet, which can include milk if requested. Parents, however, should limit the amount of fruit and fruit juice, and fatty, rich, and spicy foods until the child's stools are back to normal.

Constipation

Constipation is a condition that is not easily defined because bowel habits vary greatly from individual to individual. The term, however, is used most commonly to describe a change in *normal* bowel habits: a decrease in frequency of bowel movements, the passage of small hard stools, or pain during defecation occurring after the newborn period. Most cases of constipation can be related directly to diet; however, other causes include lack of exercise, medications, and physiologic and psychosocial factors.

For infants who are constipated, increasing the amount of water they drink may help. The addition of corn syrup or prune juice to formula also may alleviate constipation. Older infants should be encouraged to eat cereal, fruits, vegetables, and to drink plenty of water and fruit juice (especially prune juice).

An increase in fluids and dietary fiber (good sources include whole-grain breads and cereals, fruits, and leafy vegetables) will alleviate the symptoms of constipation for most children. Enemas and laxatives should *never* be used unless advised by a physician. If constipation persists, parents should contact their child's pediatrician.

ATHLETIC CHILDREN

Exercise is important for all children. Exercise builds muscle, regulates metabolism, strengthens the body's systems (especially respiratory and circulatory), and helps control appetite. Strenuous or competitive exercise may call for certain changes in diet.

The most important consideration when feeding athletic children is to make sure they get enough calories. The number of additional calories hinges upon age, growth status, and the type of exercise and its duration and intensity. Extremely athletic children who are 7 to 10 years old may need 3,000 to 4,000 calories a day when the energy needed for activity is added to that needed for normal growth. Adolescent athletes who undertake rigorous workout schedules may need as many as 5,000 calories

Table 8.2
FEEDING THE ATHLETIC CHILD

If an athletic child needs 3,000 calories to maintain weight, the distribution of these calories can be found by multiplying calories needed by the recommended percentages and then dividing by calories per gram. For example:

55 percent (.55) carbohydrates
3,000 calories × .55 = 1,650 calories from carbohydrates
1,650 carbohydrate calories ÷ 4 calories per gram
    = 413 grams of carbohydrates a day*

30 percent (.30) fat
3,000 calories × .30 = 900 calories from fat
900 fat calories ÷ 9 calories per gram
    = 100 grams of fat a day*

15 percent (.15) protein
3,000 calories × .15 = 450 calories from protein
450 protein calories ÷ 4 calories per gram
    = 113 grams of protein a day*

*Labels usually provide the number of grams of carbohydrate, fat, and protein in a product.

a day. Obtaining enough calories usually is not a problem because activity makes appetite and calorie consumption increase.

The recommended distribution of calories is 55 percent from carbohydrates, 30 percent from fat, and 15 percent from protein. Table 8.2 may provide parents some help to determine how much carbohydrate, fat, and protein their athletic child needs.

The best way to increase the number of calories is to add more carbohydrates, especially starches, and fat to the diet. Carbohydrates are stored in the liver and in muscle tissues in molecules called glycogen, and can be a source of energy. Excess carbohydrate, however, is also deposited as fat. Both carbohydrate and fat are used during exercise, and the proportions vary with intensity, duration, and availability of stored fuel. For example, at low rates of activity, fat supplies a larger proportion of necessary energy. During heavy exercise, the main fuel is glycogen.

Contrary to popular belief, adding extra protein to the diet is not necessary because protein is not a primary source of energy during exercise. While protein, in conjunction with exercise, is important when the goal is to increase muscle mass, the key to muscle development is repeated exercise. Adolescents who are trying to increase muscle mass for sports such as weightlifting, wrestling, or football may want to increase the amount of protein by 20 to 45 grams or more a day above the RDA. Excessive quantities of protein, however, are not needed. Adding more protein to the diet without increasing exercise will *not* increase muscle mass.

Athletes also need more water, enough to replace fluids lost through perspiration and to prevent dehydration. This applies to all athletes: little girls who are dancing or performing gymnastics as well as to adolescent boys who are playing varsity football or basketball. Children should be reminded to drink because a loss of as little as 3 percent of body water could result in exhaustion and dehydration or, less dramatically, cause a child to become tired and less effective during activity.

The American College of Sports Medicine recommends that children and adults drink 13 to 17 ounces of fluids 15 minutes before exercising to reduce the risk of dehydration. In addition, exercise should be interrupted every 20 minutes to drink 6 ounces of fluids, especially if the climate is hot or dry and windy. People should not wait until they are thirsty to get a drink because during exercise, thirst is not a reliable monitor of the body's need for water.

Several types of sports drinks are advertised as the perfect way to replace water and electrolytes (sodium, potassium, and chloride) lost during exercise. Most of these drinks, however, are high in sugar, usually about 5 percent. Sugar increases the amount of time that fluids remain in the stomach, and this can cause cramps, stomachaches, nausea, and diarrhea. In addition, when fluids are in the stomach they cannot get into the muscles and other body systems, where they are greatly needed during exercise. If sports drinks are used they should be diluted with equal amounts of water. *Again, water is the best way to replace fluids lost during exercise.*

Some sports drinks manufacturers claim that the electrolytes in their products can increase muscle performance and decrease the incidence of muscle cramps; however, there is no evidence to support these claims. In addition, they claim that these drinks will replace sodium that is lost in perspiration. Sodium loss, however, usually is small (one gram of sodium for every quart of sweat). The average diet contains too much salt; therefore, most people have more than enough sodium in their bodies to spare a little bit for perspiration. Replacing salt usually is not necessary unless the exercise was so long or so vigorous that 5 or more pounds were lost. Adding a little extra salt to food immediately after exercise is usually the best way to replenish the body's reserves, if needed.

Taking salt tablets also is not advised because they put too much salt in the body too fast. High concentrations of salt can draw water out of muscles. Taken frequently, salt tablets increase the risk of heatstroke and heart and kidney problems.

When children and adolescents compete in sports in which they must qualify for a specific weight class, such as wrestling, horseracing, or rowing, they often go on crash diets that severely restrict calories. Insufficient calorie intake, however, weakens the body and leads to decreased performance during competition.

In rowing competition in the United States, for example, lightweight crews weigh in the night before the event. In order to meet weight requirements it is not unusual for team members to crash diet and intentionally let themselves become dehydrated by running in the heat wearing heavy clothes. After weighing in they have that evening and a few hours the next day to replenish themselves.

The weigh-in procedure for rowing competition in the Soviet Union, however, is a little different. The first USA lightweight crew to compete there learned they had to weigh in at race time. The rowers, therefore, were dehydrated just before they competed, and they attempted to race while in this condition. As a result, many of them ended up in a Moscow hospital receiving intravenous fluid replacements. As this example shows, crash dieting, taken to such extremes, can be dangerous. In fact, it can be fatal.

Another problem with crash dieting before an athletic event is that many adolescents go on eating binges immediately after competing. If this starving-binging pattern is repeated, it could lead to problems with growth and development and poor eating habits. The best way for athletic children to lose weight is to increase exercise while maintaining a lower-calorie diet, although it never should include fewer than 2,000 calories a day.

HYPERACTIVE CHILDREN

Much controversy exists regarding a link between diet and hyperactivity — a behavioral problem that involves increased, and often inappropriate, activity. Hyperactivity is a medical diagnosis and should be made *only* by a physician. Just because a child seems overly active to a family member does not mean that he or she is hyperactive. Hyperactivity is a serious and pervasive problem that can interfere greatly with home, school, and social life of children. Parents frustrated with problems associated simply with an overly energetic child are often too quick to accept the label of hyperactivity.

A change in diet, if recommended, usually is just one component involved in treating hyperactive children. Behavior modification, family counseling, special education, psychotherapy, and drug therapy also may be involved.

The most common dietary plans used to control hyperactivity are the Feingold diet, sugar-reduction diets, allergy-elimination diets, and megavitamin therapy. All of these plans, however, are controversial, and evidence showing the effectiveness of any nutritional therapy when dealing with hyperactivity is inconclusive (see Chapter 7 for a more detailed discussion of some of these special diets).

The Feingold diet has attracted more attention than any other dietary treatment for hyperactivity. This food plan involves eliminating from the child's diet all artificial colorings, artificial flavorings, aspirinlike compounds (salicylates), and several antioxidant preservatives.

Continued experiments with the Feingold diet have shown that it benefits only a small number of hyperactive children. Most of the success stories among Feingold followers can be attributed to parents' heightened interest in diet coupled with an overall change in the family life-style. Children on this diet may have trouble receiving enough of some vitamins and minerals, especially vitamin C. Parents who use it must be careful to make sure it is well-balanced, nourishing, and not overly restrictive.

A high level of refined sugar in the diet is another factor that has been linked with hyperactivity. The idea is that some children digest and absorb sugar improperly. When these children eat too much sugar, abnormal behavior is the result. While studies on glucose tolerance and activity level, however, have so far been inconclusive, keeping the level of refined sugar down is a good idea.

Food allergy (discussed in Chapter 7) also has been suggested as a cause of hyperactive behavior among children. According to the theory, if a physician diagnoses allergies or intolerances to specific foods such as milk, wheat, eggs, soybeans, or chocolate, then hyperactive behavior should improve when the offending substances are eliminated from the diet. This has been true in some cases, but there is much doubt about whether hyperactivity is an actual symptom of an allergy or whether a child may become overly active as a way to deal with other uncomfortable symptoms. The hyperactivity-allergy link is still being studied.

Experiments with megavitamin therapy (also discussed in Chapter 7) among hyperactive children have been inconclusive. Most physicians and registered dietitians consider the use of megavitamins a potentially dangerous treatment for health problems.

With the possible exceptions discussed above, until more is known about the relationship between diet and hyperactivity, parents should continue to feed hyperactive children nourishing, well-balanced diets. Common sense would dictate that if a child's behavior seems to grow worse when a particular food is eaten, parents should try to reduce the amount of that substance or eliminate it. If it is an important part of the diet, it should be replaced with other foods that are rich in the same vitamins and minerals.

ACNE

When the first pimple pops up on an adolescent's face, fear of acne may cause him or her to shy away from candy bars, sugary soft drinks, and greasy french fries. While this may be a sensible change in eating habits, the role of diet in acne has not been proved.

Most dermatologists maintain that the type of acne that typically plagues teenagers is caused by hormones that stimulate glands, increasing the production of oil. The condition can be aggravated by stress, the stage of menstrual cycle, and picking or squeezing the affected areas.

Taking large doses of vitamin A, which is necessary for healthy skin, at one time was thought to be a way to reduce acne. Megadoses of vitamin A, however, have never proved to be effective in treating most cases of acne. In fact, excess amounts of this fat-soluble vitamin can cause a variety of health problems (see Table 2.20 and Chapter 7). Some dermatologists treat acne with topical vitamin A medications or vitamin A derivatives, which are applied directly to the skin. The results of these treatments, however, have been mixed. Because of the dangers of vitamin A toxicity, teenagers with acne should not use vitamin A internally or externally without consulting a physician.

Teenagers with acne (as well as teenagers with clear skin) should eat a variety of nourishing foods to maintain smooth function of all the body's systems, including the skin. Careful gentle washing and shampooing and some over-the-counter medications, such as benzoyl peroxide, may help reduce acne. A physician should be consulted if the acne problem is severe or if there are questions about the need for therapy.

PREVENTING CAVITIES

Cavities, also called dental caries, are common among children. Research indicates that 90 percent of the children in the United States have had at least one cavity by the time they reach 12 years of age. The incidence of cavities, however, is declining because of widespread fluoridation of drinking water (see Chapter 2), improved dental treatments, and increased public awareness of the link between certain types of food and cavities.

Cavities are caused by a breakdown of enamel, the hard, white outer covering of teeth. Tooth enamel can weaken when food particles, especially fermentable carbohydrates such as sugar, adhere to a tooth's surface. Bacteria, which are naturally present in the mouth, combine with food and saliva to form a substance called plaque. Bacteria in plaque react with carbohydrates, turning them into acid. If allowed to remain on the teeth, this acid can destroy the calcium, weaken the enamel, and produce a cavity.

Diet continues to play a key role in preventing and reducing the risk of cavity development. Sweets that stick to tooth enamel — gum with sugar, caramels, dried fruits, and hard candy — are more likely to cause cavities than soft drinks, fruit juice, and ice cream, which are cleared from the mouth quickly. Children should be encouraged to brush and floss their teeth immediately after meals and snacks, especially when sticky sweets are consumed. If brushing is impossible, they should rinse out their mouths with water.

Eating coarse, raw foods — carrots, celery, lettuce, and most other vegetables and fruits — that do not stick to tooth enamel can help prevent tooth decay. These foods promote production of saliva, which rinses teeth. Cheese, meats, and nuts also are saliva stimulators, and if eaten after sweets these foods have been found to reduce the risk of cavities. In addition, adequate amounts of calcium and phosphorus, the two primary minerals in enamel, are important to maintain sound teeth.

Fluoridated water, toothpaste, and mouthwash also may help strengthen enamel. In areas where the water is not fluoridated, children should receive regular fluoride supplements. Many dentists apply fluoride directly to the surface of teeth. In addition, surface sealants (liquid plastic applied to teeth and allowed to harden to form a protective coating) have been found to be effective in preventing cavities.

Infants and young children who are allowed to go to sleep with a bottle of milk or sugar-containing liquid, such as fruit juice, may develop serious tooth problems commonly called nursing bottle caries. The sugar in the liquid pools in the mouth where it remains in contact with teeth for extended periods of time, providing an ideal media for bacterial growth and acid development. Swallowing and saliva production decrease when the child is asleep, so these natural protective mechanisms become less effective in preventing cavities.

Young children should not be allowed to fall asleep with a bottle in their mouths. Once this habit is established it may be difficult to break. To prevent the risk of tooth decay, parents who feel they must give their children bottles at bedtime should fill them with water rather than formula, milk, fruit juice, or other liquids that contain sugar.

Parents will confront many other special situations and problems that require changes in the meals they offer their children. The best rule of thumb is good information, enough exercise, and a sensible diet. A well-nourished, well-exercised body has the best chance of remaining healthy, and a healthy body has the best chance for normal growth, development, and performance.

9

FOOD AND HEALTH

"Had I known I would live so long,
I would have taken better care of
myself."

Winston Churchill

Food and health go hand in hand. An unbalanced diet — one which lacks the essentials already described, or involves eating too little or too much — over a long period of time invariably leads to developmental and health problems. This has become clear over the past two centuries as greatly increased understanding of nutrition has contributed significantly to healthier, longer lives.

THE GROWING SCIENCE OF NUTRITION

A century ago, scurvy, rickets, goiter, and other diseases caused by undereating and unbalanced diets were common. Today, most of these diseases rarely occur in developed nations. This does not mean, however, that people's diets have improved significantly. Instead, new problems have developed, particularly problems related to overeating. The rates of high blood pressure, strokes, heart disease, and obesity, for example, are much higher today than they were 100 years ago.

Ancient physicians such as Galen, a pioneer in healing who lived in Greece from 131 to 201 A.D., claimed that they could modify patients' behavior by prescribing certain diets. Modern nutritional knowledge, however, did not really begin until the 17th and 18th centuries. Antoine Laurent Lavoisier is called the father of nutrition because in the late 18th century he discovered that respiration and consumption of oxygen are directly related to the metabolism of food.

During that period, other important facts about the body and the chemical properties of food were being identified. René Reaumur, for example, discovered in the early 18th century that enzymes in the stomach convert food into smaller, absorbable substances. Before then, the function of the stomach was unknown.

Gerardus Johann Mülder, in 1838, coined the term proteins for the nitrogen-containing substances in foods. Vitamins were discovered early in the 20th century after a number of experiments revealed that certain diseases could be cured by eating specific types of foods. In 1906, Christiaan Eijkman showed that a water-soluble extract from rice polishings could cure beriberi. James Lind, in 1853, proved that scurvy could be cured by eating oranges and lemons, although vitamin C was not crystalized until 1932. Cod-liver oil and sunlight were known to cure rickets long before the reasons were identified. In 1912, Casimir Funk gave the name "vitamines" to the still mysterious substances that were necessary to human life, and he connected them to beriberi, scurvy, and rickets. Individual vitamins were separated and named during the next 40 years.

In 1896, W. O. Atwater published the first table of food values, which then included only protein and calories. In 1916, only 20 years later, E. V. McCollum made popular the idea of "protective foods," foods important for their vitamin and mineral content. At the same time, Graham Lusk made the argument that adolescents need as much, if not more, food as adults, a concept universally accepted today.

The knowledge about nutrition, accrued over the last two centuries, has had a profound effect on the American diet. After World War I, for example, the consumption of leafy vegetables, citrus fruits, and milk increased. One of the primary reasons for this was the popularity of McCollum's protective-foods theory, although other contemporary technical advancements, such as the kitchen icebox and pasteurization of milk, contributed greatly.

In the late 1960s and early 1970s, teachers discovered that children who were restless and listless often had come to school with no breakfast. As a result, the federal government launched a School Breakfast Program, which supplies a nourishing breakfast to some children at a reasonable cost, or at a reduced cost or free to those children from low-income families who qualify. This program, together with the National School Lunch Program (see Chapter 6), which started in 1946, allows eligible school-aged children, who are growing rapidly and, therefore, are particularly vulnerable to nutritional deficiency diseases, to have two-thirds of the daily requirements available to them on school days. In addition, nutrition has become part of education; almost every child learns about the Basic Four Food Groups and three square meals a day.

The Food Stamp Program, begun in 1964, increases the food-buying power of the poor. It does not, however, supply enough food to adequately nourish a child. The Supplemental Food Program for Women, Infants, and Children (WIC), which provides nourishing food supplements and nutrition education to limited numbers of pregnant and lactating women and children to 5 years of age, began in 1974. Unfortunately, all these programs have been affected by government budget cuts.

Following World War II, the National Research Council of the National Academy of Sciences began publishing the Recommended Dietary Allowances (RDA) (see Chapter 2). Since then, the RDA have been revised every four to six years to reflect current scientific knowledge. The 1980 set of guidelines, or the ninth edition, gives the latest RDA. New RDA figures were expected in 1985 but disagreement on some figures kept the tenth edition from being approved and published.

In 1977, the Senate Select Committee on Nutrition and Human Needs published the original *Dietary Goals for the United States* and then a revised edition, which clarified some, though not all, of the controversies surrounding the first edition. One problem with this document is that the guidelines are written for adults and do not address the needs of children. Table 9.1 summarizes the committee's findings.

Three years after these goals were published, the Department

Table 9.1
DIETARY GOALS FOR THE UNITED STATES (SECOND EDITION)

Goal 1. To avoid overweight, consume only as much energy (calories) as is expended. If overweight, decrease energy intake and increase energy expenditure.

Goal 2. Increase the consumption of complex carbohydrates and "naturally occurring" sugars from about 28 percent of energy intake to about 48 percent of energy intake.

Goal 3. Reduce the consumption of refined and processed sugars by about 45 percent to account for about 10 percent of total energy intake.

Goal 4. Reduce overall fat consumption from approximately 40 percent to about 30 percent of energy intake.

Goal 5. Reduce saturated fat consumption to account for about 10 percent of total energy intake, and balance that with polyunsaturated and monounsaturated fats, which should account for about 10 percent of energy intake each.

Goal 6. Reduce cholesterol consumption to about 300 milligrams a day.

Goal 7. Limit the intake of sodium by reducing the intake of salt to about 5 grams a day.

(*Source:* Select Committee on Nutrition and Human Needs, U.S. Senate, *Dietary Goals for the United States, Second Edition*. Washington, D.C.: U.S. Government Printing Office, 1977.

of Agriculture and the Department of Health and Human Services jointly published a report entitled *Nutrition and Your Health: Dietary Guidelines for Americans*. The seven guidelines were broad-based, emphasizing moderation in diet and variety of food. The second edition of these guidelines was published in 1985. The seven guidelines remained the same. Table 9.2 outlines these guidelines.

Also in 1980, the Food and Nutrition Board of the National Academy of Sciences published *Toward Healthful Diets*, a report that was similar to the goals and the guidelines. The major difference in the *Toward Healthful Diets* report was that it made no recommendations for reducing saturated fat or decreasing the level of cholesterol in the diet.

Table 9.2
NUTRITION AND YOUR HEALTH: DIETARY GUIDELINES
FOR AMERICANS

Guideline 1.   Eat a variety of foods.

Guideline 2.   Maintain desirable weight.

Guideline 3.   Avoid too much fat, saturated fat, and cholesterol.

Guideline 4.   Eat foods with adequate starch and fiber.

Guideline 5.   Avoid too much sugar.

Guideline 6.   Avoid too much sodium.

Guideline 7.   If you drink alcohol, do so in moderation.

(*Source:* U.S. Department of Agriculture and Department of Health and Human Services, *Nutrition and Your Health: Dietary Guidelines for Americans.* Washington, D.C.: Home and Garden Bulletin No. 232, 1985.)

NUTRITION-RELATED DISEASES

Nutrition-related diseases are of two kinds: diseases of undernutrition, caused either by multiple- or single-nutrient deficiencies, and diseases of overnutrition or overconsumption.

Undernutrition

Multiple-nutrient deficiencies occur when a person has too little to eat or suffers from a disease that prevents the absorption of food, increases nutrient requirements, or causes essential nutrients to be improperly absorbed. The most common result of this form of undernutrition is weight loss.

A healthy adult of average weight can lose about 25 percent of his or her body weight and survive. Losing much more than that usually is fatal, although there have been extraordinary cases of people losing 50 percent of body weight and surviving. Undernourished people expend less energy, conserving their energy reserves for basic life processes.

At its most extreme, undernutrition — or starvation — leads to death. This occurs regularly to large segments of populations around the world during famines, which can be caused by natural disasters such as earthquakes, droughts, or floods; by human disasters, such as wars; or by combinations of natural and political events. This kind of disaster happened in Ethiopia and other parts of Africa during the terrible drought of the early and middle 1980s. Death from starvation also can occur as a result of psychological disorders such as anorexia nervosa, a condition that primarily afflicts teenaged girls who are obsessed with their weight and so stop eating (see Chapter 8).

When hunger does not lead to visible emaciation, as it has in Ethiopia, it is often "invisible." Its effects, however, are shockingly present in the United States. In 1984 the Citizens' Commission on Hunger in New England, Harvard School of Public Health, published a report entitled *American Hunger Crisis: Poverty and Health in New England.* This study documented the scope of hunger and malnutrition in one region of the country and raised serious questions about the nutritional status of people in other regions of the country.

As a result of these findings, the Physicians' Task Force, an independent fact-finding body of (primarily) physicians, was established to assess the extent of hunger and malnutrition in the nation, to analyze why hunger is a problem, and to make recommendations. They concluded that hunger in America is a public health epidemic. Many Americans were shocked by the assertion in the report, *Hunger in America,* published in 1985, that some 20 million Americans — roughly one in 12 — are hungry.

Undernutrition contributes to the high infant mortality rates seen in poor communities throughout the country. For example, in New York City, the infant mortality rates in the wealthy Sunset Park section of Brooklyn and in Manhattan's Silk Stocking section are 5.8 per thousand and 7.5 per thousand, respectively. These rates are among the lowest in the world. By contrast, in low-income areas, such as New York's central Harlem and Brownsville, Texas, the rate is 25.6 per thousand and 25.3 per thousand. Low birthweight is one cause of infant mortality and one of the direct results of poor maternal health and nutrition.

Hungry children suffer from growth retardation more frequently than well-fed children. The Physicians' Task Force estimated that some 500,000 children in the United States are "experiencing growth delays and other impairments generally associated with inadequate diet." Hungry children, or children whose mothers were undernourished while pregnant, particularly during the second trimester, also perform less well on standard assessment tests, particularly on the physical, social, and intellectual tests. Undernourished children are often listless, apathetic, disinterested in their environment, less able to pay attention, and restless. These characteristics can severely limit achievement in school.

Vitamin-deficiency-related diseases were the curse of the past, but they rarely occur today in the United States. Scurvy, caused by the lack of vitamin C, devastated the populations of sailors, soldiers, adventurers, and even the forty-niners during the California gold rush. Although, as mentioned earlier, the cure for scurvy has been known since 1853, soldiers in World War I died of this disease. Vitamin C was crystalized in 1932, but deficiencies of this vitamin are common among the poor today, although they rarely are severe enough to cause scurvy.

Rickets, a disease caused by vitamin-D deficiency, is uncommon today because this vitamin is added regularly to milk. Other vitamin deficiency diseases that have, for the most part, been eliminated in the United States are pellagra and beriberi. Pellagra occurs when not enough niacin (a B vitamin) is eaten. Beriberi is caused by a deficiency of thiamin (another B vitamin). Thiamin and niacin are among the vitamins now used to enrich white flour.

The major mineral-deficiency diseases also have become rare. Goiter, a disease that affects the thyroid, is caused by a deficiency of iodine. This disease has been recorded since early Egyptian times. In fact, the slightly rounded neck that characterizes moderate goiter was at one time considered a mark of beauty; it can be seen in the portraits of many elegant women. Goiter rarely is found in the United States today because iodine is added to salt.

Iron-deficiency anemia, however, continues to persist. Children and menstruating and pregnant women, all of whom need extra iron, are especially vulnerable to this disease, which is associated with fatigue and weakness. The Centers for Disease Control, which collect health statistics of the United States population, found in 1982 that 7 percent of children under 6 years of age were anemic. The rate was higher for children from 6 to

9 years old. Iron supplements often are prescribed for this condition when food sources are insufficient. Many infant formulas and cereals are fortified with iron. All varieties of liver and other organ meats are excellent sources; red meats, poultry, shellfish, and egg yolks also are good sources of iron.

Deficiency of protein, which is necessary for normal growth, building and repairing tissues, and maintaining red blood cells, is rare in the United States but common in many parts of the world. Protein-energy malnutrition (PEM) is graded mild, moderate, or severe. Severe PEM is further divided into diseases called marasmus and kwashiorkor.

Marasmus occurs as a result of a severe calorie deficiency. Children with this disease are recognized by their small size for age; "skin-and-bones" appearance because of absence of normal fat layers; thin, dull hair that falls out easily; apathy; and extreme sensitivity to temperature.

Kwashiorkor occurs after prolonged protein deficiency. The disease may cause children to be small for their age, irritable, and temperature sensitive. In addition, kwashiorkor sufferers often have depigmented hair that breaks off easily; discoloration of skin that usually peels, denuding large areas; and edema, the presence of large amounts of fluid in tissues, particularly the legs.

PEM is associated with changes in many body processes, resulting in adaptation to protein and/or calorie deficiencies. Because of the limited food intake, a person with PEM often has several other nutrient deficiencies such as iron, vitamin A, and vitamin C. In developed nations, severe PEM generally occurs because of an underlying illness, fad diets, self-induced starvation, or as a result of child abuse. Mild and moderate PEM, however, occurs in developed nations among poorer segments of the population and may reflect the inadequacy of a country's social programs to care for its people.

Overnutrition or Overconsumption

While undernutrition continues to plague the poor, health problems related to overnutrition and overconsumption now affect a major portion of the United States population. Overnutrition can be as dangerous as malnutrition or undernutrition. In adults, some of the consequences of overindulgence are heart disease, high blood pressure, atherosclerosis (hardening of the arteries), and strokes.

Obesity has been called the killer disease. While it is true that Americans overemphasize the slim, lean look, for too many people excessive weight has become a serious health problem. Obesity occurs when more calories are consumed than expended. It is often the result of eating patterns that are excessively high in fats and carbohydrates, and a sedentary way of life that includes little exercise. The cure for obesity involves reducing the number of calories consumed and increasing the amount of exercise (see Chapter 8).

Obesity is associated with high blood pressure, heart disease, atherosclerosis, diabetes, and gall-bladder disease. Obese women also are more likely to develop cancer of the uterus and breast. Unfortunately, obesity leads to greater inactivity, which in turn leads to greater obesity. It is a vicious cycle, often yielding devastating results.

Heart disease, directly related to overnutrition, is the leading cause of death in the United States today. Table 9.3 summarizes the Senate Select Committee's findings about risk factors that could lead to heart disease, which are outlined in the report *Dietary Goals for the United States*. The connection is clear: Eating too much in general and eating too much saturated fat, cholesterol, and/or salt can contribute to physical conditions that lead to heart disease.

Atherosclerosis, a condition in which plaques, or fatty deposits, attach to the artery wall (generally at juncture points), is one of the causes of heart attacks. It also causes strokes and gangrene (death of a body part because of circulation failure to that area) in the legs. Atherosclerotic plaques narrow blood vessels, making it difficult for the heart to pump blood through them. Sometimes the thickening closes the vessel entirely. More often, a piece of the plaque breaks off and lodges in a smaller channel, thereby blocking it. When this happens in the coronary artery, the result is a heart attack; when in the brain, a stroke; and when in the lower extremities, gangrene.

Two of the major causes of atherosclerosis are overconsump-

Table 9.3
RISK FACTORS ASSOCIATED WITH HEART DISEASE

Risk Factors	Physiological Result	End Result
Eating and drinking too much	Overweight	
Not exercising enough		
High total fat consumption	Elevated blood cholesterol	
High saturated fat consumption		
Low polyunsaturated : saturated fat level		Higher risk of heart disease
High cholesterol consumption	Elevated blood pressure	
High salt consumption		
Overweight	Accelerated atherosclerotic process	
Diabetes		
Smoking		

(*Source:* U.S. Senate Select Committee on Nutrition and Human Needs, *Dietary Goals for the United States,* Second Edition. Washington, D.C.: U.S. Government Printing Office, 1977.)

tion of saturated fats and cholesterol. Because estrogen, a female hormone, inhibits atherosclerosis, the incidence of this disease in males under 55 years of age is far greater than in women. A total of 35 percent of the young men killed in the Korean War, with an average age of 22 years, were found to have significant narrowing of their coronary arteries as a result of atherosclerosis.

High blood pressure, or hypertension, is another major cause of heart disease. It contributes to kidney disease, strokes, and edema (swelling of tissues). High blood pressure often occurs when the body is unable to eliminate excessive dietary salt, which retains water in the body. When salt is not eliminated properly, the volume of blood to be transported increases. The heart then has to work harder to pump this extra fluid throughout the 60,000 miles of blood vessels. The blood vessels contract to reduce the blood flow and ease the heart's work; therefore, the heart then has to pump even harder.

Hypertension occurs more often in obese people than in people of normal weight. This is because an extra mile of blood vessels is required for every extra pound of body fat, and the heart is required to work harder and harder.

The exact cause of cancer remains a mystery. Recent evidence, however, suggests that cancer may be linked with diet. Colon cancer, the most life-threatening cancer in the United States, and breast cancer, the leading cancer among American women, may be associated with diets high in fats and dairy products. Cancers of the breast and uterus may be associated with obesity. Cancers of the colon, rectum, breast, and uterus may be associated with high-fat and low-fiber diets. Other forms of cancer that have been linked to diet are cancers of the stomach, liver, prostate, and large and small intestines. Cancer also has been associated with a number of additives used in processed foods, and even to some methods of processing (see Chapter 11).

Cancer also may be associated with alcoholism — the habitual, excessive drinking of alcoholic beverages. Specifically, cancers of the head and neck, esophagus, liver, and large intestine (the colon) are thought to be causally linked with overconsumption of alcohol. Heavy drinking is known to cause liver and heart diseases (including abnormal heart rhythms), digestive problems, and weight problems.

While a relatively small percentage of teenagers and very few children may be considered alcoholics, it is alarming that a growing number of Americans between 10 and 20 years of age regularly consume alcoholic beverages. Alcohol is a toxic drug; it has both a poisonous and anesthetizing effect on body tissues and processes. In particular, the liver, stomach, and small intestine are prime targets of the damaging effects of alcohol.

From the standpoint of healthy eating, alcoholic beverages can cause problems for children and teenagers. Although beer and wine, for example, are relatively high in calories, alcoholic beverages provide extremely little nutritional value. For example, a single ounce of spaghetti or potato contains more nutrients than a 12-ounce glass of beer. Physicians find that the calories from alcohol often are consumed at the expense of nourishing food, which supplies essential vitamins and minerals. In addition, alcohol increases the body's need for some nutrients.

People who consume too much alcohol are more likely to develop a variety of nutritional deficiencies. Individuals who drink regularly find that their appetites and hunger are suppressed. It is common for regular drinkers to eat poorly. In addition, when alcohol is consumed, the body has difficulty using nutrients from those foods that are eaten. In particular, stores of B vitamins (especially niacin and thiamin) are depleted by the metabolism of alcohol in the liver, and it becomes more difficult for the body to absorb folic acid, vitamin B_{12}, thiamin, and vitamin C. Alcohol also increases the output and flow of urine, possibly leading to some loss of essential minerals that are water soluble, such as potassium and magnesium.

Many adults who drink are able to do so in moderation. Use of alcohol by teenagers and children, however, is a different matter and should be actively and consistently discouraged, without exception. Education in the schools, in newspapers and magazines, and on radio and television about the obvious hazards of drinking and driving needs to be supplemented by calm, reasoned explanations at home about the multiple self-destructive effects of alcohol on bodies and minds. *Alcohol and growing children do not mix.*

While these are the major diseases of overnutrition and overconsumption, there are many more. The possible harmful effects of high levels of the fat-soluble vitamins and of minerals are reviewed in the vitamin and mineral tables in Chapter 2. As these tables indicate, overconsumption of vitamin A and vitamin D can lead to serious illness. (See also Chapter 7.) The consequences of overconsumption of minerals are similarly harmful.

While millions of Americans suffer from diseases of poor nutrition — both undernutrition and overnutrition — many more millions are eating well. In fact, Americans as a whole are becoming more diet conscious, eating more nutritionally balanced diets than ever before.

The rising interest in nutrition has many causes. Knowledge about nutrition has increased over the last century, and information is being disseminated more effectively to the public. Many adults and young people now have a general idea of the fundamentals of a sound diet and are interested in learning more. The growing number of factual newspaper and magazine columns devoted to food is one indication of the media's response to great public interest in this topic.

Public interest and the demand for reliable information about nutrition has made an impact on the medical community as well. Today, approximately one-third of the medical schools in the United States require that students take a course in nutrition. By comparison, before the late 1970s, medical schools virtually ignored nutrition, other than its relationship to courses such as biochemistry, physiology, pathology, and hematology. In addition, many of the medical schools that do not require nutrition courses now are encouraging students to take a variety of elective courses and seminars exploring the important link between diet and health.

The growing number of registered dietitians is another indication of the increased interest in and recognition of the importance of nutrition. Registered dietitians have been trained to use diet as a means of enhancing health and preventing or controlling disease, and they are among the best, most reliable sources of nutrition information. To become registered to practice, dietitians must complete an approved nutrition program at an accredited college or university; gain practical, firsthand experience through approved internships; and pass a comprehensive registration examination given by the Commission on Dietetic Registration of the American Dietetic Association. Currently there are approximately 50,000 registered dietitians in the United States. Most work in hospitals, nursing homes, schools, military services, and public health programs. There are, however, more than 4,000 registered dietitians in private practice, where they counsel about food and nutrition and plan diets for individuals, often through referral from or in consultation with physicians.

Registered dietitians are nutritionists, but not all nutritionists are registered dietitians. Anyone can call himself or herself a nutritionist. Some nutritionists, such as registered dietitians, people with Ph.D.s in nutrition, and some physicians, can provide reliable, sound information. Unfortunately, the public's interest in nutrition has spawned some so-called "nutritionists" who actually know little about food and diet planning. These self-styled diet "experts" often are not as interested in nutrition and health as they are in their clients' ability and willingness to follow an unconventional diet and to pay the bill.

The best way to find a reputable registered dietitian is through local hospitals' dietary or nutrition departments; the state health department; the state dietetic association; the public relations department of the American Dietetic Association (see Resources section at the end of this book) or in the telephone book Yellow Pages, under "Dietitian."

Nutrition, indeed, is an expanding, changing field. Enough reliable information, however, currently is known to enable parents to feed their families confidently, knowing that they are providing a balance of foods that will promote their children's mental and physical well-being.

10

THE BEST FOOD: PROVIDING, PREPARING, AND PROTECTING IT

Food may look beautiful and its taste
may be very attractive, but that alone
does not make it acceptable to Gas-
tronomy. It must above all be absolutely sound and fresh.

Andre Simon

A nineteenth-century housewife
would find the modern supermarket truly overwhelming. Not
only is there an endless smorgasbord of canned, boxed, bagged,
frozen, and convenience foods, dairy products, fresh produce,
meats, and breads, but today what the shopper sees is not always what the shopper gets. Inside a can with a label showing
colorful, perfectly cut, crisp-looking green beans may be some
pitiful, gray-green, limp specimens. A bag of green beans in the
frozen-food section may be more nutritious than canned beans
but may still lack some nutrients found in the fresh variety.

Choosing the most nourishing forms of the best food is only
the first step toward good nutrition. Once the shopping has
been done and the food is in the house, proper storage methods
are necessary to retain vitamins and minerals and prevent the
possible spread of harmful bacteria. Then, practical preparation
and cooking methods are needed to keep food appetizing and
wholesome.

FINDING THE BEST FOODS

Most American consumers buy food in one of the major supermarkets, which in the past 50 years have spread throughout
the country, replacing the old-time general and specialty stores.
Today's supermarkets stock more than 10,000 different items,
which can make grocery shopping a confusing task.

Choosing the best food requires knowledge, practice, and
some luck. As shoppers examine mounds of green beans, piles
of peaches, or stacks of tomatoes, they may search for color,
firmness, size, or ripeness. As they compare one package of
chicken breasts to another, they may look for color or meatiness.
As they scan loaves of bread, they may test for softness, type of
grain, texture, or size of the slices. Other shoppers may be more
interested in the price, quantity, and the number of additives in
a product.

In general, it is best to shop the periphery of the grocery store.
This is where fresh fruits and vegetables; fresh meat, poultry,
and seafood; dairy products; and freshly baked breads usually
are located, because of the need for refrigeration and frequent
turnover. The market's rim, therefore, contains the foods with
the least processing, the fewest additives, and often the most
vitamins, minerals, and food value. (See the upcoming discussion in this chapter for a comparison of the food values of fresh,
frozen, and canned food.)

Vegetables

When choosing fresh vegetables, avoid those that are limp
and tired looking. "Old" vegetables cannot be revived by stir-
frying, boiling, steaming, or baking.

Although most of the common vegetables are available year
round, in season they tend to have the best food value, flavor,
texture, and price.

In general, vegetables are good sources of vitamins, minerals,
carbohydrates, and fiber. Most vegetables are composed mainly
of water and carbohydrates. There is little or no fat in vegetables
and, with the exception of legumes, they are low in protein.
Most varieties of vegetables also are low in calories.

Yellow vegetables such as carrots and some varieties of
squash provide valuable vitamin A (the deeper the color, the

higher the vitamin content). Green, leafy vegetables, such as spinach and kale, are rich in vitamins A, C, K, and riboflavin, as well as iron, calcium, and fiber. Flowering vegetables, especially broccoli, are valuable sources of vitamins A and C, riboflavin, iron, and phosphorus.

Table 10.1 reviews common vegetables and tips on how to buy the best. (*Note:* In parts of the country with warm climates, the seasons mentioned in Table 10.1 may be longer.)

Table 10.1
CHOOSING FRESH VEGETABLES

Artichokes: Artichokes are best from March through May. Select heavy, tightly closed heads with green stems and firm, unblemished leaves. Spread-out, brownish heads may be tough.

Asparagus: Peak asparagus season is March to June. Choose spears with green color extending two-thirds down the stalk. Good asparagus is firm and green with tightly closed tips. Open tips generally mean a tough stalk, while soft, wrinkled spears mean the asparagus is not fresh.

Beets: Beets are available year round, but they are best from June to October. Choose beets that are smooth, round, and firm. The small or medium-sized ones tend to be most tender. Beets should be deep red; leaves should be green and unwilted.

Broccoli: Broccoli is in season and available year round in most areas. Buy firm broccoli stalks with small, unwilted leaves. The best broccoli is topped with dark green or purplish flowerets that have compact and tightly closed buds. Avoid loose, yellowish buds because these usually are tough and old.

Brussels sprouts: The best season for Brussels sprouts is late fall and winter. Choose unblemished, tightly closed heads. The best Brussels sprouts are bright green. Avoid ones that are soft, dull-looking, or have a yellowish color.

Cabbage: Good cabbage is available year round. It comes in many varieties — smooth green, crinkly green Savoy, red, and Chinese. The best heads are crisp, firm, and heavy. Avoid heads with loose, yellowish outer leaves and blemishes.

Carrots: Carrots are available year round. Buy carrots that are well-formed, firm, smooth, and bright orange. Smaller ones usually are tastier and easier to work with. Avoid carrots that are rubbery, grayish, or have a lot of cracks and greenish color at the top.

Table 10.1
Continued

Cauliflower: The peak of cauliflower season is fall and winter. Choose heads that are crisp and white with compact, tightly closed flowerets. Outer leaves should be firm and bright green. A purplish tinge on the heads (caused by sunlight) will not affect taste. Avoid heads with brown spots, bruises, and spreading flowerets.

Celery: Good celery is available year round. The mildest celery is light green in color, while stronger-tasting celery is darker green. Buy firm, unwilted stalks with crisp leaves. Avoid celery that is flexible or split.

Corn: Fresh corn is available in the late spring, summer, and early fall, depending on the area of the country. Buy ears that have plump, yellow or white kernels that extend from top to bottom in straight lines and do not look dry. The best ears are those that are medium sized. Husks should be moist and bright green. Local corn, which has not spent much time in transport, is much tastier than corn that has been shipped from other parts of the country.

Cucumbers: Cucumbers are available year round, but they are especially good in summer. The best are firm and slender with uniform dark-green color. Avoid those with soft spots. Many people prefer cucumbers that are not coated with wax, although sometimes unwaxed cucumbers are difficult to find.

Eggplant: August and September are the best months for eggplant. Select the heaviest and firmest ones, with surfaces that are shiny and smooth. The most common variety is the large, gourd-shaped, purple eggplant; however, white eggplant and tiny purple eggplant are sometimes available.

Green and wax beans: These vegetables are available year round, but they are especially good in the late spring and summer. The best beans are those that are crisp, firm, and bright green or yellow. Beans should snap crisply when broken. Avoid beans that are limp, wrinkled, or have brown spots.

Greens (beet, collard, dandelion, kale, mustard, Swiss chard, and turnip): Most greens are available year round, but they are especially tasty in the late summer and fall. Select greens with bright green, crisp, unwilted leaves. Avoid those with brown edges, variations in color, and thick stems.

Lettuce (iceberg, Bibb, Boston, garden, red-leaf, escarole, chicory, watercress, endive, romaine, arugala): Most types of lettuce are available year round. Iceberg, the most popular salad lettuce,

Table 10.1
Continued

should be large, compact, and heavy. In general the darker leaves of all types of lettuce will have a stronger flavor (and more vitamins and minerals) than the lighter leaves. Choose crisp lettuce that is fresh looking with a good green or sometimes reddish-green color.

Lima beans: Fresh lima beans are available in the spring and summer. They usually come in the shell, which must be broken before the beans are squeezed out. Select fresh, firm, bright green pods that are slightly flexible and have a velvety texture.

Mushrooms: Fall and winter are the ideal times for fresh mushrooms. Of the commonly sold variety, the best are firm, white, and velvety with caps closed around the stem. Avoid mushrooms that are dark, spotted, or soft. Some less common varieties, such as morels, may be available locally. Unless well trained in identifying mushrooms, people should eat only store-bought varieties. Some wild mushrooms are poisonous.

Okra: The okra season runs from May to October. Okra pods should be bright green, tender, and pliable. The best tasting pods are small — anywhere from two to four inches long.

Onions: All kinds of onions — yellow, sweet, Spanish, Bermudas, white, shallots, and scallions — are available year round. For bulb-type onions, choose ones that are unsprouted, very firm, and rounded with dry, thin skins. Select scallions with crisp, tender, bright green tops and firm, white bottoms.

Peas: Fresh peas are best in the spring and early summer. They usually are sold in the pod and, like lima beans, require shelling. Choose firm, bright green pods. It is difficult to determine the quality of peas without cracking open a pod and tasting a pea. It should be tender and sweet. Snow peas, also called sugar or Chinese peas, are eaten pods and all. Buy flat, bright green, firm snow pea pods.

Peppers (green bell, red bell, Italian, green chili, and red chili): Most pepper varieties are available year round. Choose peppers that have a good color and a natural shine rather than a waxed surface. The sides should be smooth, firm, and unwrinkled. Red bell peppers are sweeter than green bell peppers. Sometimes, orange and yellow ones are available. Italian peppers have thinner skins and a sweet, delicate flavor. Red and green chili peppers are extremely hot.

Potatoes: Most varieties of potatoes — Idaho, russet, red new, white new, sweet, and yams — are in stores year round. The best

Table 10.1
Continued

potatoes are firm, smooth, round or oval, and blemish free. Avoid potatoes with sprouts, too many eyes (tiny buds in the skin), green blotches, large cuts, growth cracks, bruises, discolored areas, or a musty smell. Sweet potatoes and yams should have an orange color and be smooth and tapered at the ends.

Radishes: Radishes are available year round. Bunches usually are best because each radish can be inspected. Select dark red, hard radishes with fresh, green leaves. Prepackaged radishes should be inspected carefully, and bags with cracked, off-color, or soft radishes should be avoided.

Spinach: Spinach is available year round. Loose, bulk spinach usually is better than the spinach that is prewashed and prepackaged. Select leaves that are crisp and medium to dark green with small, tender stems. When buying packaged spinach, make sure the leaves are fresh and not too wet or too powdery.

Squash: Summer squash (yellow, zucchini, and pattypan) is available most of the year but is best from late spring to early fall. Winter squash (acorn, Hubbard, butternut, buttercup, green and gold delicious, banana, pumpkin, and spaghetti) is available in the fall and winter months. Select summer squash that is small, firm, and smooth with bright green or yellow, shiny surfaces. Winter squash should have a hard, possibly rough, surface with few blemishes.

Sprouts: Mung bean and alfalfa sprouts, the two most common varieties, are available all year. Choose sprouts that are fresh looking, resilient, and crisp. Avoid those that are wet and slimy with a moldy smell.

Tomatoes: The best tomatoes are available in July, August, and September, but tomatoes grown in hothouses are available year round. Locally grown, vine-ripened tomatoes provide the best taste, texture, and juice. Packaged hothouse tomatoes usually are pale with hard skins and mealy textures. Small cherry tomatoes, which also are grown in hothouses, may offer better flavor in the off season. Select firm, smooth, bright red tomatoes. Avoid those with soft spots, cracks, or breaks.

Turnips and rutabagas: White turnips are available year round, and rutabagas (also called yellow turnips) are available in the fall and winter. Choose turnips that are hard and round with smooth, unblemished skins. A coating of paraffin wax may mean that a turnip has been stored for a long time.

Fruit

Science and modern technology, including improved transportation methods and better refrigeration, have made many
popular varieties of fruit available year round. Exotic and tropical fruits also appear routinely in supermarkets. The best
choices, however, are local, seasonal varieties, which offer good
flavor and high nutrient value at a low cost.

Most fruits are rich sources of natural sugar, vitamins, minerals, and fiber. With the exception of olives and avocados, fruits
are virtually fat-free. Fruits, which are composed of a high percentage of water, provide little protein to the diet.

Vitamin C is found in varying quantities in all fresh fruit, but
citrus fruits such as oranges and grapefruit are the richest
sources of this important vitamin. Also, citrus fruits, as well as
strawberries and figs, supply limited amounts of calcium. Yellow fruits such as cantaloupes and peaches provide some vitamin A, and figs, plums, and dried fruits supply B vitamins,
especially thiamin. Dried fruits, bananas, grapes, berries,
peaches, and apricots contain some iron. All fruit provides varying amounts of potassium and magnesium.

Below is a list of fruit with tips on selecting the best of the
batch. (*Note:* In some parts of the country with a warm climate,
the seasons mentioned in Table 10.2 will be longer.)

Table 10.2
CHOOSING FRESH FRUIT

Apples (Baldwin, Cortland, Yellow and Red Delicious, Granny Smith,
Gravenstein, Grimes Golden, Jonathan, McIntosh, Melrose,
Newtown Pippin, Northern Spy, Rhode Island Greening, Rome
Beauty, Russet, Spitzenberg, Stayman, Wealthy, Winesap, York
Imperial): Apple season is late summer and fall, but many varieties
are available year round. Look for firm, brightly colored fruit.
Some apples, such as Granny Smiths and Rhode Island Greenings,
are green when ripe. A few varieties, such as Golden Delicious
apples, should be bright yellow. Red apples, such as Jonathan, Red
Delicious, and Winesap, should be bright scarlet; others, such as
McIntosh, Newtown Pippin, and Gravenstein, are best with a
greenish-red background. Too greenish a tinge, however, may
mean that the apple is hard, starchy, and flavorless. Fruit that is

Table 10.2
Continued

too yellow may be soft and mealy. Smaller varieties tend to be less mealy. Avoid apples that are bruised or shriveled. Local tree-ripened varieties usually are tastiest for eating raw and best for cooking and baking.

Apricots: Apricot season is June and July. Select fruit that is small, firm, and plump with an orange-yellow color. Ripe apricots should yield slightly when pressed gently. Avoid shriveled apricots, as they may lack flavor.

Avocados: Avocado season is November through May. Two varieties are available — a smooth green-skinned fruit, and a darker fruit with rough skin. Most avocados are sold slightly underripe, but they ripen within a few days if unrefrigerated. Ripe avocados should yield slightly to gentle pressure but not be too soft.

Bananas: Bananas are available year round. Often the bananas sold in the produce department are underripe — hard and slightly green at the ends. These will ripen quickly. Ripe bananas are bright yellow with brown flecks, and firm but not hard. Remember that these will become overripe quickly at home. Red bananas are brown-red in color and slightly softer than the common yellow banana.

Blueberries: Wild blueberries are available in midsummer; cultivated berries are in season from spring to fall. Buy blueberries that are plump, dry, firm, and bright blue with a slight frostlike coating. Cultivated berries are fatter and fleshier than the wild variety, and less intense in flavor.

Cantaloupes: Cantaloupes are in season from June through November. Look for a smooth, shallow depression at the stem end (which means it was ripened on the vine). No part of the stem should remain on the fruit. Netting on the skin should be thick, coarse, and raised over a yellow-beige rind. Ripe cantaloupes will have a pleasant smell, and the skin will yield slightly to pressure on the end. Avoid green, bright yellow, or soft rinds.

Cherries: Cherries are in season during the summer months. The most common types — Bing, Black Tartarian, and Napoleon — should be deep red, and plump to the point of near bursting. Sour cherries, which are used primarily in baking, are smaller and pale red.

Cranberries: Peak season for cranberries is September through January. Look for firm, plump berries that bounce like rubber balls

Table 10.2

Continued

when dropped on a hard surface. Color differences generally do not affect taste.

Grapes: Green and local varieties of grapes are available in the summer and fall. Most red, purple, and black grape varieties are in season in the late summer, fall, and winter. (Seedless varieties are better for young children. For older children and adults, the seeds provide a boost of fiber.) Select grape bunches with plump, unblemished, brightly colored grapes. The clusters should be firmly attached to the stems. Avoid bunches that are off-color or have deteriorating stems.

Grapefruit: This fruit usually is available year round, but it is best in the fall, winter, and spring. Choose firm, heavy, well-rounded fruits. The thinner the skin, the juicier the fruit. Grapefruit that narrows at the stem end may be less juicy and have less flavor. Scars on the rind will not hurt the fruit. Avoid soft or dented fruit.

Honeydews, casabas, and Cranshaws: These melon varieties are in season in the late summer and fall. Look for ones without green rinds. When ripe, the blossom end should yield to pressure. Honeydews and Cranshaws should have a sweet smell.

Lemons: Lemons are available year round. Choose fruit that is heavy and firm — but not hard — with a bright yellow, shiny, thin rind. Avoid greenish lemons with rough, thick skins.

Limes: Limes are available year round. Look for full, heavy fruit with a bright green color, and shiny, thin skin. Avoid limes that are yellowish and thick-skinned.

Oranges, tangelos, and tangerines: Most varieties of oranges are available year round, but they are best in the fall, winter, and spring. Tangerines and tangelos are in season in the winter. Look for heavy fruit with a glossy skin that is not too thick or coarse. Greenish tinges or skin blemishes usually do not affect the taste. Discoloration around the stem end, however, may be a sign that the fruit is overripe. Spoiled oranges develop soft spots and a dull white or green mold.

Papayas: This tropical fruit is in season in May and June. Papayas should be pear shaped with a smooth-textured surface. Ripe papayas are firm, yet should yield slightly to pressure. Medium-sized orange or yellow papayas are best.

Peaches and nectarines: These fruits are available from late spring through the fall, but they are at the peak of flavor in the summer.

Table 10.2
Continued

Peaches should be golden to orange, well rounded, fuzzy, and slightly soft when pressed. Nectarines should be orange-yellow with patches of red. The area along the seam should be soft. Avoid fruits with tan or brown spots.

Pears: Bartlett pears are in season in the late summer and fall. Other varieties, such as the Anjou, Bosc, and comice, are available in the winter. Ripe pears will yield slightly to gentle pressure. It may be better to buy them when they are firm and allow them to ripen at home. Bosc pears are best eaten while they are somewhat firm. Color will vary with the variety. Blemishes on the skin usually will not affect taste. Avoid pears with soft brown spots.

Pineapples: Tropical pineapples are in season year round, but they are best in the spring months. Look for large, heavy fruit with no soft spots. A small, compact crown usually denotes good fruit. Ripe pineapples emit a dull, solid sound when thumped with the finger. Protruding eyes and a sweet, delicate aroma also indicate ripeness. Avoid those from which the leaves can be pulled off easily.

Plums: Plum season is July and August. Choose fruits that are of good color — whether purple, red, blue, yellow, or green — and even round or oval shape. Ripe plums should be plump and slightly soft with smooth, unshriveled skins. Choose medium-sized plums; larger ones generally have a blander taste.

Pomegranates: These fruits are available in the fall months. Choose pomegranates that are brightly colored — ranging from yellow-red to brilliant crimson — with slightly flattened ends. Ripe ones should be firm, plump, heavy, and about the size of a large orange. Avoid those that are blemished or shriveled.

Raspberries: Some types of raspberries are in season in June and July, and other varieties in the early fall. Look for fresh, clean berries that are shiny and brightly colored. Red raspberries should be bright red, and black raspberries are blackish-purple. Avoid berries with green spots, whitish fuzzy mold, or dampness.

Rhubarb: This fruit is available from January through June from warm climates, or in the late summer in cooler areas. Choose firm, thick, bright reddish stalks that are not overly stringy or fibrous.

Strawberries: Hothouse berries or berries grown in warm climates are available year round, but strawberry season in most of the country is May, June, and sometimes in September. Select bright red, shiny, well-formed berries of medium size. Large berries may have less flavor. Avoid those that are soft, moldy, or damp.

Table 10.2
Continued

Watermelon: The height of watermelon season is summer. Look for firm, well-shaped melons with bright green color. The surface of a ripe watermelon can be scraped off easily with a fingernail. The flesh should be juicy and deep pink with no white streaks, and the seeds should be dark and shiny.

Meat

Meat, one of the more expensive items routinely purchased in supermarkets, consumes the greatest percentage of the average person's food dollar. Although consumption of beef, lamb, pork, and veal has declined recently, meat remains the featured attraction on the dinner plate in most American households.

The United States Department of Agriculture inspects and grades meat sold in interstate commerce. The most expensive grade is *PRIME,* found mainly in gourmet butcher shops, restaurants, hotels, and clubs. Prime meat is marbled (flecks of fat throughout the meat), extremely tender, and juicy with a fine texture.

The highest quality meat carried in supermarkets usually is *CHOICE.* Choice grade means that the meat is tender and juicy with a good texture, but it is not as well marbled as prime meat. Meat that receives a *GOOD* grade from USDA inspectors is less fatty and juicy than prime and choice meats. It can be a good buy, and it usually is tender if cooked slowly in moist heat. *STANDARD* and *COMMERCIAL* grades of meat, which are from low-quality or older animals, generally are not available in supermarkets. These grades are given to meats that have little marbling and thin layers of exterior fat. The flavor may be bland, and the meat tends to be coarse, tough, and dry.

Listed below are tips for buying beef, lamb, pork, and veal.

Beef: Expensive cuts of beef are not necessarily better than less expensive cuts — at least nutritionally speaking. Highly marbled cuts such as Porterhouse steaks and standing rib roasts usually cost more per pound than leaner cuts, such as chuck or rump. (The exception is hamburger. Lean ground beef — 10 to 15 percent fat — is more expensive than regular ground beef — 20 to

---

Figure 10.1

CUTS OF BEEF

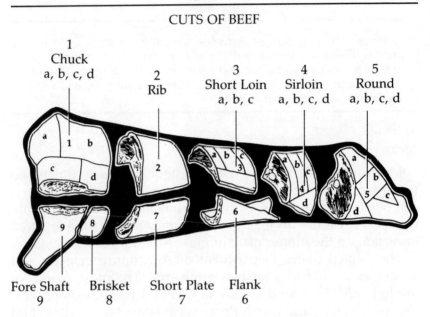

30 percent fat.) But more than three-fourths of the calories in expensive cuts come from fat, and most of this is saturated fat and cholesterol, which has been linked to heart disease. (See Figure 10.1 for information on the various cuts of beef.)

The best buys from the point of view of food value are the lean, inexpensive cuts that may need to be tenderized or cooked slowly in moist heat. Lean, bright pink to red meat with light-colored bones usually has the best flavor. Fat casing around the exterior of the beef should be creamy, white, and crumbly.

Veal: Veal is meat from calves slaughtered before they are 8 months old. The most expensive veal, milk-fed veal, comes from calves that are slaughtered at 3 to 5 months, before they have been weaned.

With the exception of the breast, cuts of veal are quite lean, with a thin layer of exterior fat and little visible marbling. (See Figure 10.2 for information on the various cuts of veal.)

The most expensive veal is white or very pale pink. This meat usually comes from calves that have been confined in narrow

Figure 10.1
Continued

1 — CHUCK
Ground Chuck (a)
Stew Meat (a)
Cross Rib Pot Roast (d)
Boneless Shoulder Pot Roast (c)

Blade Roast or Steak (b)
Arm Pot Roast or Steak (c)
Boneless Eye Roast (b)
Chuck Short Ribs (c, d)

2 — RIB
Rib Eye Roast or Steak
Boneless Rib Steak

Rib Steak
Rib Roast

3 — SHORT LOIN
Filet Mignon (b, c)
Boneless Top Loin Steak (a, b, c)
Porterhouse Steak (c)

T-bone Steak (b)
Top Loin Steak (a, b, c)

4 — SIRLOIN
Boneless Sirloin Steak (a, b, c)
Wedge Bone Sirloin Steak (c)
Tip Roast (d)
Tip Steaks (d)

Flat Bone Sirloin Steak (b)
Pin Bone Sirloin Steak (a)
Cubed Beef Kabob Chunks (d)

5 — ROUND
Eye of Round (b)
Bottom Round Roast or Steak (b)
Top Round Steak (b)
Round Steak (b)
Tip Roast (d)
Cubed Beef Kabob Chunks (d)

Ground Beef (a, b, c, d)
Cubed Steak (b)
Boneless Rump Roast (a)
Heel of Round (c)
Tip Steak (d)

6 — FLANK
Flank Steak
Ground Beef

Rolled Flank Steaks

7 — SHORT PLATE
Short Ribs
Ground Beef

Stew Meat

8 — BRISKET
Fresh Beef Brisket

Corned Beef Brisket

9 — FORE SHANK
Shank Cross Cuts

Stew Meat

Figure 10.2

CUTS OF VEAL

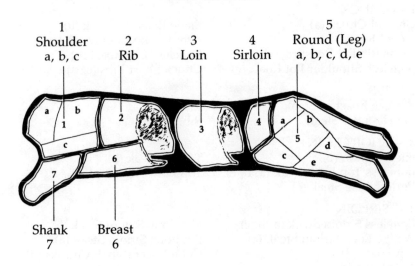

stalls so that their flesh remains undeveloped and tender. Veal that is dark pink or red usually comes from older calves or calves that have been allowed to roam and graze in the field.

Pork: Most cuts of pork contain a high percentage of fat. The least fatty parts are the tenderloin strip, center-cut leg ham, and loin chops. The fattiest cuts are the rib roast, bacon, feet, hocks, picnic shoulder, and shoulder butt. (See Figure 10.3 for information on the various cuts of pork.)

The most flavorful pork usually will be light in color — light pink, approaching white — with pinkish bones and firm, white exterior fat. A grainy look in pork may affect the tenderness slightly, but generally not the flavor.

Lamb: Meat from sheep that are from 3 to 5 months old is called baby or spring lamb. Spring lamb is tender and has a mild fla-

Figure 10.2
Continued

---

1 — SHOULDER
Arm Roast (c)   Arm Steak (c)
Blade Roast (b)   Blade Steak (b)
Boneless Shoulder Roast (b, c)

2 — RIB
Rib Roast   Rib Chops
Crown Roast   Boneless Rib Chops

3 — LOIN
Loin Roast   Loin Chop
Kidney Chop   Top Loin Chop

4 — SIRLOIN
Sirloin Roast   Sirloin Chop
Boneless Sirloin Roast   Cutlets

5 — ROUND (LEG)
Rump Roast (a)   Round Steak (b, c)
Round Roast (b, c)   Cutlets (b, c)
Boneless Rump Roast (b)   Veal Choplets (d, e)

6 — BREAST
Veal Breast   Boneless Riblets
Stuffed Breast   Stuffed Chops
Riblets

7 — SHANK
Shank   Shank Cross Cuts

Note: Stew Meat or Ground Veal is made from any cut. Cube Veal Steaks are made from thick, boneless cuts.

vor. Meat from animals 5 months to 1 year old is called winter lamb or simply lamb. Meat from older lamb usually is less tender and has a stronger flavor.

The fattier cuts of lamb, such as the loin, shoulder, rack, and rib chops, are more expensive than leaner cuts, such as leg, shank, and breast. Like beef, the most expensive cuts offer the

Figure 10.3

CUTS OF PORK

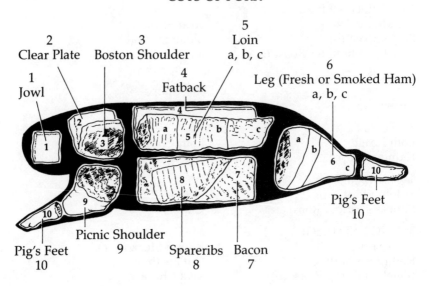

same nutrients as the least expensive cuts, but higher-priced lamb often means a higher saturated fat content. (See Figure 10.4 for information on the various cuts of lamb.)

Lamb should be lean and bright pink with creamy white exterior fat, and pinkish bones. If flesh and bones are approaching a red color, it may be a sign that the lamb was slaughtered at an older age, and it may be tough.

Poultry

The most common types of poultry are chicken, turkey, and Rock Cornish game hens. These birds provide more protein and less fat than identical amounts of red meat. The dark meat in poultry is higher in fat and cholesterol than white meat. On rare occasions, duck and goose also may be available in supermarkets. These birds, however, have higher levels of fat and cholesterol.

Figure 10.3
Continued

1 — JOWL

2 & 4 — CLEAR PLATE AND FAT BACK
Lard   Fatback

3 — BOSTON SHOULDER
Blade Boston Roast   Blade Steak
Boneless Blade Boston Roast   Pork Cubes
Smoked Shoulder Roll

5 — LOIN
Boneless Top Loin Roast (a, b, c)   Center Loin (b)
Canadian Bacon (a, b, c)   Smoked Loin Chop (b)
Back Ribs (a, b)   Top Loin Chop (b)
Tenderloin (b, c)   Loin Chop (b)
Butterfly Chop (b, c)   Rib Chop (b)
Blade Loin (a)   Sirloin (c)
Country-style Ribs (a)   Sirloin Cutlet (c)
Blade Chop (a)   Sirloin Chop (c)

6 — LEG (FRESH OR SMOKED HAM)
Boneless Leg (a, b, c)   Smoked Ham, Rump (a, b)
Sliced, Cooked, Boiled Ham   Smoked Ham, Shank (c)
  (a, b, c)   Boneless Ham Slice (b)
Boneless Smoked Ham (a, b, c)   Center Ham Slice (b)
Canned Ham (a, b, c)

7 — BACON (SLAB OR SLICED)

8 — SPARERIBS
Spareribs   Salt Pork

9 — PICNIC SHOULDER
Fresh Arm Picnic   Fresh Hock
Smoked Arm Picnic   Smoked Hock
Arm Roast   Neck Bones
Ground Pork   Arm Steak

10 — PIG'S FEET

Note: Cubed Steak, Sausage, and Ground Pork are made with Boston Shoulder, Picnic Shoulder, Loin, or Leg cuts.

Figure 10.4

CUTS OF LAMB

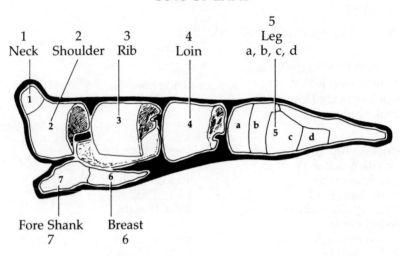

The USDA inspects poultry that is sold in interstate commerce. Most of the poultry in supermarkets is top grade or Grade A poultry. This means that the poultry should be tender, meaty, and should have a good appearance. Poultry that receives grades B or C generally is tough and is reserved for soup, stews, or commercial use.

Listed below are tips on selecting chicken, turkey, and Rock Cornish game hens.

Chicken: Smaller chickens tend to be leaner than large ones. Capons (castrated males) and stewing chickens have higher fat contents than broilers and fryers. Roasting chickens also are slightly higher in fat than broilers and fryers.

The legs and wings on chickens should spring back quickly when gently pulled away from the bird. A flexible breastbone is a sign of a young, tender chicken. The tip of the breastbone should bend readily. If it is stiff and fails to yield easily to pressure, the bird may be old and tough.

Figure 10.4
Continued

1 — NECK
Neck Slices

2 — SHOULDER
Boneless Shoulder   Boneless Blade Chops
Cushion Shoulder   Blade Chops
Square Shoulder   Arm Chops

3 — RIB
Rib Roast   Rib Chops
Crown Roast

4 — LOIN
Loin Roast   Boneless Double Loin Chop
Boneless Double Loin Roast   Loin Chops

5 — SIRLOIN and LEG
Sirloin Roast (a)   Boneless Rolled Leg (a, b, c, d)
Boneless Sirloin Roast (a)   American-style Leg (b, c, d)
Sirloin Chop (a)   Center Leg (b, c)
French-style Leg (a, b, c, d)   Leg Chop or Leg Steak (b, c)
Sirloin Half Leg (a, b)   Hind Shank (d)
Shank Half Leg (c, d)

6 — BREAST
Breast of Lamb   Boneless Riblets
Rolled Breast   Spareribs
Stuffed Breast   Stuffed Chops
Riblets

7 — FORE SHANK

Note: Lamb Stew Meat or Ground Lamb is made from any cut. Cubed Lamb Meat
or Cubed Lamb Steaks and Patties are made from thick, boneless cuts.

The color of the skin makes little difference in the taste or texture of the chicken. Yellow skin simply means that the chicken
was fed primarily corn, while white-skinned chicken has been
fed other types of grain. Chicken with skin that is rough, overly
dry, broken, bruised, or tinged with purple should be avoided.

It generally is more economical to buy a whole chicken and
cut it into parts at home than to buy prepackaged parts. But if

everyone in the family prefers drumsticks, for instance, these can be bought packaged separately.

Turkey: Fresh turkeys, when available, usually have a better flavor and texture than frozen turkeys. Frozen birds often are self-basting, which means they have been injected with butter and other fats. This, of course, adds calories. Male and female birds (toms and hens) usually are identical in flavor, juiciness, and tenderness, but hens tend to cost slightly more per pound. The size of the turkey makes little difference in taste, texture, or tenderness.

Plump, large-breasted birds with meat extending well over the breastbone usually have the best flavor. The skin should be creamy white to pale yellow, smooth, and damp. Turkeys with skin that is purplish, dry, or broken should be rejected.

Rock Cornish Game Hens: Breeding Cornish gamecocks with Plymouth Rock chickens has produced small birds called Rock Cornish game hens. They contain all white meat, and when the skin and visible fat are removed, they are quite low in fat and cholesterol.

The best game hens are plump with yellowish, smooth skin. The most tender hens are young, from 5 to 7 weeks old. Hens that are more than two pounds tend to be tougher and dryer than smaller birds.

Seafood

Seafood, like chicken, has increased in popularity in recent years because, in general, it is a good source of protein and supplies less fat and fewer calories than red meat. Many types of fresh, frozen, and canned fish and shellfish are available in supermarkets.

Some kinds of seafood are higher in fat content. Examples are albacore, bloaters, butterfish, bluefish, chub, eel, herring, mackerel, pompano, salmon, sardine, shad, smelt, sprat, canned tuna in oil, trout, and whitefish. Sardines, anchovies, caviar, fish roe, and canned tuna in oil are high in cholesterol as well as fat. Leaner varieties of fish include sole, flounder, red snapper, turbot, grouper, halibut, and canned tuna in water.

Mollusks (clams, oysters, mussels, scallops) and crustaceans (crabs, lobsters, shrimp, crawfish) are higher in cholesterol than most types of fish, but shellfish generally are low in fat.

Below are hints for buying fish and shellfish.

Fish: The key to good fish is freshness — the fresher the better. Fresh fish do not have an offensive fishy odor. Saltwater fish tend to have a slightly stronger smell than freshwater fish.

The best, freshest fish will have glossy, bright skin with good color. The scales should be shiny and stick tightly to the body of the fish. The flesh should be firm, yielding slightly when pressed gently, but the meat should spring back into place when pressure is released. The eyes of fresh fish should bulge from the head, and the gills should be clear red. Freshness can be tested by placing the fish in cold water. Fresh fish will float.

Fish with sunken eyes, an unpleasant smell, or soft flesh should be avoided. Loose scales, a dull color, or a whitish film covering the skin may mean that the fish has been allowed to dry out. Fish with any of these characteristics should be rejected.

Mollusks: Most of the common mollusks are bought while still alive. Bivalves (mollusks with two shell halves that are hinged together), such as clams, oysters, and mussels, should be bought only if the shell is tightly closed. Bivalves with open, broken, or cracked shells should be avoided.

Live, fresh clams should not float when they are placed in cold water. Mussels can be tested for freshness by trying to slide the two halves of the shell against each other. If they move, the mussel usually is filled with mud.

Tiny bay scallops or larger sea scallops (both members of the bivalve family) usually are sold out of the shell. The part that is eaten is the muscle that controls the hinge of the shell. Fresh scallops should have a sweet smell, and little liquid should be in the container. Fresh bay scallops should be shiny, moist, soft, and light pink in color. Sea scallops should be firmer in texture and filmy white in color.

Abalone is the foot of a large single-shell mollusk. It is popular in California and available fresh primarily on the West Coast. Light-colored abalone steaks that are flexible, shiny, and moist usually are the most flavorful.

Crustaceans: Fresh crabs, lobsters, crawfish, and shrimp often are available in supermarkets depending on the region and the season. Live crabs, lobsters, and crawfish sometimes are displayed in large tanks in supermarkets. Live shrimp rarely are available in grocery stores, but in saltwater areas they often can be found in bait shops or at roadside stands.

When buying crabs, lively ones that have all their claws and legs intact are the best. Crabs that are heavy for their size usually have more white meat inside, and the larger the claw, the more meat it will contain. Crabs that have an ammonia-like odor or a lot of mud on their shells should be avoided.

Live lobsters and crawfish also should be active and heavy for their size. They should be dark blue-green in color. The females usually have sweeter, more tender, more flavorful meat than males. Lobsters and crawfish should have large tails, and the best lobsters have large claws.

Shrimp should also be bought when it is as fresh as possible. Fresh shrimp should be dry, firm, and olive green in color. Shrimp tends to go bad quickly, so smell and texture usually are good indications of freshness. There is little difference in taste between large shrimp (sometimes called prawns) and small shrimp.

Eggs and Dairy Products

Important vitamins and minerals abound in the dairy case at the grocery store. This is where milk, cheese, butter, yogurt, and eggs are stored in refrigerated units.

Milk and milk products are primary soures of calcium, riboflavin, high-quality protein, vitamin D, and phosphorus. Milk also supplies vitamin A, thiamin, and niacin. Eggs are good sources of high-quality protein, iron, copper, phosphorus, vitamin A, riboflavin, vitamin B_{12}, vitamin D, and thiamin.

Eggs: At one time thought of as one of nature's perfect foods, eggs recently have come under attack for their high cholesterol content. The yolk of one egg contains approximately 275 milligrams of cholesterol, a figure that approaches the 300-milligram-a-day maximum recommended by most registered dietitians for older children and adults. *Egg WHITES are excellent sources of high-quality protein, and they are low in cholesterol and calories.*

Eggs are graded by the United States Department of Agriculture depending on their cleanliness and soundness of shell, the amount of air in the shell, and the way the yolk and white hold together. The top-ranked eggs, Grade AA, are found mainly in fancy restaurants and gourmet shops. Grade A eggs are the kind generally carried in supermarkets. Both grades AA and A are used for frying, poaching, and boiling because the white and yolk stay together well and produce attractive egg dishes. Grade B eggs have thinner yolks and more white, and they tend to spread out when cooked. These eggs are used for commercial baking and scrambling.

Egg size, which has nothing to do with grades, ranges from peewee to jumbo, with large and extra large being the most popular sizes. When looking for the best egg buy, compare prices with sizes. If the price difference between any two egg sizes is more than 8 cents, then the smaller eggs usually are the better buy.

Although freshly laid eggs have more flavor, supermarket eggs are sufficiently fresh. Freshness of egg can be judged by placing it in cold water. If the egg floats or tips upward, it is an old egg and should not be used.

The yolk and white of a fresh egg will hold together well when the egg is cracked open onto a flat surface. The yolk should form a high yellow dome, and the white should be thick and translucent. As the egg gets older, the yolk flattens and the white becomes thin. A dark red speck in the yolk simply means the egg has been fertilized. Fertile eggs are not more nutritious than others. Unless the red speck is undesirable for the sake of appearance, there is no need for concern and no need to remove it.

The color of the shell — white, cream, or brown, depending on the breed of chicken — does not affect the taste, texture, or nutritional value of the egg. Also, yolk color, which can range from light yellow to vivid orange, will not affect flavor. Color of the yolk is influenced by the type of feed and heredity.

Milk: The variety of milks offered in supermarkets is wide. Milk sold in stores has been pasteurized to destroy microorganisms, and homogenized to keep the fat globules (cream) from separating from the milk. Most milk also has been fortified with vitamin D, and skim milk usually has been fortified with vitamin A, which is present naturally in the fat of whole milk.

Whole milk is at least 3.25 percent fat and 8.25 percent protein, lactose, and minerals. Low-fat milk and skim milk contain similar amounts of protein, lactose, and minerals but less fat. Non-fat dry milk solids have been added to some brands of low-fat milk to increase the protein content. This might be listed on the label as "high protein," or "protein fortified." Low-fat milk contains 1 or 2 percent fat, and skim (or nonfat) milk contains less than 0.5 percent fat.

When shopping for milk for children older than 2 years of age and adults, the less fat the better. Very young children need the fat that whole milk supplies; however, after the age of 2 years, fat in milk does little but add extra calories and cholesterol. Low-fat and skim milk supply the same nutrients as whole milk but with less fat and cholesterol and fewer calories.

Cream: The percentage of fat in commercial cream varies greatly. Half and half, a mixture of milk and cream, contains anywhere from 10.5 to 18 percent fat. Fat content of light cream ranges from 18 to 30 percent. Light whipping cream contains from 30 to 36 percent fat, and heavy cream contains from 36 to 40 percent fat.

Cultured Milk Products: Buttermilk usually is made from pasteurized skim or low-fat milk that has been treated with bacteria cultures to produce a heavy consistency. Yogurt, made with whole, low-fat, or skim milk, also is treated with bacteria cultures to produce a thick texture. Sour cream or sour half and half are made by adding cultures to homogenized cream or half and half.

Butter: Butter is made from fresh cream and is available in two varieties: sweet (unsalted) butter and lightly salted butter. Butter, by law, must have a fat content of at least 80 percent. The majority of this is saturated fat and, as a result, butter is high in cholesterol.

Margarine: Recently, many people in developed countries have begun eating less butter, relying more on margarine, which has no cholesterol, less saturated fat, and more polyunsaturated fat. Margarine has the same caloric value as butter — and it usually costs less. Diet margarines, which generally have a higher water content and lower calorie content than regular margarines, also are available. Margarines also may contain salt, dyes, preservatives, and other additives.

Those who think the taste of margarine cannot compare with the taste of butter but are concerned about cholesterol, may combine butter and margarine. Some companies package such combinations, but it is easy and more economical to soften a stick of each and blend them together at home.

Cheese: Supermarkets usually carry a variety of bulk cheeses in their deli sections as well as prepackaged cheese in the dairy section. The large assortment of cheeses can be placed into three general categories: unripened cheese and ripened cheese (both of which are called natural cheese), and processed cheese.

Unripened cheese is produced when heat or lactic acid is added to milk to separate it into chunks of curd and liquid whey. The whey is drained off, and varying amounts of cream or milk are added to the curd to make cottage cheese, farmer's cheese, pot cheese, and ricotta cheese. This process also is used to make feta, mozzarella, and cream cheese.

Ripened cheese, such as cheddar, Swiss, Muenster, and Parmesan, is made by adding bacteria culture to the curd and allowing the cheese to ferment. The consistency of the cheese depends on the amount of whey left in it (less whey leads to a firmer cheese), and the flavor depends on the type of milk used, the length of aging, and the humidity and temperature of the cheese as it ages.

Processed cheese begins as natural cheese but it is chopped, blended, and pasteurized. Various additives often are introduced to provide the desired consistency. American cheese is the most commonly used processed cheese.

Other processed cheeses, such as "cheese food," contain a variety of natural cheeses, thickeners, stabilizers, flavors, and colors. "Cheese spreads" are processed cheeses to which gums, fats, and liquids have been added.

Most cheeses are high in fat and cholesterol. Hard cheeses

and processed cheeses usually contain more saturated fats than most soft and natural cheeses.

Unripened cheeses, such as cottage cheese, are the most nutritious varieties for everyday use. The most healthful cottage cheese is the low-fat or uncreamed variety. Most farmer's, mozzarella, and ricotta cheeses are made with skim milk. Some are made with whole milk. Other kinds of cheese with the word "imitation" on the label have vegetable fats added.

Breads and Cereals

The bakery section of the market offers a wide array of white, whole-wheat, rye, pumpernickel, sour-dough, raisin, pita, and assorted-grain breads from which to choose. For the past half century, white bread (made with wheat flour that was milled after the germ and bran were removed) has been the most popular. But whole-grain breads (made with all parts of the grain, including the germ and the bran) have surged in popularity as more emphasis is placed on fiber in the diet.

Whole-grain breads provide the best source of carbohydrates, vitamins, minerals, and fiber. "Wheat," however, does not always mean whole wheat. Appearance of the loaf alone will not tell the full story. For example, bread that is darker in color may appear to be whole-wheat bread, but it may be made with refined flour to which caramel coloring or molasses is added. Certain brands, advertised as high in fiber, contain wood pulp, sometimes identified on the label as alpha cellulose. The shopper, therefore, should be sure to read the labels on breads closely.

If a family prefers white bread, it should be enriched with some of the nutrients (B vitamins, in particular) that were removed during the refining process. Enriched white bread may contain most of the nutrients found in whole-grain breads, but it will lack the fiber.

Whole-grain cereals, like whole-grain breads, are more nutritious than their refined counterparts. Many cereals contain high levels of sugar or salt (see Tables 2.13 and 2.28). Granola, thought of as a healthful cereal choice, usually has a high percentage of sugar and, therefore, calories.

Rice is available in many forms and varies greatly in nutritional value. Rice loses nutrients as it is polished from brown rice to white rice. While the protein in polished white rice may be more digestible, some of the protein and many of its B vitamins and minerals are lost in the process. Parboiled or converted white rice contains less nutrients than ordinary rice but more than instant white rice, which contains less nutrients than all other categories.

FOOD LABELING

Shopping involves one choice after the other, and consumers need as much information as possible to make the best selections. Some of that information can be found on food labels. Although food labels continue to have limitations, great progress has been made in the past decade in addressing consumers' needs for information and their demands for learning what is in the food they buy. Labels can be a valuable resource for careful shoppers, but they must know how to read and understand them.

Federal law requires that most manufactured foods carry specific information on their labels. The name of the product, the variety or style of the product, the net weight of the food itself, and the name and address of the manufacturer or distributor must be included. Also, federal regulations require that all ingredients used in the manufacturing of a product be listed on the label. Specific quantities of each ingredient are not listed. (See Figure 10.5, a sample label.)

Ingredients are listed on labels in decreasing order by weight.

This means the item listed first is the predominant ingredient, by weight. For example, if the ingredients list on a can of beef stew indicates "carrots, potatoes, beef, gravy, salt," then this product contains more carrots than potatoes, more potatoes than beef, more beef than gravy, and more gravy than salt. A shopper who wants a meaty stew should be aware that the predominant ingredient in this product is carrots. On the sample

Figure 10.5

SAMPLE LABEL

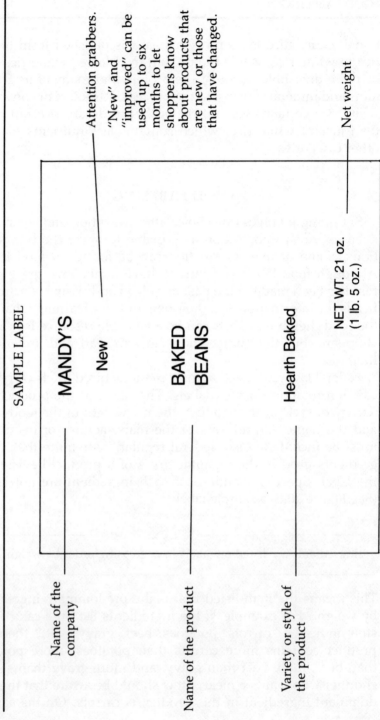

Name of the company

Attention grabbers.
"New" and "improved" can be used up to six months to let shoppers know about products that are new or those that have changed.

MANDY'S

New

BAKED BEANS

Name of the product

Hearth Baked

Variety or style of the product

NET WT. 21 oz. (1 lb. 5 oz.)

Net weight

Nutritional information (needed only on "enriched" or "fortified" food, products that claim to affect health, and those that give calorie and/or fat content on label)

Nutritional Information

Serving Size	8 oz.
Servings Per Container	2⅝
Calories	330
Protein	16 g.
Carbohydrate	49 g.
Fat	8 g.
Sodium	770 mg.
Potassium	849 mg.

Percentage of U.S. Recommended Daily Allowance (USRDA)

Protein	25	Calcium	10
Vitamin A	*	Iron	40
Vitamin C	*	Phosphorus	25
Thiamin	2	Magnesium	25
Riboflavin	6	Zinc	10
Niacin	6	Copper	20
	* = less than 2%		

INGREDIENTS: Small pea beans with pork in sauce containing water, brown sugar, salt, white sugar, and mustard.

Ingredient list (listed in decreasing order by weight)

Mandy's Food Company
1000 Shadow Street
Hagerstown, MD 21740

Name and address of the manufacturer

label in Figure 10.5, small pea beans are listed first and, thus, are the predominant ingredient.

The ingredient list also must tell the shopper what type of fats or oils are used in the product. Sometimes the label lists the specific oil, such as corn oil or soybean oil, but often information on fats is vague. For example, some manufacturers list "vegetable oil" and do not indicate which vegetable oils were used. Other manufacturers list many types of oil — some polyunsaturated and some saturated — and state that one or more of these oils were used. Consumers who are trying to lower cholesterol have no idea whether the food is high or low in saturated fat.

A major problem with the current labeling regulations is that the Food and Drug Administration exempts more than 300 food items from the ingredient-labeling requirement. These food items have standard recipes upon which the food manufacturers and the government have agreed. Cocoa products, flour, pasta, cheese, canned fruits, jellies, tomato products, and margarine are among those foods exempted from the labeling laws. The ingredients can be listed on the label, but the manufacturer is not required to provide this information unless the "official" recipe is changed in some way.

Another problem with labeling regulations is that variations of the same ingredient may be included in the list. Sugar, for example, may be disguised in several forms — honey, sucrose, corn syrup, dextrose, lactose, and molasses. Even if sugar is not listed as the first ingredient in a product, it may be the most plentiful when all its forms are added together.

The labels of three categories of foods are required to include nutritional information in addition to the ingredient list. These categories are: products that claim to be "fortified" or "enriched"; products that claim on the package or through advertisements to affect health or growth; and products that give the fat or caloric content on the label. Many food manufacturers voluntarily place nutritional information on packages as a service to consumers even if it is not required.

Nutritional information includes the size and number of servings in the package, number of calories in a serving, and amount of protein, carbohydrates, and fat in a serving. (The Food and

Table 10.3
LABELING DATES

Pull date	Found commonly on breads, dairy products, and deli meats. This represents the last day the store should sell the product. It usually is denoted by a phrase such as, "Sell by Jan. 1."
Freshness date	Used on meats and some packaged snack foods. This date tells shoppers when the product may become stale. Phrases such as, "Better if used by Jan. 1," or "Remains fresh at least one week after date stamped," carry this information.
Expiration date	Used on milk and yeast. This date tells the consumer that the product may be spoiled or ineffective after the stamped date. Phrases such as, "Do not use after Jan. 1," are expiration dates.

Drug Administration, however, allows the label amounts to vary as much as 20 percent higher or lower than the actual amounts.) Nutritional information also includes the percentage of the USRDA for adults (see Chapter 2) for protein, vitamins, and minerals. Some manufacturers, however, do include the sodium, potassium, cholesterol, or sugar content of the product as well. Beginning in July 1986, sodium content of foods must be listed on labels. This requirement was passed in response to strong consumer pressure.

When comparing nutritional information of one brand to another, shoppers must consider the size of a serving. A brand that appears to have more protein, vitamins, and minerals may have a serving size that is twice as large as most other brands. In addition, a product that appears to be lower in sodium or calories than other brands may simply have a smaller serving size.

Dates often are printed on labels or somewhere on the package to let shoppers know they are buying fresh foods, to let distributors know when to take certain perishable items off the shelf, or to indicate when the product may spoil or lose taste or nutrients. Table 10.3 describes three types of labeling dates that are used commonly today.

In general, the Food and Drug Administration and food manufacturers have been responsive to consumer needs. During the past decade the information provided has improved considerably. A decade ago a consumer knew more about the nutrient composition of dog and cat food than about food for people. Fortunately, this is not the case today.

A wise consumer will read labels carefully and make decisions based on the information provided.

FOOD PREPARATION

All the careful shopping described above can result in a kitchen full of nourishing, fresh, and wholesome food. But these foods must be prepared sensibly to keep their flavor and food value. Unwise preparation and cooking methods can destroy valuable vitamins, ruin food texture, or add too much unnecessary fat, sugar, or salt.

One of the most common, unnecessary cooking practices is adding salt or sugar to food. Many cooks automatically pour salt, or sometimes sugar, into boiling water before vegetables or pasta are added. Many people shake salt on or rub it into meat before it is broiled or roasted. (The potential disadvantages of too much sugar and salt are discussed in Chapter 2.) Children will not miss these if they do not become accustomed to them early. A delicate hand with salt and sweeteners will make meals more healthful and flavors more subtle. Salt, for example, draws water out of foods, and valuable vitamins, minerals, protein, and carbohydrates dissolved in the water end up in the salted cooking water or in the pan. Too much also can disguise the natural flavors and sweetness of vegetables.

Fruits and Vegetables

Most fresh fruits and many vegetables are delicious when served raw, and they keep most of their nourishment this way. Raw fruit or vegetables can be mixed together in a salad, served in small pieces with a dip, or eaten whole as a snack.

Even washing can destroy some valuable vitamins and minerals. Fresh fruit and vegetables, therefore, should be rinsed quickly under running water and not soaked. If fruit or vegetables, however, are caked with dirt, have pesticide or fertilizer residues on the surface, or have been coated with wax they should be scrubbed well under running water. It may be necessary to remove the peel before using them. In addition, breaking apart fresh fruit and vegetables initiates an enzyme reaction that can destroy vitamin C; therefore, cutting, tearing, or chopping should be delayed until just before they are to be used.

Cooking fresh fruit and vegetables decreases their food value, but the loss can be kept to a minimum if wise cooking methods are practiced. For example, the less water used and the less time the produce is cooked, the more nutrients are retained. Many important vitamins and minerals dissolve in water, so when food is placed in water, some nutrients are drawn out of the food and into the water.

Cooking vegetables and fruits in a microwave oven is a good way to save vitamins and minerals because little or no water is used. Pressure cooking and steaming produce also are good cooking methods because the food does not come into direct contact with water. Some vitamins and minerals, nevertheless, are lost in the steam. If the cooking water is used in that same meal — in soups, gravies or sauces, for example — then the nutrient loss is decreased. Stir frying (cooking food quickly in hot oil) is another cooking method that leads to minimum vitamin and mineral loss. The fat adds extra calories to the vegetables, so only small amounts of polyunsaturated fats should be used if this cooking method is chosen. (See Chapter 2.)

If fruits and vegetables must be boiled, they should be cooked for a short time in as little water as possible, and the cooking water used during the meal. Vegetables and fruit cooked in the skin keep more of their vitamins and minerals than if they are peeled first. Potatoes, beets, carrots, turnips, and other root vegetables, which may have some dirt on the surface, can be scrubbed well rather than peeled.

Fewer vitamins and minerals are lost if vegetables or fruit is cooked whole or cut in large pieces. They should be cooked just before they are to be served and should not remain in the cooking water for a long time because vitamins and minerals will

Table 10.4
THE EFFECTS OF FREEZING AND CANNING
Sample: 100 grams of green beans (3½ oz.)

	Sodium (mg)	Vitamin A (RE)*	Vitamin C (mg)
Product type			
Fresh, raw	7	120	19
Fresh, cooked in a small amount of water without salt and drained	4	109	12
Frozen, cooked without salt, drained	1	115	5
Canned			
(Solids and liquid)	237	58	4
(Drained solids)	236	93	3

*Retinol Equivalents.

leach out. Baking soda (sodium bicarbonate) added to cooking water may keep vegetables bright green, but it destroys much of the vitamin C and thiamin in the food.

Frozen fruits and vegetables are the next best thing to fresh. Defrosting them before cooking loses vitamins and minerals. As with fresh, frozen fruit and vegetables should be cooked in as little water as possible, for a short period of time, and the cooking water should be used in the same meal whenever possible.

Vitamin and mineral loss is greatest with canned fruit or vegetables because they usually are packed in water. If the liquid from the can is added to a gravy or boiled down into a sauce and poured over vegetables, some of the vitamins and minerals can be recaptured.

Almost any kind of processing, such as refrigerating, freezing, canning, or cooking, will lead to loss of some valuable vitamins and minerals in food. In addition, processing often adds undesirable ingredients, such as sodium, to food. Table 10.4 shows how processing and preparation can affect green beans.

As Table 10.4 shows, fresh, raw green beans are low in sodium, high in vitamin A, and contain some vitamin C. Canned green beans have considerable sodium and less vitamin C, which is water soluble. The vitamin A content changes little because this vitamin is fat soluble. Fresh cooked and frozen cooked green beans are comparable.

If fresh beans are to be used immediately, then they probably have higher food value than frozen. If they will sit in the refrigerator for several days before they are cooked, then the level of some vitamins and minerals may decrease; therefore, the frozen variety may be better. Vegetables for freezing are picked when they are ripe, which is when they are at the peak for vitamin and mineral content, and then quickly frozen to preserve nutrients.

Meats, Poultry, and Seafood

Cooking meats gently enough to retain vitamins and minerals while reducing the saturated fat content is tricky business. The leanest cuts of red meats, which are the most healthful, usually are prepared using long cooking times and moist heat, such as pot roasting, stewing, and braising. These methods result in greater loss of thiamin, niacin, and riboflavin into the cooking liquid. (Many of these water-soluble vitamins, however, can be obtained from other sources, such as whole-grain breads.) If the cooking liquid is used as a gravy or sauce, some of the vitamins are saved. If time permits, the liquid should be cooled so the fat can be skimmed off. Faster cooking methods, such as broiling, frying, and roasting allow the meat to retain more of its vitamins.

Thiamin and several other minerals are sensitive to high heat, so meats that are rare may be richer sources than well-done meats. Pork, however, should never be served rare because it must be cooked long enough to kill harmful organisms. (Pork must reach a core temperature of 150 to 160 degrees F.)

Excess fat should be trimmed off of red meat before and after cooking. With poultry, the skin, which is primarily fat, and the fatty deposits under the skin and around the tail can be removed before cooking if a moist, slow method is used. Skin can also be removed before serving. Skin, however, is often considered a tasty part of a chicken. The choice of whether to eat it could depend on the amount of fat in the rest of the meal or the family's diet in general. Serving chicken dishes that use cheese, tomato sauce, herbs and spices, sauces, vegetables, and pasta can be a good way to get rid of the skin and fat and still serve a nourishing chicken dish the family will enjoy.

Charcoal broiling is another way to reduce the fat content of meats. Research shows, however, that charcoal smoking (as opposed to broiling) for a long time may lead to the formation of carcinogens in red meat, chicken, and fish. Meats can be partially baked or parboiled before they are placed on the grill to reduce the amount of smoking. This is especially effective for chicken, which takes a long time to cook on the grill. Keeping the lid of the grill open while charcoal broiling meats decreases the amount of smoke.

Other Food Preparation Tips

Rice and pasta should not be rinsed with fresh water after they are cooked because many of the vitamins and minerals that are released into the cooking water cling to their surface as the water is absorbed.

The amounts of sugar, salt, shortening, and oils that are called for in recipes usually can be reduced significantly without affecting the final product. Also, when recipes require milk or cream, skim milk, low-fat milk, or buttermilk often can be used to reduce the level of saturated fat. Careful experimenting will show how this can be done.

Low-fat yogurt can be substituted for sour cream for most dishes.

When cooking with eggs, it is a good idea to use more egg whites and fewer egg yolks. Yolks are high in cholesterol and fat, while egg whites are low in cholesterol, fat, and calories and are good sources of high-quality protein (albumin). (The unused raw egg yolks can be fed to cats and dogs and will help keep their coats shiny and healthy.) Again, whether to eat a lot of egg yolks can be put into the context of a family's overall fat and cholesterol consumption.

Cooking in microwave ovens is fast and will lead to small vitamin and mineral losses.

Heavy cookware generally will distribute the heat more evenly and help prevent burning. Skillets made of iron may destroy some vitamins in food; however, cooking in this type of pan will add iron to the diet. Copper and brass pots must be well lined because food can absorb these metals, and large amounts can be harmful. In addition, copper and brass can destroy valuable vitamins. Glass pots let in light, and small amounts of riboflavin, which is sensitive to light, can be lost. Using nonstick cookware can be a good way to decrease the level of fat in the diet because pots and pans do not have to be greased before they are used. Stainless steel, a mixture of iron and other metals, can cause problems for people who are allergic to some kinds of metal. Also, starchy foods can stain the surface, and salt residues can slowly eat through the surface.

Aluminum pots and pans should not be used to cook salty, acid, or alkaline foods because the metal may dissolve and get into food. In addition, aluminum can cause vegetables, such as cabbage, Brussels sprouts, cauliflower, and broccoli, to take on too strong a smell during cooking. Aluminum also can hurt appearance by turning food that is supposed to be white to yellow, orange, or brown. Although some have suggested a link between Alzheimer's disease and aluminum, studies so far have failed to show a strong connection.

FOOD STORAGE

Air, light, moisture, and heat can make food spoil and break down nutrients. Knowing the best way to store foods can preserve food value, reduce spoilage, and prevent formation of harmful bacteria that can make foods toxic — and, sometimes, fatal.

Refrigeration

In general, the shorter the storage time and the cooler the temperature, the less vitamin and mineral loss. When fresh foods are to be used within a few days, the best place to store them is in the refrigerator. Table 10.5 provides guidelines on refrigerator storage times for a variety of food. Refrigerators should be kept between 32 and 40 degrees F to prevent the rapid growth of bacteria, molds, and yeasts. The meat and dairy keepers are the coldest areas and should be kept between 32 and 35

Table 10.5
HOW LONG WILL IT KEEP IN THE REFRIGERATOR?
(32–40 degrees Fahrenheit)

Food	Storage Time
Meat, poultry, seafood	
Uncooked meat and fish	
Roasts, steaks, chops	3 to 5 days
Ground beef, stew meat	1 to 2 days
Organ meat (liver, kidney)	1 to 2 days
Chicken, turkey	2 to 3 days
Fish	2 days
Shellfish	2 to 3 days (30–32 degrees)
Cooked or smoked meat, poultry, seafood	
Ham, uncanned	1 to 3 weeks
Ham, canned	1 year
Hot dogs, opened package	1 week
Cooked meat or poultry dishes	4 days
Fruits and vegetables	
Fruit, fresh, ripe	
Apples, oranges, grapefruit	2 weeks
Apricots, bananas, berries, cherries, grapes, nectarines, pears, peaches, plums	1 week
Pineapples, ripe	5 days
Cooked fruit, most varieties	1 week
Vegetables, fresh, raw	
Asparagus, broccoli, Brussels sprouts, green beans	3 days
Cauliflower, spinach, rhubarb	5 days
Lettuce, green peppers, tomatoes	1 week
Cabbage, carrots, beets, radishes	2 weeks
Green peas (shelled), lima beans, corn	2 days
Green peas (unshelled)	10 days
Cooked vegetables	4 to 5 days
Milk, dairy products, eggs	
Milk, whole, low-fat, skim, buttermilk	5 days
Cream, half and half	5 days
Yogurt	1 to 2 weeks
Butter, margarine	1 to 2 weeks
Cheese	
Cottage, ricotta, farmer's, pot	5 days
American, cheddar, Swiss, mozzarella, Colby, Brie	2 weeks

Table 10.5
Continued

Food	Storage Time
Eggs, in shell, raw	4 weeks
Eggs, hard boiled	2 weeks
Breads, cereals	
Cornmeal, oats, whole-wheat flour (should be refrigerated if not used in two months)	1 year
Biscuits, coffee cake, corn bread	3 days
Pies	
Cream, custard, chiffon, meringue	2 days
Fruit	3 days
Cakes	
Cream fillings, whipped cream	2 days
Baby foods	
Expressed breast milk	1 day
Formula	
Opened powdered	1 to 2 months
Opened liquid	2 days
Baby food, commercial, opened	3 days
Home pureed	2 days

degrees F. In most refrigerators, the areas at the bottom and on the door are the warmest.

Meats, poultry, and fish should be stored in the refrigerator. They should be wrapped loosely in paper or foil to allow air to circulate. This will keep moisture at a low level and retard bacteria growth. Meats should be stored in the coldest part of the refrigerator.

Large cuts of fresh red meat, such as roasts, usually remain fresh up to five days in the refrigerator. Chopped meat should be used within two days. Smoked and cured meats, on the other hand, can remain in the refrigerator for several weeks. Fresh fish should not be kept in the refrigerator longer than two days. Shellfish will not keep in the refrigerator more than a few hours but can be kept in an ice chest sitting directly on ice cubes or below 32 degrees F for two or three days. Fresh poultry should not be refrigerated for more than three days.

Leftover cooked vegetables should be stored in the refrigerator in tightly covered containers. Fresh vegetables should remain in the vegetable drawer, where they will stay crisp for several days. As time passes, the vitamins and minerals as well as the flavor of vegetables will decrease. Fresh peas and lima beans should be refrigerated in their pods and shelled just before they are used.

Potatoes and sweet potatoes should not be refrigerated. Instead, they should be kept in a cool, dry, dark place. Onions (except scallions) also should be kept in a cool, dry, dark place when whole, but they need to be refrigerated once they have been peeled or sliced. Tomatoes should not be refrigerated until they have ripened completely.

Fruit can be left out at room temperature until fully ripe, then refrigerated to slow down the ripening process. Fruit should be stored with sufficient air circulation. Fruit that is bruised or has soft spots should not touch other fruit. The skin of bananas will blacken when in the refrigerator, but the fruit inside will remain firm and fresh for up to a week.

Dairy products and eggs also should be stored in the refrigerator. Milk and cream retain more nutrients for longer periods of time when stored in opaque containers. (For this reason, it is better to buy milk in paper cartons than plastic jugs.) Soft cheeses should be kept in the refrigerator. Hard cheeses can be refrigerated but usually remain fresh for several weeks if kept in a cool, dark place.

Bread remains fresh when wrapped well in foil or plastic and stored in opaque containers in a cool, dark place such as a bread box or pantry. Refrigerating yeast breads will delay the formation of mold but may cause the bread to dry out. Biscuits, muffins, and coffee cakes stay fresh for several days when wrapped tightly in aluminum foil or plastic and stored in the refrigerator. Cakes and pies with cream fillings or whipped cream toppings must be refrigerated. Plain cakes can be kept in a cool place under a large inverted bowl.

Freezing

When food is to be stored for extended periods of time, extra care must be taken to prevent spoilage and retain as many nutrients as possible. In most cases, freezing is the best way to accomplish this. Freezing usually helps maintain good food color, texture, and flavor. Uncooked meats, fish, poultry, hard cheeses, milk, and bread, keep well in the freezer. Most fruit and vegetables — either cooked, blanched (plunged into boiling water for several minutes), or uncooked — freeze well.

Table 10.6 provides guidelines for storing food in the freezer.

Fresh lettuce, cabbage, carrots, cucumbers, radishes, celery, tomatoes, onions, potatoes, and bananas will not freeze well. Breads, cakes, and pastries made with egg whites may not hold up in the freezer. Other foods that should not be frozen include cream sauces, soft cheeses, meringue, and gelatin.

Freezers should be kept at 0 degrees F. Even at these cold temperatures, vitamin loss will be greater for some foods than for others. The vitamin C content of broccoli, spinach, cauliflower, and peaches, for example, may be reduced to half of its original level when frozen for several months. Peas and asparagus, however, can keep more than 90 percent of their vitamin C content for a year or longer in the freezer.

All food should be as fresh as possible when frozen. While freezing will halt growth of bacteria and mold, it will not destroy these microorganisms once they are present in food.

If spoiled food is placed into the freezer, spoiled food will come out of the freezer.

Canning

Canned foods, either commercially canned or home canned, also lose vitamins and minerals with time. This loss, however, is reduced when the cans are kept slightly cooler than room temperature. Most canned foods can be stored for a year if they are kept in a temperature between 50 and 70 degrees F. After opening a can, the unused portion should be refrigerated. Canned meats, fish, and poultry should be used within 2 days of opening; fruits within 1 week; and vegetables within 3 days.

Fruits and vegetables are the most commonly canned foods. Pickles, olives, jellies, jams, and preserves remain fresh and ap-

Table 10.6
HOW LONG WILL IT KEEP IN THE FREEZER?
(0 degrees Fahrenheit)

Meat, poultry, seafood	
Uncooked	
Beef and lamb	9 to 12 months
Pork	4 to 8 months
Veal	4 to 6 months
Sausage, ham, bacon	1 to 3 months
Calves liver	3 to 4 months
Ground beef, stew meat	4 to 6 months
Ham, uncanned	1 to 3 months
Chicken (whole)	8 to 12 months
Turkey (whole)	6 to 9 months
Fish	4 months
Cooked or smoked meat, poultry, seafood	
Ground beef, lamb, veal	4 months
Hot dogs, bacon, cold cuts	1 month
Fish	2 months
Chicken, turkey	3 months
Fruits and vegetables	
Most fresh and cooked fruits	1 year
Fresh juice concentrates	1 year
Fresh and cooked vegetables	
Asparagus, corn, broccoli, Brussels sprouts, squash, green beans, lima beans, green peas	10 months
Milk, dairy products, eggs	
Milk, whole, low fat, skim, cream	3 months
Ice cream, ice milk, sherbet	1 month
Butter, margarine	9 months
Cheese	
Cottage, ricotta	3 months
Cream cheese	1 month
American, cheddar, other hard cheeses	3 months
Eggs, raw, out of shell, whites and/or yolks	6 months
(whole eggs and egg yolks should be mixed with ¾ teaspoon sugar per whole egg or ¼ teaspoon sugar per yolk before freezing)	
Breads, cereals	
Quick breads	
Banana, zucchini, carrot, pumpkin	2 months
Cookies	3 months
Yeast breads and rolls	2 months

Table 10.6
Continued

Baby foods	
Expressed breast milk	2 weeks
Formula, liquid	1 month
Home purees	
Fruit	1 year
Vegetables	1 month
Meats	2 months

petizing for long periods of time when properly canned. Canned meats, poultry, and fish are available commercially, but these foods rarely are home canned today. Freezing is a better method for retaining vitamins, minerals, texture, and flavor.

In canning, the goal is to maintain the desired appearance, flavor, and texture of the food while preventing the growth of harmful bacteria, yeasts, and molds. It is very important to follow instructions or learn from an experienced person. Serious food poisoning can be the result of improper canning.

FOOD POISONING

Caution and common sense are the best protection against food poisoning. Food that has been improperly processed or stored provides an ideal environment for the growth of bacteria, molds, and yeasts. Most of these microorganisms will simply cause food to spoil; a few, however, can lead to uncomfortable, sometimes dangerous, illness. Toxins (poisons) in bacteria can create a variety of problems in the body.

Salmonella and staphylococcus are the two most common causes of food poisoning. The symptoms — diarrhea, nausea, vomiting, cramps, and fever — may be uncomfortable, but rarely are serious or life threatening. Clostridium perfringens, a less common form of food poisoning, usually does not last long and is not serious. In severe cases of food poisoning, such as clostridium botulinum, trichinella spiralis, and paralytic shellfish poisoning, organ function or entire body systems may be affected.

Salmonella

The most common type of food poisoning, salmonella is esti-mated to affect more than 2 million people a year. It is caused by one of the more than 150 various strains of *salmonella* micro-organisms that are toxic to the human gastrointestinal tract.

Salmonella toxins often are found in meats — especially pork — when eaten raw or undercooked. The bacteria also can pen-etrate eggshells that are slightly cracked, as well as unrefriger-ated egg yolks and whites. Dairy products that have been un-refrigerated for several hours and fish and shellfish taken from contaminated waters are potential sources of salmonella. House-hold pets, rodents, turtles, and other animals, including those that are slaughtered for food, also can be carriers of the bacteria. Salmonella most often spreads to humans through poor sanita-tion and improper cooking and storage of food.

Washing hands with soap and water before handling food is *always* necessary.

The first symptoms of salmonella usually appear 6 to 48 hours after eating the contaminated food. Abdominal cramps, fever, headache, vomiting, diarrhea, and chills are the most common signs. These usually subside within one to five days. Severe cases of salmonella poisoning can result in dehydration, espe-cially among young children.

Salmonella bacteria are killed by thoroughly cooking foods in temperatures of more than 140 degrees for at least 10 minutes. Cooked foods, especially meats, fish, shellfish, poultry, eggs, and dairy products, should be served immediately after cooking or else refrigerated after they have cooled slightly.

The bacteria thrive in temperatures between 44 and 115 de-grees F, and they multiply quickly when cooked food is cooled slowly and later warmed. Poultry stuffing is an ideal breeding ground for the bacteria, so after the first roasting all stuffing should be removed from the bird and fully reheated before being served again.

To prevent food poisoning from salmonella, leftovers should

be stored in a refrigerator that is between 32 and 40 degrees F. Leftover foods, especially pork, sausage, and poultry, should be completely reheated before serving. Milk, eggs, coleslaw, potato and macaroni salad, and gravy should be discarded if they are unrefrigerated for more than three hours. Thorough washing of dishes, pans, and utensils in hot, soapy water also helps reduce the risk of salmonella.

Staphylococcus

Staphylococcus food poisoning is caused by a microorganism that multiplies rapidly in dairy products, meats, sandwich spreads, and prepared salads that have been improperly refrigerated. The bacteria find their way onto food from secretions from the nose, throat, pimples, or open staph wounds (a cut or scrape that is infected with staph bacteria).

Symptoms of staph bacteria infection are nausea, vomiting, cramps, fever, and diarrhea. The symptoms can occur from 30 minutes to 8 hours after the contaminated food is consumed, and they usually last for one or two days.

Because the staph toxin is heat resistant, cooking will not destroy it. It is important to prevent staph bacteria from forming in foods. Identifying possible staph-infected foods may be difficult because the bacteria usually cause no odors or discoloration.

Likely sources of staph bacteria are foods that have been left unrefrigerated for several hours, especially dairy products, meats, sandwich spreads, coleslaw, mayonnaise-base salads, sauces, and gravies. *Any foods that have been inadequately stored should be discarded.*

To reduce the risk of staph bacteria, foods should be refrigerated at temperatures between 32 and 40 degrees F. When picnicking, foods, especially those most susceptible to the bacteria, should be stored in insulated coolers that will keep them at a safe temperature until they are eaten. Children's lunch-box sandwiches (especially those made with sandwich spreads, mayonnaise, or deli meats) left for several hours in a warm room, cold cuts displayed in inadequately cooled cases, and food that has remained on warming tables or under heat lamps for long periods of time also may cause staph bacteria to multiply.

Botulism

Clostridium botulism, an extremely dangerous and sometimes deadly form of food poisoning, is quite rare. When eaten, active botulism spores can release a poison that affects the nervous system. The first symptoms usually are nausea, vomiting, dizziness, blurred vision, lethargy, and weakness. Later symptoms may include difficulty in swallowing and breathing, and paralysis. Death can result if paralysis affects the muscles that control breathing. Symptoms set in from one to eight days after the contaminated food is eaten.

Botulism spores are widespread in the environment, but they remain dormant and present no danger when exposed to oxygen. In fact, inactive spores are frequently consumed with foods. These inactive spores, however, can germinate in environments that are free of oxygen and low in acid, such as within cans containing low-acid produce or in packages of vacuum-packed meat. The active spores can be destroyed when high heat is applied to foods. Boiling the contents of a can for 10 minutes, for example, will kill botulism spores. Prolonged exposure to air also will destroy the spores.

The most common source of botulism is low-acid home-canned foods that are improperly processed. (Most vegetables, and all meats, poultry, and seafood are low-acid foods. Most fruits are high acid.) Low-acid home-canned foods should be boiled for at least 10 minutes before they are served.

Commercially canned goods and vacuum-packed meats rarely are sources of botulism because of strict processing regulations and the addition of nitrites and nitrates. Nonetheless, some botulism cases have been traced to commercial foods. Foods that are contaminated with botulism have no offensive odor. Botulism, however, may cause a can or a jar to bulge or leak. *Cans that appear to be defective should be discarded immediately.*

Honey should not be given to children younger than 1 year of age.

Infant botulism, usually caused by feeding honey to children under the age of 1 year old, is a sometimes fatal form of botulism. Symptoms of infant botulism include weakness in sucking, constipation, and listlessness.

Infant botulism is caused by the dormant clostridium botulinum spores that may be present in honey, whether home-gathered or commercial. If an infant is given honey, the spores may germinate in the intestinal tract, and toxic substances may be released from the spores. Apparently, some substance is present in infants' intestines that is not present in older children or adults.

Clostridium Perfringens

Clostridium perfringens is caused by spores that survive the cooking process and multiply in foods when they stand for several hours at temperatures between 45 and 120 degrees. The most common sources are cooked meats, gravies, and casseroles containing meat that are improperly refrigerated.

Symptoms of clostridium perfringens include diarrhea and nausea. Vomiting and fever are not associated with this type of food poisoning. Symptoms usually occur nine hours to one day after eating contaminated food, and they may last one or two days.

To reduce the risk of clostridium perfringens, cooked meats should be cooled rapidly and refrigerated immediately in temperatures no higher than 40 degrees F.

Trichinosis

Trichinosis is caused by tiny worms *(trichinella spiralis)* that find their way into meat, especially pork. Humans can be infected when they eat this meat raw or undercooked. Trichinella worms enter the digestive system and move to the bloodstream and muscles. Symptoms, which occur three to 30 days after exposure, include fever, diarrhea, aches, and swelling. The worms are killed by high, prolonged heat. Pork and pork products, such as sausage and bacon, should be cooked until the core temperature of the meat is 150 to 160 degrees F.

Paralytic Shellfish Poisoning

Toxic microorganisms that live in the sea can cause what is known as red tide, a condition in which great numbers of fish and shellfish die after being infected with bacteria. When humans consume clams, scallops, mussels, or oysters that have been taken from red-tide areas, paralytic shellfish poisoning may result.

Symptoms, which set in within 30 minutes of eating the contaminated shellfish, include a burning sensation in the nose, facial numbness, difficulty in breathing, and sometimes paralysis in one or more parts of the body.

The best way to prevent paralytic shellfish poisoning is to avoid shellfish that has been harvested in red-tide areas. When buying shellfish, especially during red-tide alerts, people should be sure the dealer is reputable.

If parents are careful and knowledgeable about buying, preparing, and storing food, they should find it easy to provide meals that are attractive and nourishing, as well as safe.

11

ADDITIVES

Looks can be deceiving —
it's eating that's believing.

James Thurber

Consumers hold high expecta-
tions of the foods they buy and eat. They demand freshness and
firmness. They demand consistency in taste, texture, color, and
shape. They expect their foods to be clean and bacteria free.
When they open a package they expect the food inside it to be
the same as the food in another package of the same product.

In an effort to satisfy these demands and expectations, food
manufacturers routinely add extra ingredients to their products
during preparation and processing. These extra ingredients, or
food additives, are intended to perform a variety of useful functions. They prevent the growth of microorganisms that cause
spoilage. They preserve food, enhance flavors and colors, create
textures, and prevent separation of ingredients. They keep
foods fresh for long periods of time, and allow seasonal foods
to be offered year round. They make food wet, dry, firm, soft,
foamy, or nonfoamy. And they help reduce food costs.

Additives can also make food more nourishing. Vitamins and
minerals are lost during processing, and manufacturers put
them back into the food in a process called "restoration." Thiamin, niacin, and iron, for example, are lost when whole grains
are processed into cereal. These nutrients are replaced to make
the food value of the final product equal to that of the original.
In addition, manufacturers of flour, bread, whole-grain cornmeal, corn grits, and white rice "enrich" their products with vi-

tamins and minerals according to federal standards. Thiamin and niacin lost during milling are added back to the original levels, but riboflavin is added in greater amounts than in the whole grain. Calcium and vitamin D also may be added.

Many foods are "fortified," which means that vitamins and minerals have been added to make the product more nourishing than it was originally. Often the vitamins and minerals added would not naturally have been in the food. Milk, for example, is fortified with vitamin D, which helps the body absorb calcium; iodine is added to salt; and vitamin A is added to margarine, skim milk, and nonfat dry milk.

Additives also have disadvantages. In recent years, they have been called poisonous, carcinogenic, toxic, and dangerous — and, in fact, some additives have proved to be harmful. Such global statements, however, are misleading because there are more than 3,000 additives, and no single catch-all phrase can be applied to all of them. There are many different additives doing many different things to many different kinds of foods.

Some additives are extracted from natural sources, while others are synthetic compounds created in laboratories. Some synthetic substances can enhance the value of a processed food. For example, calcium propionate, which inhibits the growth of mold, provides some calcium; and synthetic vitamins added to white bread make it more nourishing. Conversely, certain natural substances, such as safrole (a flavoring derived from sassafras), can be harmful. Research has shown that safrole can cause cancer, and its use has been banned.

"Natural" is not always good, and "synthetic" is not always bad.

Additives can be placed into food by the manufacturer, or they can find their way into food accidentally. Unintentional additives, such as pesticide residues, detergents, or molecules of wax, glue, plastics, or metals, often end up in foods as a result of farming practices, handling, packaging, or environmental conditions.

The United States Food and Drug Administration (FDA) is responsible for public safety regarding the use of additives. Prior to 1958, food safety regulations tended to be weak and ineffective. The government shouldered the entire burden of testing additives. This was done infrequently, however, and only after a questionable additive had been used in food for a long time. Often it took legal action to ban a food.

The 1958 Food Additives Amendment to the Food, Drug, and Cosmetic Act strengthened food safety regulations by requiring the food industry to prove the safety of all additives used in processing before a product became available. The amendment, however, excluded additives that were in common use before 1959. These additives were placed on the list of substances deemed Generally Recognized as Safe (GRAS).

Included in the Food Additives Amendment was the Delaney Clause, which calls for the discontinuation of any additive found to produce cancer. This provision does not apply to additives that are on the GRAS list. The FDA, however, has the option of removing any additive's GRAS designation and invoking the Delaney Clause. This clause led to the elimination of cyclamate in 1969 and nearly brought about the elimination of saccharin, nitrates, and nitrites in the 1970s.

In the case of nitrites and nitrates, the food industry lobbied Congress to exempt these two additives from the Delaney Clause, arguing that their role in preventing botulism (see Chapter 10) outweighed other possible health risks. Saccharin also was saved by Congress after industry representatives and many consumers said that the sweetener was necessary for dieters and diabetics.

Additives that have come into use since 1959 and have met the FDA's safety requirements are on the GRAS list. Some others are allowed in food but have not been studied enough for GRAS designation. These additives, such as saccharin and brominated vegetable oil, are allowed on an interim basis. Additives that have been found to be harmful, such as cyclamate, coumarin, and safrole, are on a list of substances prohibited in food.

For some additives, the FDA sets limits on the level that can be used in processing. Usually, this level is the minimum amount required to produce the desired effect, and no more than one-hundredth the amount found to cause health problems. Other additives have no specific limitations. Two of these substances — sugar and salt — are the most commonly used of all additives. Overconsumption of either can be harmful.

Sugar (including table sugar, fruit sugar, corn syrup, honey, and molasses) represents approximately 85 percent of all additives. It is the chief cause of dental disease. Many sugar-laden foods tend to be high in calories and low in nutrients. Filling up on too many of these sugary foods can mean eating less of the foods that contain valuable nutrients. (See Chapter 2 for more information about sugar.)

Salt, which constitutes an additional 10 percent of all additives, has been linked to high blood pressure, heart and kidney disease, and headaches. (See Chapter 2 for more information about salt.)

A growing awareness about the importance of good nutrition and the strong link between some forms of cancer and diet has prompted many questions and concerns about additives. Because additives, though valuable, are seldom essential components of foods, and because they can be controlled and regulated, they have been the focus of much public pressure.

Research continues to reveal possible adverse effects as well as possible benefits of many different additives. This information changes frequently, making it difficult to offer firm recommendations about which additives are safe and which are not. This chapter, therefore, provides information about some of the most common, yet controversial, food additives. Keeping informed about what goes into food is the best way for parents — and all consumers — to decide whether the benefits of eating a food containing certain additives outweigh the risks involved.

COMMON FOOD ADDITIVES

Brominated Vegetable Oil (BVO)

This additive stabilizes oils in fruit-flavored liquids. It is used in some baked goods, carbonated citrus beverages, and some ice creams. BVO is made from vegetable oils — corn, cottonseed, olive, sesame, or soybean — that are blended with bromine. Flavoring oils, which are less dense than water, are combined with BVO to keep them evenly distributed in a product.

Before 1970, BVO was on the GRAS list. The FDA removed that designation when a Canadian study reported a variety of health problems in rats that had been exposed to high doses of BVO for several months. As a result, BVO was placed on the list of additives approved on an interim basis. The FDA allows its use to be no greater than 15 parts per million.

In the body, BVO accumulates in fat tissues. Hazards of prolonged exposure to BVO include damage to the heart, liver, and thyroid. It also has increased the fatty deposits in livers and kidneys, stunted growth, and caused lethargy in test animals. In some laboratory studies, BVO caused defects in the reproductive organs of male animals.

Butylated Hydroxyanisole and Butylated Hydroxytoluene (BHA and BHT)

These two additives are used as antioxidant preservatives, increasing the shelf life of fats and oils by preventing them from becoming rancid. Both additives, which often are used together, are found in many shortenings, vegetable oils, potato chips, potato flakes, cereals, enriched rice, chewing gum, baked goods, beverages, candy, gelatins, ice cream, and many oil-based foods. BHA and BHT, both of which are synthetic compounds, are generally recognized as safe for use in food when the level of each is no more than .02 percent of the total fat or oil content.

When consumed, BHA and BHT are absorbed into the digestive tract, processed in the liver, and excreted. Some residues, however, may accumulate in fat cells. At high levels these residues are suspected of causing enzyme changes that could make the body more susceptible to some types of cancer. Birth defects are another risk of excessive BHA and BHT use. BHA and BHT also are suspected of enlarging the livers and kidneys of some laboratory animals. But the level necessary to produce such a reaction is at least 500 times greater than the amount to which a human would be exposed.

On a positive note, BHA and BHT may help protect the fat-soluble vitamins (vitamins A, D, E, and K) in foods. There is some indication that antioxidants may delay the aging process and increase life span. Fragmentary evidence also indicates that BHA and BHT may lessen the effects of some cancer-causing agents.

Caffeine

Caffeine is a stimulant that occurs naturally in coffee, tea, chocolate, and kola nuts. It is also used as an additive in other food, such as soft drinks, especially cola-based beverages. Much of the bitter-tasting caffeine from kola nuts is removed during the processing, and extra caffeine often is added to produce a tangy flavor. (See Table 3.3 for the caffeine content of selected foods.)

Caffeine is a drug and can be addictive. It stimulates the central nervous system, increases cholesterol in the blood, dilates the arteries to the heart, constricts blood vessels to the brain, and causes blood-sugar levels to rise then rapidly fall. This roller-coaster effect stimulates the desire for more caffeine. Caffeine can produce insomnia, irritability, slight fever, and shakiness. It also has been associated with behavioral changes, especially in children. Caffeine causes some children to be overly active, nervous, and prone to temper tantrums.

High levels of caffeine increase production of stomach acid, which has been linked to the development or irritation of peptic ulcers. Some studies have reported a slight correlation between caffeine consumption and heart disease. Caffeine also has been associated with fibrocystic breast disease. Animal experiments with caffeine have shown that it can cause birth defects and miscarriages. Most physicians recommend that pregnant women avoid caffeine-containing foods and beverages.

Carrageenan

Carrageenan, a natural product derived from a seaweed called Irish moss, is used primarily in dairy products to stabilize, thicken, and gel. It is found in some cheese spreads, chocolate, evaporated milk, ice cream, heavy cream, sour cream, candy, and syrups. It also is used to thicken jellies, add body to carbonated beverages, and prevent excessive foaming in beer.

The additive, which is poorly absorbed by the body, has no

nutritional value. When high doses of carrageenan were administered to test animals over a period of time, the result was fetal damage and death. Experiments with carrageenan have produced intestinal ulcers. There also is some evidence that it could cause cancer.

Until recently, most infant formula manufacturers used carrageenan to increase the shelf life of their products. Although there have been no reported incidents of harmful effects of carrageenan among human infants, most formula companies have removed this additive.

Ethylanediamine Tetracetic Acid (EDTA)

EDTA is an antioxidant agent found primarily in salad dressings, carbonated beverages, canned shellfish (crab, clams, and lobsters), mayonnaise, margarine, processed fruit and vegetables, fruit drinks, and beer. This additive prevents various metal and mineral impurities — which can find their way into food during processing or packaging — from spoiling or altering the taste, color, or odor of a product. EDTA works like a claw to trap contaminants. The additive also can prevent oxygen from reducing the level of vitamin C in processed fruit and vegetables.

Although considered safe at normal levels of use for most people, EDTA has been known to cause severe reactions in people with certain allergies or asthma. At high doses the additive can cause zinc deficiencies and kidney damage. At extremely high doses, EDTA has caused chromosome damage in plant and animal cells.

Monosodium Glutamate (MSG)

This additive has no particular taste of its own, but when combined with other flavors, MSG enhances, intensifies, and brings out subtleties that liven tastes. MSG is found commonly in Chinese food, pastries, candy, condiments, meat, pickles, soups, stews, sauces, and seasonings. Although MSG can be extracted from proteins present in many natural sources, most comes from specially fermented sugar crystals. Corn and seaweed, which are rich sources of glutamic acid, also provide some of the MSG produced today.

Problems with MSG first came to light in 1968, when a physician of Chinese descent described symptoms he experienced after eating a Chinese dinner. These symptoms included headache, a burning sensation in the nape of the neck and forearms, numbness, and tightening of the chest. He named this series of strange sensations Chinese Restaurant Syndrome. A team of physicians traced the source of the symptoms to MSG, which frequently is used in abundance in Chinese cooking, especially soups. Researchers believe that MSG is absorbed rapidly by the bloodstream and travels into nerve endings, causing discomfort.

While the specific ill effects of eating Chinese foods are temporary, excessive consumption of MSG for long periods of time may be associated with permanent health problems. For example, large doses of MSG fed to animals damaged nerve cells in the part of the brain that controls appetite, body temperature, and other key functions. The additive also was found to damage reproductive organs. It has caused female animals to conceive less frequently and to give birth to smaller litters. Some evidence also links MSG with learning disabilities in laboratory animals.

The additive once was used commonly in baby foods, mainly to make these foods more pleasing to parents' palates. Public pressure in the late 1960s and early 1970s caused baby food manufacturers to remove MSG from their products. An FDA review panel concluded in 1980 that MSG, when used in moderation, was not harmful to adults, but nonetheless food manufacturers were advised to reevaluate the quantities used as well as the need for any MSG in processed food.

Nitrites and Nitrates

These multipurpose additives prevent the growth of botulism-causing microorganisms while enhancing food flavor and color. They are added to bacon, corned beef, ham, hot dogs, sausage, smoked fish, smoked poultry, and beer.

Most human exposure to nitrites and nitrates comes not from food additives, but from natural sources. Nitrites are produced in human saliva, and nitrates are found naturally in many vegetables, such as spinach, lettuce, celery, collard greens, turnip greens, beets, radishes, potatoes, turnips, and carrots. Nitrates also may be in drinking water supplies that have been contaminated by fertilizer residues.

Nitrates themselves are not particularly harmful. Most nitrates are excreted from the body. A small percentage of the nitrates consumed, however, can be changed into nitrites by digestive juices. Nitrites may react with hemoglobin (the oxygen-carrying substance in red blood cells) and change it to methemoglobin (a substance that cannot transport oxygen).

Eating nitrites, in most cases, will not alter blood chemistry significantly. But if the percentage of methemoglobin in the blood rises too high, the result may be skin discoloration and shortness of breath. In extreme cases, death may occur. Babies are more susceptible to this condition — known as methemoglobinemia — than adults. For this reason, nitrates and nitrites have been removed from almost all baby foods.

Nitrates and nitrites also can lead to the formation of nitrosamines, which are potent cancer-causing agents. This chemical conversion can occur inside or outside the body. Nitrites combine with byproducts of amino acids called amines, which are found in meat, fish, and other proteins, to produce nitrosamines in the stomach. Nitrosamines also can form inside a food before the product is eaten. This occurs when natural amines in food combine with nitrites during processing. Cooking nitrites at high temperatures (such as frying bacon) also can produce nitrosamines.

Studies show that nitrosamines can affect reproduction. Small fetuses, birth defects, and prenatal death have been observed in lab tests as a result of large doses of nitrosamines.

Phosphoric Acid and Phosphates

Phosphorus is a mineral found naturally in many protein-rich products. The body needs phosphorus to build bones and teeth; break down carbohydrates, proteins, and fats; and form genetic material and cell linings. Phosphorus is needed in equal amounts with calcium to perform these functions. (See Chapter 2.)

When used as an additive, phosphorus usually takes the form of phosphoric acid or one of the common phosphate compounds

— calcium phosphate, sodium phosphate, iron phosphate, sodium acid pyrophosphate, sodium aluminum phosphate, and ammonium phosphate. Phosphoric acid makes beverages more acidic, while phosphates serve as nutrients, emulsifiers, and color retainers. Phosphorus additives are found in many soft drinks, cheeses, cereals, breads, cakes, pastries, powdered foods, dehydrated potatoes, syrups, and cured meats.

Phosphates themselves are not toxic, but because the body needs phosphorus and calcium in equal amounts, an overabundance of phosphorus can create a calcium deficiency. This condition can lead to poor development of bones and teeth in children.

Calcium shortages also may cause osteoporosis in adults. Phosphorus-calcium imbalances most often occur in children and teenagers who drink large quantities of soft drinks and in adults who consume few dairy products.

Propyl Gallate

This synthetic additive is an antioxidant added to vegetable oils, meat products, potato sticks, chicken soup, and chewing gum. It often is used in conjunction with BHA and BHT to retard the spoilage of oils, thus increasing shelf life.

Propyl gallate in large doses is suspected of affecting growth and development. Tests also have shown it to be harmful to the kidneys and livers of test animals. Although no tests have shown a definite connection between propyl gallate and cancer, a 1981 long-term feeding study suggested that the additive could have cancer-causing properties.

Quinine

Quinine is a bitter flavoring in food and drinks. It is found in tonic water, bitters, bitter lemon, and quinine water. Made from the bark of the cinchona tree, quinine has been in common use since the early 1600s, when it was found to be a cure for malaria. It also was used long ago to induce abortions.

Overconsumption of quinine may cause birth defects, particularly fetal deafness or hearing damage. Use of quinine also has been linked with nausea and vision problems. This additive can cause severe allergic reactions in people who are sensitive to it. Quinine water consumed to excess has been found to cause a rare disease known as purpura, in which blood leaks from small blood vessels near the skin, giving the skin a purplish tinge.

Sulfiting Agents

These synthetic additives, derivatives of sulfur, are used in many foods to bleach, preserve, maintain color, and prevent the growth of harmful bacteria. The most common sulfiting agents are potassium bisulfite, potassium metabisulfite, sodium bisulfite, sodium metabisulfite, sodium sulfite, and sulfur dioxide. Sulfiting agents are found in many fresh-sliced and processed fruits and vegetables (in restaurant salad bars), wine, grape juice, carbonated drinks, dehydrated potatoes, and powdered soup mixes.

Sulfite additives can destroy thiamin in food. They restore pink color to meats that age has turned brownish-gray. Some meat producers have used sulfites to deceive customers into buying old, poor quality meats. To curb this practice and to protect vitamin content of foods, the FDA has placed limits on the use of sulfiting agents, prohibiting their use in meats and in foods that are recognized as valuable sources of thiamin.

Sulfites have been controversial recently because they can cause severe reactions in people with asthma or allergies. In fact, sulfites have been linked to death in a number of cases. The FDA has proposed a ban on the use of sulfites on fresh fruits and vegetables. This ban would apply to almost all fruits and vegetables sold in supermarkets, restaurants, and salad bars.

On the positive side, sulfites can help increase the stability of vitamin C. Sulfur dioxide, in particular, helps preserve both vitamin C and beta carotene, which the body converts to vitamin A.

FOOD COLORS

Of all the food additives, food colors are the most controversial. Their use in foods is cosmetic. They give foods a brighter, more appealing appearance. But by doing this they also may mask poor quality, decrease use of more desirable, natural ingredients, or tempt people to eat foods that are nutritionally inferior.

Some added colors are derived from natural sources and actually may enhance nutritional value. For example, ferrous gluconate, which is used to dye black olives a uniform color, is a source of iron; beta carotene, which the body converts to vitamin A, is used as a yellow color in some margarine, butter, and cake mixes.

Concerned consumers have argued that if food colors pose any health risk, these substances should not be used in food products. Food manufacturers counter that shoppers would not purchase pale maraschino cherries, white sticks of margarine, or green oranges. The synthetic food dyes are the targets of most criticism. These dyes, which are the most numerous of all color additives, are highly purified chemicals derived from coal tars.

Currently, the FDA permits the use of nine synthetic dyes in foods. These are Blue 1, Blue 2, Green 3, Red 3, Red 40, Yellow 5, and Yellow 6. Use of a dye called Citrus Red 2 is limited to the skins of oranges, and Orange B can be used to color only the skins of bologna, hot dogs, and other processed meats.

If artificial colors are used in foods, that information must be included on the label. The specific dyes that have been added, however, need not be specified by name. The one exception to this is Yellow 5, which is called tartrazine. The FDA requires that Yellow 5 be identified because it can cause allergic reactions in aspirin-sensitive people.

All of the artificial colors have been indicted for a variety of adverse health effects. Red 40, which is the most commonly used dye today, has been found to cause tumors in test animals. Red 3 may interrupt normal function of the brain and affect behavior. Also, research has shown a link between this dye and thyroid tumors in rats. Studies with Blues 1 and 2 suggest that both could be cancer causing. Green 3, which is rarely used, has caused severe allergic reactions, and it has produced malignant tumors and bladder cancer in laboratory animals. Yellow 6 may affect eyesight when used in extremely high quantities.

Experiments with Citrus Red 2 have shown that it can damage the organs of laboratory animals. The color also can cause cancer. Because it is permitted only on orange rinds and does not seep into the fruit, the FDA continues to allow it. Orange B is permitted, yet it is used rarely today. The dye remains at the surface of food, so small amounts produce the desired color. This dye is suspected of causing cancer, and large amounts have produced liver nodules in dogs.

FLAVORINGS

The FDA recognizes thousands of flavorings — both natural and artificial — for use in foods. In fact, the list of substances in this category is, by far, the lengthiest of any other additive group. Flavorings are found in almost all processed foods. Their most common uses include soft drinks, candy, cereals, desserts, cakes, pastries, condiments, canned goods, and ice cream. The FDA requires that use of artificial flavorings be stated on the label. Specific flavoring names, however, do not have to be listed.

Flavorings sometimes compensate for the lack of the natural, more expensive ingredients. Almost all synthetic flavors mimic natural flavors. The chemical makeup of some synthetic substances, in fact, is identical to the natural ingredients.

Artificial flavors make possible alternatives for food that people cannot eat. Persons who cannot digest milk, for example, can enjoy the taste of ice cream made from artificially flavored soybean powder. Vegetarians who enjoy the taste of meat can eat soyburgers, soya chicken, or vegetable bacon.

As a group, synthetic flavorings have come under criticism because many are not well tested. Some, such as ethyl methyl phenylglycidate, which is a berry flavoring, are suspected of causing reproductive and developmental problems.

Some natural flavorings are harmful. Safrole, as mentioned previously, was banned for use after it was found to produce liver cancer. Nutmeg and mace, both of which come from the myristica tree, can cause intoxication and hallucination when consumed in very large quantities. Smoke flavor, which is made from the condensation of hickory or maple smoke, is suspected of causing cancer. This flavoring is found in some barbecue sauces, cheese, smoked fish and nuts, processed meat, and baked beans.

SWEETENERS

Refined sugar, or sucrose, is by far the most common of all food additives. Other natural sugars, such as corn syrup, honey, and molasses, also constitute a high percentage of the sweet taste that is introduced into many foods during processing. As people have become more and more weight conscious, low-calorie, non-nutritive sweeteners have come into greater use.

Saccharin

Saccharin is the best known, and most controversial, of all non-nutritive sweeteners. In 1984, Americans used more than 1.84 million tons of saccharin, an increase of nearly 70,000 tons from the previous year. Saccharin is found commonly in dietetic foods, particularly sugar substitutes, dietetic canned fruits, low-calorie preserves, frozen foods, and some diet soft drinks.

Saccharin is approximately 400 times sweeter than sugar, and the same amount of sweetness can be obtained for about one-tenth the cost of sugar. One major drawback is saccharin's bitter aftertaste. Food manufacturers, however, have found that adding certain amino acids can help mask the bitterness.

The sweetener was discovered in the late 1800s when a chemist tasted a petroleum derivative and found it to be incredibly sweet. He took out a patent on his sweet discovery, dubbing it "saccharin." It has been available since the early 1900s, but because of the bitter aftertaste, saccharin was not used extensively until 1969. That was the year cyclamate, saccharin's no-calorie, no-aftertaste cousin was banned as a possible cancer-causing additive.

The FDA currently allows saccharin to be used in foods, but it is no longer included on the GRAS list. Instead, it is contained in a section of the Federal Code that allows additives to be used in food pending further study. Saccharin's GRAS designation was removed after studies showed the substance may cause cancer. The FDA tried to ban saccharin in the late 1970s, but responding to public pressure, Congress overruled the decision.

The first hints of saccharin problems arose in the 1950s, when experiments revealed that feeding high doses of saccharin to test animals or implanting saccharin pellets into their bladders caused tumors. These findings were all but ignored until studies in the early 1970s confirmed saccharin's cancer-causing properties. The FDA ordered all products containing saccharin to include a warning stating it is a "non-nutritive sweetener for persons who must restrict their intake of ordinary sweets."

In 1977, a Canadian study concluded that feeding high levels of saccharin to pregnant rats produced bladder cancer in their male offspring. As a result, saccharin was banned in Canada. In the United States, a stronger warning was ordered on all products containing saccharin. This warning, which continues to be required today, reads: "Use of this product may be hazardous to your health. This product contains saccharin, which has been determined to cause cancer in laboratory animals."

Further testing has shown that saccharin may stimulate the appetite and interfere with blood-sugar regulation. Thus, the substance may prove counterproductive to its two main users — diabetics and dieters. Also, scientists have advised pregnant women and young children to avoid saccharin because developing fetuses and growing children may be more vulnerable to its harmful effects.

Aspartame

Aspartame, which is marketed under the name NutraSweet when used as an additive and Equal when used alone as a sweetener, is found mainly in low-calorie soft drinks, breakfast cereals, chewing gum, gelatins, puddings, hot chocolate mixes, and ice cream. It is not used in anything baked because high heat makes it lose its sweetness.

The sweetener has approximately 180 times the sweetening power of sugar, and the same sweetness can be obtained at one-tenth the calorie cost. Aspartame, unlike saccharin, has no aftertaste and requires no cancer risk warning.

The FDA approved aspartame for use in dry foods in 1981, and since that time the substance has enjoyed one of the sweetest success stories among all additives. Aspartame's sales in 1982 reached $74 million, and this figure exploded to $600 million in

1984. The huge jump was attributed to a 1983 FDA decision permitting aspartame in soft drinks.

There has, however, been some bitter with the sweet. Although its manufacturer, G. D. Searle & Co., has claimed that aspartame is one of the most tested additives in history, critics of the substance say that the FDA's decision to approve the sweetener was premature. They cite studies that link severe reactions to the use of aspartame and point to thousands of consumer complaints about the additive.

Aspartame is composed of two amino acids, aspartic acid and phenylalanine. Amino acids are natural substances, and form the basic structures of protein. Most protein molecules are large and are digested slowly. Aspartame molecules, however, are small and are absorbed quickly into the bloodstream.

Some people lack the enzyme necessary to process phenylalanine properly. This enzyme deficiency is an inherited condition known as phenylketonuria (PKU), which causes phenylalanine to accumulate in the bloodstream. (In the United States one out of every 10,000 babies is born with PKU, and one out of every 50 people is a carrier of the PKU trait, although unaffected by the disorder.) Pregnant women who have the PKU trait and have high levels of phenylalanine in their bloodstreams run a great risk of giving birth to brain-damaged babies. Newborns with PKU must be placed on a restricted diet to prevent mental retardation. Aspartame must be avoided by anyone with PKU. Labels of food containing aspartame must bear the statement "Phenylketonurics: contains phenylalanine."

Consumption of aspartame also has been associated with such symptoms as menstrual difficulties, aggressive behavior in some children, severe headaches, vision problems, seizures, depression, and sleep disorders. Animal experiments suggest that aspartame may alter brain chemistry in infants and children.

Aspartame's effectiveness in helping people lose weight also has been challenged. The additive may block production of a vital appetite-controlling brain chemical called serotonin. As a result, consumption of aspartame may make the body crave more sweets.

The FDA has decided that aspartame is safe for consumers' use. Only time and more research will reveal the truth.

Sorbitol

Sorbitol is a sugar alcohol that contains approximately 60 percent of the sweetness of sugar and an equivalent number of calories. It is used in candy, jellies, chewing gum, cakes, pastries, shredded coconut, and frozen desserts.

Because sorbitol is absorbed into the bloodstream slowly, diabetics can consume it. The additive remains in the intestinal tract until it is fermented by natural bacteria. The byproducts of the fermentation process, however, may lead to cramping, diarrhea, and stomach upset.

Unlike saccharin and aspartame, sorbitol must be added in large quantities to obtain the desired sweetness. People who have gastrointestinal problems and children whose digestive systems may be unable to properly process the sweetener may be more vulnerable to its adverse effects. The FDA requires that products containing more than 50 grams of sorbitol be labeled with a statement saying, "excessive consumption may have a laxative effect."

Xylitol

Xylitol, a sugar made from birchwood, will not increase blood-sugar levels as much as most other sugars. As an additive it is used only in sugarless chewing gum, and it apparently causes fewer problems with dental decay than refined sugars. When used in large quantities, xylitol has been known to have a diuretic effect (an increase in the flow of urine). Some studies have suggested that the additive may cause tumors and organ damage in test animals.

UNINTENTIONAL ADDITIVES

Foods go through many steps from the time they are harvested or slaughtered to the time they land on the dinner table. At each step of the journey they can come into contact with a variety of nonfood substances that end up in the finished products, usually in tiny amounts. All of these, including pesticide residues, molecules from packaging materials, solvents, lubricating oils, defoamers, plastics, textile fibers, adhesives, hormones, and antibiotics are known as indirect additives. The FDA regulates the quantities of these allowed in foods.

According to a 1984 survey conducted by the Food Marketing Institute, more than three-fourths of all people in the United States believe that chemical residues pose a serious health hazard. Pesticides and herbicides caused the most concern.

Chlorinated insecticides are used less frequently today than in the recent past; however, residues remain in the environment, and traces of these insecticides are found in the tissues of most plants and animals. Dicholo-diphenyl-trichloroethane (DDT) is the best known of the insecticides.

DDT has produced cancer in laboratory animals and is suspected of causing cancer in humans. Such findings prompted the FDA to ban DDT in 1972, except for a few specific uses. The insecticide, nonetheless, remains a health threat. DDT and many other potent pesticides and herbicides, such as arsenic and lead and mercury compounds, decompose slowly. When plants are dusted or sprayed with these chemicals, residues fall on the leaves and into the soil. These chemicals dissolve in the soil and are carried into plant cells. Residues remain in the soil for many years, so any future produce grown in the treated area will contain the chemical.

The contamination problem multiplies when livestock eat grass that contains residues. Birds may consume insects and seeds that have been exposed to the chemicals, and fish can absorb pesticides through water that has received runoff from treated fields. These pesticides accumulate in the fat cells of animals. The pesticide contamination moves up through the food chain until those living things at the top are involved. Humans, therefore, may be exposed to pesticides through meat and fish, as well as fruit and vegetables.

Pesticides, however, play a key role in agriculture. Currently, farmers lose nearly one-third of their crops to insects, animals, and disease. It is estimated that without pesticides crop losses would double — and so would the cost of food. Research into less dangerous pesticides continues to be important.

Pesticides are just one of the threats to the food supply. Another major environmental problem is industrial chemicals, which have been dumped carelessly into the environment. Polychlorinated biphenyls (PCBs) are the most toxic of these industrial chemicals. PCB compounds can cause cancer and were banned in the United States. Like pesticides, PCBs are slow to break down and will be found in food supplies for many years. These compounds have been identified in fish, poultry, wild birds, beef cattle, milk, and human breast milk.

Another major concern is the use of hormones. Hormones and synthetic hormonal-type products are used to fatten livestock before slaughter. Hormones stimulate production of lean meat and reduce the need for large amounts of expensive grain, thus keeping down the cost of meat. Diethylstilbestrol (DES), a synthetic chemical that has hormonal effects, was used extensively in beef cattle before 1979. The chemical, however, was found to cause a rare form of cervical and vaginal cancer in young women whose mothers had taken DES to prevent miscarriage. In 1979, the FDA banned DES in livestock.

Only a few hormones currently are used on livestock, and most of these are natural hormones including estrogen, progesterone, or testosterone. These hormones usually are implanted in the ears of cattle. In food for human consumption, the FDA allows no more than one six-hundredth the hormone level that would be expected in milk of pregnant cows.

Today, a substance called zeranol is the only synthetic hormonal implant allowed in beef cattle. Derived from moldy corn, zeranol has been controversial because it is suspected of having a connection with thelarche, a condition in which children's reproductive organs develop prematurely.

Another concern is the routine use of antibiotics, which are added to animal feed to reduce infections that may inhibit growth and development. Antibiotic residues may accumulate in meat, causing problems for people who are sensitive to penicillin and other antibiotics. Also, scientists have contended that the consistent use of antibiotics leads to the development of infectious organisms that are resistant to the medications. Use of antibiotics in cattle is not allowed in Canada and many European countries, and some countries will not import meat from the United States for this reason.

IRRADIATION

Irradiation, a process in which food is exposed to radioactive gamma or X-rays to kill bacteria and insects, has gained much attention recently as an experimental way of protecting and preserving food. Irradiation is considered an additive in food, and it is regulated by the FDA. When food is irradiated, this information must be listed on the label.

Currently, irradiation is permitted only on a few foods. It can be used to control microorganisms in spices, control insects in wheat, prevent sprout development in white potatoes, and kill *trichinella spiralis* in pork (see Chapter 10). The FDA, however, is considering the use of irradiation for fresh fruit, vegetables, and several other foods.

Irradiation, as might be expected, is a controversial issue. Its proponents argue that the process keeps perishable food, such as meat, fruit, and vegetables, fresh for longer periods of time and increases the shelf life of unrefrigerated food by killing bacteria, yeasts, and molds that cause spoilage. Irradiation, therefore, could reduce the amount of wasted food and could help decrease world hunger. Unlike some other methods of preserving food, such as canning and smoking, the temperature of the product remains fairly uniform during the irradiation process, so there is little vitamin and mineral loss. In addition, irradiation kills insects and bacteria without leaving pesticide or herbicide residues on food. Proponents point to the fact that military personnel, astronauts, and hospital patients with immune disorders have eaten irradiated food for many years, and no harmful effects have been reported.

Opponents, however, say that there is need for more research on the effects of irradiated food. Only a few studies have been conducted, and some of these have found that animals fed irradiated food have a higher incidence of kidney problems, chromosome damage, and testicular tumors than animals fed non-irradiated food.

Irradiation also has been criticized by consumer groups, who say that the amount of radiation needed to kill insects, such as fruit flies, would harm the flavor and texture of fruit and vegetables. Also, irradiation kills only those insects that are in food when it is treated. Insects can find their way back into food, such as grain, which often is stored for long periods of time.

Irradiation critics argue that there are safer, better tested, and less expensive methods for controlling bacteria and insects. The recent approval of irradiation to kill trichinella spiralis in pork, for example, was unnecessary because there are tests that can detect this parasite in animals. In addition, only a handful of cases of trichinosis from contaminated pork are reported each year. Finally, many people are concerned that if irradiation becomes widespread it could add to the problem of transporting and disposing of radioactive waste.

LIVING AND COPING WITH ADDITIVES

The number of food additives continues to grow, and the number of foods containing additives is rising correspondingly. Few people can lead an additive-free life. Staying informed about additives remains the best way to determine whether the benefits of consuming a certain substance outweigh the risks involved.

Labels can be helpful when selecting foods. The FDA requires that additives be included in the ingredients list of most food items. *A potentially harmful additive used in one brand does not mean that all brands contain the additive.* For example, most hot dogs and bacons contain nitrites, but some producers now make nitrite-free varieties of these meats.

Eating more fresh fruits and vegetables will eliminate many additives from people's diets. Frozen food usually has fewer additives than the canned variety. Artificial flavorings and colors easily can be eliminated from home-prepared foods. Using real meat juices instead of stock cubes eliminates much extra salt. Natural fruit juices are preferable to synthetic fruit flavors. If coloring must be added to foods, natural colorings are usually a better choice than synthetic colors.

Eating a wide variety of foods also will limit exposure to additives. If a food containing a harmful additive is consumed every now and then, the risks will be less than if that food is eaten every day. Cutting down on soft drinks, sweets, and highly processed convenience foods will eliminate a substantial portion of the additives consumed. Replacing these foods with fresh fruits and vegetables, whole-grain breads and cereals, and lean meat, fish, and poultry will not only cut down on additives but will also lead to a more nutritious, well-balanced diet.

12

MYTHS AND TRUTHS ABOUT NUTRITION: A QUIZ FOR PARENTS

You'll have to eat oatmeal or you'll dry up. Anybody knows that.

Kay Thompson
Eloise

Information about nutrition is everywhere today: food columns in newspapers, a torrent of diet books, radio and television talk shows about health and eating well. Friends and relatives swap recipes and stories about food bargains and good eating places. Many popular beliefs about nutrition and health are true; others contain an element of truth that has been twisted and exaggerated. Unfortunately, misinformation often is all too easy to find and can be tempting to accept without critical examination. In some cases, half truths or gross deceptions are promoted knowingly for profit by unprincipled food manufacturers, self-styled diet or fitness "experts," and unscrupulous publishers, among others.

As the public's interest in health issues increases, separating fact from fiction or truth from half truth grows more difficult. Mistaken ideas about nutrition sometimes even originate from the well-meaning attempts of nutrition experts to translate complex ideas into easy-to-understand language for the general public. It is helpful to remember that the field of nutrition is complex and complicated primarily because scientific research is often conflicting. Many of the truths about eating and health are still evolving.

To satisfy parents' curiosity and to heighten general awareness about nutrition, a quiz follows. Of the 40 familiar statements about food and diet, some are true, some false; others are partly true, and some are simply confusing. Answers are given, followed by brief explanations, which refer readers to other chapters where they can read more about the subject.

THE NUTRITION QUIZ

Mark each of the following statements in one of these four ways:

T   for true

F   for false

TF   for partly true, partly false

U   for unclear or confusing

_____   1. Cow's milk can be given to babies instead of breast milk or infant formula.

_____   2. Most healthy babies can regulate how much breast milk or formula they take.

_____   3. A baby about to start eating solids should be given a special transitional formula.

_____   4. Infants younger than 4 to 6 months of age should not be started on solid foods.

_____   5. Introduction of solid foods relatively early will prevent an infant from developing food allergies.

_____   6. Commercially prepared strained-meat baby foods have more protein than commercially prepared high-meat baby foods.

_____   7. Because breast milk is considered an ideal food, a baby needs no other nutrients before switching to solids.

_____ 8. Leaving a baby with a bottle in his or her crib at bedtime can be harmful.

_____ 9. Once a baby is eating solids, a good way to encourage sleep is to feed the baby a little cereal right before bedtime.

_____ 10. Skim milk is better for health at all ages than whole milk.

_____ 11. Soft drinks are more likely to cause tooth decay than raisins or other dried fruits.

_____ 12. Home-prepared baby foods are better than commercially prepared foods because home-prepared foods contain no additives.

_____ 13. Honey is lower in calories and more nutritious than sugar.

_____ 14. Margarine is better for a child than butter because it is lower in calories.

_____ 15. Brown eggs are more nutritious than white eggs.

_____ 16. Children need high amounts of protein for energy.

_____ 17. Junk foods are useless — just as the name implies.

_____ 18. Fats are unhealthy.

_____ 19. Children who do not like milk should take calcium supplements.

_____ 20. The best way for a teenager to lose weight is to eat moderately while exercising more.

_____ 21. A growing child should take vitamin supplements.

_____ 22. Vitamin A is a good remedy for teenage acne.

_____   23. Vitamin supplements should not be taken before meals because they tend to stimulate the appetite.

_____   24. A child who appears to be developing a cold should take extra vitamin C.

_____   25. Fast foods should be avoided because of their high calories and low nutritional value.

_____   26. The low-calorie sweetener aspartame (Nutra-Sweet and Equal) is harmful to young children.

_____   27. Children younger than 1 year of age should not be given honey because it has been known to cause botulism in babies.

_____   28. In general, children should avoid drinks that contain caffeine.

_____   29. Fish is "brain" food.

_____   30. There are specific foods children must eat for good health.

_____   31. It is sometimes a good idea to deny a meal to a misbehaving child.

_____   32. It is healthier for children to eat their meals in a certain order.

_____   33. Snacks can spoil a child's appetite.

_____   34. It is important to get a child used to eating breakfast foods (cereal, eggs, toast) at breakfast.

_____   35. Most of the important vitamins and minerals in a potato are found in the skin.

_____   36. Raw vegetables contain more vitamins than cooked vegetables.

_____   37. Chicken and fish are better for a child than red meat.

_____   38. Natural (organic) vitamin preparations are no better than synthetic vitamins.

_____   39. Starchy foods are best avoided.

_____   40. Sports drinks are perfect fluid replacements
                 after a vigorous athletic workout.

Answers

1. F	11. F	21. TF	31. F
2. T	12. TF	22. F	32. F
3. F	13. F	23. F	33. TF
4. T	14. F	24. U	34. F
5. F	15. F	25. TF	35. F
6. T	16. F	26. U	36. TF
7. TF	17. F	27. T	37. TF
8. T	18. TF	28. T	38. T
9. F	19. TF	29. F	39. F
10. F	20. T	30. F	40. F

DISCUSSION

1. Cow's milk can be given to babies instead of breast milk or infant formula: False

Unmodified cow's milk — the kind found in the grocer's dairy case — is not an adequate substitute for breast milk or infant formula for a baby under the age of 1 year. Cow's milk suits the needs of calves, who grow at an extremely rapid rate. It contains three times as much protein and proportionately greater quantities of minerals (such as potassium and sodium) than human milk. This excess of protein and minerals can impose enormous, unnecessary stress on the kidneys of human infants. Furthermore, when unmodified cow's milk is used for feeding human infants, the possibility of inducing iron deficiency anemia exists. Although the major ingredient in most formulas continues to be cow's milk, it is modified to match more closely the composition of human milk. (See Chapter 3.)

2. *Most healthy babies can regulate how much breast milk or formula
they take:*   True

Infants are remarkably efficient at regulating their own diets.
Left to their own devices, most healthy babies will consume just
about the right number of calories needed for normal growth
and development. Parents can take feeding cues directly from
the baby. When the baby is hungry, he or she usually makes this
very clear. (See Chapter 3.)

3. *A baby about to start eating solids should be given a special
transitional formula:*   False

Transitional formulas usually are not necessary when a baby
starts to eat solid foods. Although transitional formulas contain
the same nutrients as regular formulas, they contain fewer calories and less protein. This shift in composition makes babies
consume larger quantities in a feeding. The net result is that the
baby gets the same proportional nourishment — but at a higher
price. (See Chapter 3.)

4. *Infants younger than 4 to 6 months of age should not be started
on solid foods:*   True

Once again, babies are good at providing parents with the most
reliable cues. Babies younger than 4 to 6 months of age push
solid objects (except fingers, nipples, and other things that are
sucked on and cannot be swallowed) out of their mouths. They
are exhibiting an important inherited survival reflex called the
extrusion reflex. After 4 to 6 months, a baby gains better control
over all body coordination (such as lifting the head and hand-
eye movements) and the extrusion reflex begins to disappear.
Therefore, it is best not to introduce solids until a baby is about
6 months old. In the past, some child-development specialists
have recommended that solids be introduced in the child's first
month in order to advance a baby's development. Today, however, little or no evidence exists to show that introducing solids
early affects a baby's physical or mental capabilities in any way.
This is just as well, since parents who offer solids before a baby
is ready are likely to be frustrated by messy feeding bouts and
still-hungry babies. In addition, there is evidence that introduc-

ing solids too early may lead to future weight problems. (See Chapter 3.)

5. Introduction of solid foods relatively early will prevent an infant from developing food allergies: False

There is no evidence to indicate that introducing solids early helps prevent food allergies. In fact, early exposure to solids may be a risk factor for food allergies. The immune system, which governs tolerance to foreign or new substances (including food), is not developed fully until 12 to 24 months of age. Therefore, new foods (especially those such as wheat and eggs, which tend to cause allergies) should not be introduced until an infant is 6 or 7 months of age, and then only one at a time. In this way any allergy will show up clearly. If several different foods are given at the same time, and the child develops an allergy, it often is difficult to identify the offending food. (See Chapters 3 and 7.)

6. Commercially prepared strained-meat baby foods have more protein than commercially prepared high-meat baby foods: True

Strained-meat baby foods contain only meat. In general, meat is higher in protein than vegetables, and strained meat usually contains about twice as much protein as high-meat baby foods. High meat, a commercial, nonscientific term, in most cases means that the jar contains a combination of meat and other foods, usually vegetables. Typically, a high-meat baby food includes about 70 percent meat and 30 percent vegetables and other fillers. Careful reading of labels is always helpful. (See Chapter 3.)

7. Because breast milk is considered an ideal food, a baby needs no other nutrients before switching to solids: True and False

It is true that mother's milk is close to perfect for babies. In addition to containing the nutrients a baby needs, breast milk provides the baby with disease-fighting agents from the mother's immune system. For about the first four to six months of life, a healthy baby usually can exist on breast milk alone. At about that age, however, a baby's nutritional requirements begin to change. The baby needs increased amounts of certain nutrients, including vitamin D, fluoride, and iron. If a baby starts on solids at the age of 4 to 6 months, supplements of these nutrients may not be necessary. But if a mother continues to breast feed a baby without introducing solids, supplements are necessary. Some physicians recommend that mothers begin providing nutritional supplements to breast-fed babies even before they reach the 4-month mark. In general, mothers who are breast feeding should consult their pediatrician for advice about supplementation. (See Chapter 3.)

8. Leaving a baby with a bottle in his or her crib at bedtime can be harmful: True

Although a bottle may prevent a bout of crying at bedtime, this habit can do more harm than good by causing dental caries, gum disease, malformation of teeth, and other problems. In addition, giving a baby a bottle may establish a pattern that results in the child's needing food in the crib to fall asleep. This is not a good idea; there should be as few factors as possible interfering with the establishment of good sleeping and eating habits. (See Chapters 3 and 8.)

9. Once a baby is eating solids, a good way to encourage sleep is to feed the baby a little cereal right before bedtime: False

Parents should avoid feeding a baby right before bedtime unless the baby is obviously hungry. There is no evidence that feeding a baby cereal at bedtime will encourage sleep. In fact, this practice can lead to overfeeding. Babies can become used to eating right before falling asleep and may have trouble breaking that habit. (See Chapter 3.)

10. Skim milk is better for health at all ages than whole milk:
False

Skim milk is not better for children younger than 2 years old. Because skim milk contains fewer calories than whole milk, babies drink more of it and, consequently, consume too much protein, which puts a strain on their immature kidneys. In addition, young children need the fatty acids in whole milk. For most children past the age of 2 years, skim milk probably is better than whole milk because it contains less saturated fat. Saturated fat has been shown to increase cholesterol levels in the body, and high levels of cholesterol can contribute to adult cardiovascular disease. (See Chapter 3.)

11. Soft drinks are more likely to cause tooth decay than raisins or other dried fruit: False

Soft drinks, although high in sugar, are not a prime culprit in causing tooth decay because they pass through the mouth rapidly. Dried fruit, also high in sugar, is sticky and tends to stick to teeth. Dried fruit, however, is a good source of calories, vitamins, minerals, and fiber and a sensible, healthful snack choice for children. To prevent dental problems, children should be encouraged to brush their teeth, or at least rinse their mouths, after eating dried fruits or other sticky snacks. (See Chapter 8.)

12. Home-prepared baby foods are better than commercially prepared foods because home-prepared foods contain no additives: True and False

While homemade food tends to be more interesting and fresher tasting, there often is little nutritional difference between the two. In years past, commercial baby foods tended to contain more unnecessary additives, such as salt, sugar, and modified starch, than those that were homemade. This is no longer the case. In fact, while commercial foods now are often additive free, some parents frequently add salt and sugar to their own preparations to satisfy their own taste. Registered dietitians advise against this. There is no reason to accustom a baby to two ingredients that could contribute to future health problems (obesity or hypertension, for example). Parents who make baby food at home can control the use of all intentional additives, including sugar, salt, spices, and modified starch. Parents who use commercial preparations should read the labels carefully. (See Chapter 3.)

13. Honey is lower in calories and more nutritious than sugar:
False

Honey is a sugar. Both table sugar and honey contain 4 calories per gram. They both contain few other nutrients besides carbohydrates. On balance, there is little difference between the two, although sugar has the advantage that, unlike honey, it is not as likely to stick to the teeth and promote tooth decay. (See Chapter 2.)

14. Margarine is better for a child than butter because it is lower in calories: False

There is no difference in calories between margarine and butter. Margarine, however, is lower in saturated fats and higher in polyunsaturated fats. Studies show that saturated fats can increase the amount of cholesterol in the body which, in turn, can precipitate cardiovascular problems in later life.

There also is some evidence that polyunsaturated fats can help stem this process. Because there is a wide range of margarine ingredients, including varying amounts of polyunsaturated fat, parents should look for brands that list ingredients on the label. (See Chapters 2 and 10.)

15. Brown eggs are more nutritious than white eggs: False

The color of the shell is determined by the breed of chicken from which the egg came. There is no nutritional difference between brown and white eggs. There also is no difference in flavor, texture, or cooking performance between brown and white eggs that are equally fresh. (See Chapter 10.)

16. Children need high amounts of protein for energy: False

Protein is vital to building muscles and the structure of body cells, but it is not vital as a source of energy (calories). The nutrients that should be eaten to provide energy for the body are carbohydrates and fats. When insufficient carbohydrates and fats are consumed, protein is used as a source of energy, at the expense of muscles and cells. Therefore, children should not rely on protein as an energy source. It is important to ensure that a child eats a balanced diet that includes adequate amounts of carbohydrates and fats, as well as protein. (See Chapter 2.)

17. Junk foods are useless — just as the name implies: False

Although junk food means different things to different people, most people associate the phrase with foods that are high in sugar (candy, cakes, pies, chocolate) or high in fats (fast foods, potato chips). These foods are thought to be lacking in nutritional value — just useless junk. Actually, the phrase junk food is a contradiction in terms because all *foods* have some value. If children, however, eat so much of the sweet or fatty foods that they have no appetite left for nourishing meals, and thus do not get enough vitamins, minerals, protein, or fiber, parents' worries are justified. Junk foods, on occasion, however, will not harm a child who, for the most part, eats a balanced diet. (See Chapter 4.)

18. Fats are unhealthy: True and False

Consumers have been so inundated with negative information about fats that it is no wonder they have such a poor reputation. It is true that too much fat — especially saturated fats — can be harmful to the cardiovascular system. Also, fats contain more than twice as many calories as carbohydrates and protein. (1 gram fat = 9 calories; 1 gram carbohydrate or protein = 4 calories.) It is also true that the percentage of calories from fat in most American diets is high — about 65 percent, compared to the recommended 35 percent. These excess calories may contribute significantly to obesity. But there is good news about fats, too. For example, fats contain many important fat-soluble vitamins, including A, D, E, and K; they provide essential fatty acids; and they contain necessary materials for cell structures. Body fat pads and protects internal organs. For these reasons, no-fat diets are potentially dangerous. In sum, fat itself is good. It is *excess* fat and saturated fat that are bad. (See Chapter 2.)

19. Children who do not like milk should take calcium supplements:
True and False

A common fallacy holds that milk is the only food that contains enough calcium for a growing child. Actually, several other foods are excellent sources of calcium. They include yogurt; cottage cheese; other cheeses; buttermilk; and dark green, leafy vegetables, such as spinach. A problem arises when a child does not like milk or any of these other foods. In that situation, it is wise to consult the child's pediatrician about calcium supplements, which may be recommended. In general, parents should not give a child any kind of supplements unless they have been advised to do so by a physician after a thorough review of the child's eating habits. (See Chapter 3.)

20. The best way for a teenager to lose weight is to eat moderately while exercising more: True

There is a simple formula for losing weight: consume fewer calories than are used. The body is then forced to burn body fat for energy. Eating moderately and increasing exercise level improve mental and physical health at the same time that they produce a reduction in weight. For most teenagers, dieting can be a matter of watching portion sizes and other little things, such as sugar or salad dressing, and making exercise part of the daily routine. There is no need to go hungry. A drastic reduction in calories is a poor way to lose weight. Such crash diets are not likely to provide enough protein, vitamins, and minerals for the body. Many people who attempt such crash diets lose weight rapidly, but most of this is water loss that is put right back on. They can become depressed and often obsessed with avoiding food. Eventually, the temptation to eat becomes overwhelming, food binges follow, and weight is quickly regained. (See Chapters 7 and 8.)

21. A growing child should take vitamin supplements: True and False

If children eat well-balanced diets (a variety of foods from all food groups), they should not need vitamin supplements. Some children, however, go through phases when they will eat only one or two kinds of food, for instance milk, peanut-butter sandwiches, or cereal. These children may need vitamin supplements. Children with certain health problems, such as many allergies, also may need extra vitamins. (See Chapter 2.)

22. *Vitamin A is a good remedy for teenage acne:*   False

There is no evidence that a large dose of vitamin A (or spreading the liquid form of vitamin A on the skin) reduces acne, which is the result of hormonal changes. In fact, large oral doses of vitamin A can be harmful because the body cannot effectively metabolize excesses of most vitamins, especially the fat-soluble vitamins such as vitamin A. A prudent diet, coupled with careful washing and shampooing may reduce the symptoms of acne — but there are no guarantees. If a child has moderate to severe acne, the best advice would come from a dermatologist. (See Chapter 8.)

23. *Vitamin supplements should not be taken before meals because they tend to stimulate the appetite:*   False

This is but one of many myths about vitamins. Taking vitamins, which have no calories, before meals does not affect appetite. (See Chapter 2.)

24. *A child who appears to be developing a cold should take extra vitamin C:*   Unclear

For many years, experts have debated the finding of Dr. Linus Pauling that extra amounts of vitamin C can prevent colds or, at least, improve the course of a cold. After several further studies, it remains unclear whether vitamin C actually affects the development of colds. The balance tips slightly toward concluding that the relationship between vitamin C and preventing colds or reducing their severity is weak. Certainly a child should not receive large amounts of any vitamin on a regular basis unless prescribed by a physician. (See Chapters 2 and 8.)

25. Fast foods should be avoided because of their high calories and low nutritional value: True and False

Fast foods have a reputation for providing lots of calories and few nutrients. The first notion generally is true. Two slices of pizza indeed may be higher in calories than, say, half a cup of tuna fish served with celery sticks and an apple. But higher in calories does not necessarily mean lower in nutritional value. Pizza, for example, is made with a crust, cheese, and tomato sauce. This combination includes foods from three of the four food groups (bread, meat or milk, and vegetable), thus providing carbohydrate, protein, vitamins, and minerals. Clearly, eating only pizza could lead to a lack of many other nutrients as well as fiber. It would not be a good idea, however, to feed a child only tuna fish and an apple every day. A sensible goal for parents is to maintain balance in their children's diets so that enough calories and a range of nutrients are provided. If a child is overweight, the extra calories may be a problem. But fast foods are not inherently bad, and there is no need to avoid them for nutritional reasons. Within the menus of fast food restaurants, there are some food choices that can make meals and snacks more — or less — nourishing. (See Chapters 4 and 6.)

26. The low-calorie sweetener aspartame (NutraSweet and Equal) is harmful to young children: Unclear

Aspartame is a compound made from two amino acids (the building blocks of protein). It has become a popular replacement for saccharin for three reasons: (1) It is made from amino acids, not artificial chemicals; (2) Some people think it tastes better than saccharin; and (3) Large amounts of saccharin have been shown to cause cancer in laboratory animals. Aspartame, however, has been criticized by consumer-advocacy groups who contend that the body cannot metabolize such high concentrations of amino acids efficiently, and that health problems, even brain damage and cancer, may result if growing children use too much aspartame. The Food and Drug Administration contends that aspartame has been studied for 20 years, that it is safe for public consumption, and that the symptoms reported are mild in nature and not different from problems people experience for many other reasons. The controversy over low-calorie sweeteners is certain to continue. Although it seems unlikely that moderate amounts of aspartame will harm a child, parents may be best advised to avoid products containing artificial sweeteners unless recommended by a physician. Foods containing aspartame must not be consumed by children with phenylketonuria (PKU), a disease in which the body lacks an enzyme needed to process phenylalanine, one of the amino acids in aspartame. Most products that contain phenylalanine contain this information on the label. Parents of children with PKU should read all labels carefully. (See Chapter 11.)

27. Children younger than 1 year of age should not be given honey because it has been known to cause botulism in babies: True

Experts recommend that parents not give honey to any child less than 1 year old. Botulism is a rare but powerful food poisoning caused by an extremely dangerous toxin (poison). Within 16 hours to eight days of eating food contaminated by toxin from *C. botulinum* bacteria, a range of progressively worsening symptoms can occur, beginning with headache and dizziness, and progressing to double vision, muscle paralysis, vomiting, and difficulty in breathing and swallowing. Death may occur in severe cases because of paralysis that inhibits breathing. The symptoms of botulism in newborns are constipation and weak sucking during feeding. The infant becomes hungry and often thirsty, and a condition sometimes called floppy baby can develop, characterized by listlessness and poor muscle tone. *C. botulinum* bacterial spores can live in commercially or home-packed honey. For reasons that remain unclear, these do not affect adults but can cause severe illness when children younger than 1 year of age eat honey. (See Chapters 3 and 10.)

28. In general, children should avoid drinks that contain caffeine: True

Caffeine is an addictive, stimulant drug that tends to suppress appetite. It is found in coffee, tea, certain colas and other soft drinks. Some people enjoy caffeine for its stimulant effects, as a pick-me-up, especially in the morning. Others consume these drinks simply because they like the taste. Although small amounts of caffeine usually are not harmful for adults, children who consume caffeine regularly may experience nervousness, irritability, insomnia, and gastrointestinal disturbances. Therefore, it is a good idea not to give children caffeine, especially if they experience any of these symptoms. (See Chapters 3 and 11.)

29. Fish is brain food: False

Although fish is a good, nutritious food, it has no special power to increase anyone's intelligence level. (See Chapter 7.)

30. There are specific foods children must eat for good health:
False

Although children need to eat balanced diets, it is not important for them to eat any specific food. It is important, however, for them to eat foods from all four food groups to receive sufficient levels of the nutrients necessary for normal growth and development. If a child does not like a particular food, such as peas or turnips or pork chops or grapes, there is no reason to force him or her to eat it. It is pointless and upsetting to demand that children eat foods that are particularly distasteful to them. Children can get the essential nutrients from many food sources. There are no magic foods that children must eat for good health. (See Chapters 4 and 5.)

31. It is sometimes a good idea to deny a meal to a misbehaving child: False

Children need to eat for energy and growth, and, therefore, food should not be connected with punishment. Food is as basic for children as sleep. Withholding food from a child actually can aggravate bad behavior. Parents should never withhold food as a form of punishment. (See Chapter 5.)

32. It is healthier for children to eat their meals in a certain order:
False

The order in which food is consumed is largely a result of cultural influence. As an example, Americans and certain Europeans vary widely with regard to when salads are eaten during a meal. Americans usually eat salad as an appetizer or as a side dish with the main meal. In many European cultures, however, salad is served after the main course has been cleared from the table. Similarly, Americans will eat bread and cheese before a meal, while a cheese plate often closes a European meal. From a nutritional point of view, the order of the food matters little. From a cultural and social perspective, however, the order may be important. (See Chapter 1.)

33. Snacks can spoil a child's appetite: True and False

The number of times per day that people eat is substantially a matter of social scheduling. Indeed, the typical size of our meals — medium breakfast, light lunch, heavy dinner — is itself a matter of current practice. In many cultures there are four meals a day — light breakfast, heavy lunch, light tea, and medium dinner. The point is that it is unnecessary to adopt a rigid three-meals-a-day schedule. The average child is likely to be hungry five or six times during the day — right after waking, midmorning, noon, midafternoon, early evening, and, perhaps, midevening. There is no reason to deny a child snacks between meals. In fact, many nutrition experts advocate feeding a child six small meals a day. Some parents worry that snacks will keep a child from eating nourishing food, and this can be true if snacks always consist of caramel-coated popcorn or chocolate-covered ice-cream bars. But if children snack on cheese and fruit or nuts or yogurt or carrot and celery sticks, even if they are not hungry enough to eat the next usual meal, they will have benefited from the nutrients in the snack. (See Chapter 4.)

34. It is important to get a child used to eating breakfast foods (cereal, eggs, toast) at breakfast: False

What is eaten for breakfast is largely a matter of culture. In Japan many people eat raw fish for breakfast. Breakfast in the United States often consists of cereal, eggs, bacon, toast, juice, and milk. There is, however, no nutritional reason for eating these foods in the morning. In fact, eggs and bacon are both high in cholesterol and actually can be less nourishing than cold chicken served with a vegetable and a piece of fruit. The important thing is for breakfast to provide enough energy for the child to get through to the next meal or snack without fatigue or extreme hunger. A balanced meal in the morning can feature whatever foods the child likes. The more he or she likes the meal, the more he or she will eat — and the better prepared the child will be for the day ahead. (See Chapter 4.)

35. Most of the important vitamins and minerals in a potato are found in the skin: False

This is a common misconception. Many people believe that the skin is full of vitamins, minerals, and other nutrients, while the inside is essentially empty calories and high-calorie carbohydrates. Actually, the calorie content of an average-sized potato is surprisingly low — about 110 calories. It is the addition of sour cream or butter or margarine that makes it high in calories and potentially fattening. Nutrients in a potato are found throughout the vegetable. It is true that the skin is a good source of fiber and contains some important minerals. But the main reason the skin is important is that it holds the nutrients in the potato while it is cooking. If a potato is peeled before boiling, many vitamins will be lost in the water. Boiling or baking it in the skin, however, reduces this loss. (See Chapter 10.)

36. Raw vegetables contain more vitamins and minerals than cooked vegetables: True and False

Raw fresh vegetables generally contain more vitamins and minerals than cooked vegetables because some nutrients can escape during the cooking process. This is especially true for the water-soluble vitamins, which can leach out into the cooking water and steam. Most of these vitamins, however, can be retained by using cooking methods that require little or no water and short cooking times — steaming, pressure cooking, stir frying. If vegetables are boiled, vitamins and minerals in the cooking water can be recaptured if the water is used (boiled down into a sauce or poured into soup or stew) in the same meal. Raw vegetables can also lose vitamins over time, especially if they are stored improperly. Cooked fresh vegetables, therefore, may contain as many or more vitamins and minerals than older, raw ones. (See Chapter 10.)

37. Chicken and fish are better for a child than red meat: True
and False

The major problem with red meat is its high fat content. Chicken
and fish often are recommended because their fat content is significantly lower. Red meat, however, is a better source of iron.
If possible, parents should try to limit the amount of fatty red
meat in a child's diet, but not cut it out entirely, unless there are
other good sources of iron. (See Chapters 2 and 10.)

*38. Natural (organic) vitamin preparations are no better than
synthetic vitamins:*   True

Natural (organic) and synthetic vitamin preparations contain the
same chemical properties and offer the same nutrient value.
Consumers, however, may pay more for natural vitamins because they are more difficult to produce. (See Chapter 7.)

39. Starchy foods are best avoided: False

Starchy foods, such as rice, potatoes, bread, pasta, cereals, dried
beans, and seeds, have gained a mistaken reputation as being
high in calories and low in vitamins and minerals. In fact,
starchy foods, sometimes called complex carbohydrates, are
lower in calories than an equal amount of meat because starches
have little or no fat. In addition, certain combinations of starchy
foods can supply high-quality protein. In addition, starchy foods
are good sources of the B vitamins, vitamin C, and fiber. (See
Chapter 2.)

*40. Sports drinks are perfect fluid replacements after a vigorous
athletic workout:*   False

Most sports drinks, advertised as replacements for water, salt,
potassium, and calcium lost in perspiration, also have high
sugar contents (about 5 percent). The sugar lengthens the time
they remain in the stomach, thus increasing the potential for a
stomachache. (Canned soft drinks are worse because they contain 10 percent sugar.) The best choice is water — in moderate,
frequent quantities. If children insist upon having sports drinks,
they should be diluted with equal quantities of water. (See
Chapter 8.)

GLOSSARY

Absorption   A part of the digestive process in which nutrients pass from the human digestive tract through the intestines and into the blood stream and lymph system

Acid   A hydrogen-containing water-soluble compound, which will react with a base to form a salt

Additives   Ingredients or chemicals added to food intentionally or unintentionally during processing or preparation

Allergy   Sensitivity to certain irritating substances resulting in a reaction, such as skin rash, sneezing, or itching

Amino Acids   Nitrogen-containing organic compounds that are the chief structures of protein

Anemia   A lack or reduction of red blood cells, hemoglobin, or blood volume in the body

Anorexia Nervosa   A disorder in which a person has a distorted self-image of being overweight and, as a result, eats too little

Antioxidant   An additive that slows the process in which oxygen reacts with fats, oils, flavorings, and colors, causing them to change or become rancid

Atherosclerosis   Clogging of the arteries because of fatty deposits on the inner vessel lining

Bacteria   Microscopic one-celled organisms, which multiply by cell division; some types benefit the body while others can cause illness and disease

Base   Water-soluble compound that can neutralize an acid to form a salt

Bulimia   A disorder in which a person goes on a food binge, usually eating high-caloric items, and then self-induces vomiting because of guilt or fear of weight gain

Calories   Energy derived from food; units of heat measurement, defined as the amount of heat needed to raise the temperature of one gram of water one degree centigrade

Carbohydrates   Compounds made of carbon, hydrogen, and oxygen that form the supporting tissue of plants; in the form of sugars, starches, celluloses, and gums, they are important food for people

Carcinogen A cancer-causing substance

Carotene Yellow or red pigment in carrots, sweet potatoes, egg yolks, and other foods that the body can convert into vitamin A

Cellulose A colorless, transparent, nondigestible carbohydrate that is part of the structure of plants and serves as a source of fiber in the body

Cholesterol A fatlike substance produced in the liver and found in bile, gallstones, fat, blood, and brain tissue; it is also in eggs, animal fat, and milk

Deficiency Lack of a nutrient that could lead to illness or disease

Digestion The complex processes by which food is broken down into chemicals that can be absorbed and used as fuel for the body

Diuretic A substance that increases the amount and flow of urine

DNA Deoxyribonucleic acid, a substance in chromosomes that carries genetic information

Eczema Skin inflammation and rash, usually resulting in redness, itching, and oozing to form a crusty, scaly layer; often associated with food allergies

Edema Buildup of fluid in cells and tissues causing swelling and puffiness

Electrolyte A substance, such as sodium, potassium, or chloride, that dissolves in water (ionizes), making the solution capable of conducting the minute electrical current in the body

Enrich Replacing vitamins and minerals lost during processing or adding nutrients not present in the original food to the final product to make it more nourishing

Enzyme A protein that acts upon another substance to cause a chemical change without undergoing any change itself

Extrusion Reflex A reflex present at birth to about six months, that causes infants to spit out small solid objects that can be swallowed

Fats Greasy or oily tissue that forms soft padding between organs and stores excess energy supplies in animals; oily substance in many plants

Fat-soluble Vitamins (vitamins A, D, E, and K) Carbon-containing compounds that dissolve in dietary fats

Fatty Acids Acid resulting from the breakdown of fats; fatty acids that are essential to the body are linolenic, arachidonic, and linoleic (the body cannot produce this one and it must be obtained through food)

Fortify Improve the nutritional value of a food by adding vitamins, minerals, and other nutrients—some of which may not normally be in the original ingredients

Gastrointestinal Pertaining to the stomach and intestines

Glucose The simple sugar formed by the complete breakdown of carbohydrates; the chief source of energy in the body

Glycogen The form in which carbohydrates are stored in the liver and used when needed, as during strenuous exercise

Goiter Enlargement of the thyroid gland, which causes the front of the neck to swell; it often is caused by iodine deficiency

Hemoglobin The iron-containing pigment of red blood cells, which carry oxygen to cells

Hormone A chemical secreted into the blood stream by an organ or gland that affects the activity of another organ

Hydrogenate To introduce hydrogen into a substance, such as a liquid oil to make it more solid; the more hydrogenated the oil, the more saturated it is

Infection Growth and multiplication of harmful bacteria, viruses, parasites, or other microorganisms in the body

Insulin A hormone produced by the pancreas that regulates the levels of glucose and amino acids in the blood

Irradiation A process in which food is exposed to radioactive gamma or X-rays to kill bacteria and insects

Lactation The secretion of milk in mammals

Legumes The pod or fruit of beans, peas, lentils, and other related plants

Lipids The total group of fats and fatlike substances that are stored in the body and serve as a fuel source, protect and pad organs, and perform other functions

Malnutrition A disorder caused by an inadequate diet or faulty use of food in the body

Megavitamins High doses of vitamins, from 10 to 2,000 times the Recommended Dietary Allowances

Metabolism The sum of all the complex chemical and physical processes of matter and energy that occur within living systems

Metabolic Rate The rate at which energy is expended by the body

Minerals Inorganic (non-carbon-containing) substances that are needed in relatively small amounts to maintain good health and smooth function of the body's systems

Nutrients The substances contained in food—protein, carbohydrates, fats, vitamins, and minerals—that provide fuel and nourishment for the body

Nutrition The science that studies the processes by which the body takes in food and uses it to maintain health and sustain life

Organic Carbon-containing substances that come from plants or animals; also pertains to the use of natural fertilizers from plants and animals rather than synthetic chemicals

Pernicious Extremely severe, fatal

Polyunsaturated Fatty Acid (PUFA) Fatty acids that contain double chemical bonds; they usually are from vegetable sources; tend to lower blood cholesterol levels; usually are liquid at room temperature

Preservatives Food additives that destroy or inhibit microorganisms that cause spoilage

Protein A nitrogen-containing organic compound, which is made up of amino acids and found in all cells; it is essential for normal body functions

RNA Ribonucleic acid; a substance found in cells that is responsible for transmitting hereditary information

Saturated Fatty Acid Fatty acids containing no double chemical bonds; they usually are from animal sources; tend to raise cholesterol levels; often are solid at room temperature; and always solidify when refrigerated

Supplement Any nutrient taken in addition to those obtained through food sources to increase the body's total level of certain nutrients

Toxicity Having poisonous effects

Toxin A substance that is poisonous

Vitamin Organic (carbon-containing) substances that are found in minute quantities in food and are needed for normal functioning of body systems

Water-soluble Vitamins (vitamin C and the B-complex vitamins) Carbon-containing compounds that dissolve in water

RESOURCES

Allergy Foundation of America
801 Second Avenue
New York, New York 10017

American Academy of Pediatrics
1801 Hinman Avenue
Evanston, Illinois 60204

American Association for Maternal
and Child Health
116 South Michigan Avenue
Suite 806
Chicago, Illinois 60603

American Dental Association
Bureau of Dental Health Education
211 East Chicago Avenue
Chicago, Illinois 60611

American Diabetes Association
18 East 48 Street
New York, New York 10017

American Dietetic Association
430 North Michigan Avenue
Chicago, Illinois 60611

American Foundation for Maternal
and Child Health
30 Beekman Place
New York, New York 10022

American Heart Association
44 East 23rd Street
New York, New York 10010

American Home Economics
Association
2010 Massachusetts Avenue, N.W.
Washington, D.C. 20036

American Nutrition Society
P.O. Box 158-C
Pasadena, California 91104

American Public Health
Association
1015 18th Street, N.W.
Washington, D.C. 20036

Center for Science in the Public
Interest
1755 S Street, N.W.
Washington, D.C. 20009

Cereal Institute, Inc.
135 South LaSalle Street
Chicago, Illinois 60603

Cooperative Extension Service
Federal Extension Service
Department of Agriculture
Washington, D.C. 20250

Department of Food and Nutrition
American Medical Association
535 North Dearborn Street
Chicago, Illinois 60610

Food and Nutrition Board
National Research Council
National Academy of Sciences
2101 Constitution Avenue, N.W.
Washington, D.C. 20418

Food and Nutrition Information
  Center
National Agricultural Library
U.S. Department of Agriculture
Baltimore Boulevard
Beltsville, Maryland 20705

Food and Nutrition News
National Livestock and Meat Board
Chicago, Illinois 60603

Food and Nutrition Section
American Public Health
  Association
1790 Broadway
New York, New York 10019

La Leche League International
9616 Minneapolis Avenue
Franklin Park, Illinois 60131

Maternity Center Association
48 East 92 Street
New York, New York 10019

National Committee for Children
  and Youth
1401 K Street, N.W.
Washington, D.C. 20005

National Dairy Council
620 North River Road
Rosemont, Illinois 60018

National Health Systems
P.O. Box 1501
Ann Arbor, Michigan 48106

National Institute of Child Health
  and Human Development
U.S. Department of Health and
  Human Services
Bethesda, Maryland 20014

Nutrition Foundation, Inc.
99 Park Avenue
New York, New York 10016

Nutrition Foundation, Inc.
Office of Education and Public
  Affairs
888 17th Street, N.W.
Washington, D.C. 20006

Nutrition News
National Dairy Council
Chicago, Illinois 60606

Poultry and Egg National Board
250 West 57th Street
New York, New York 10010

Society for Nutrition Education
2140 Shattuck Avenue
Suite 110
Berkeley, California 94704

State Departments of Health,
Nutrition Division

United Fresh Fruit and Vegetable
  Association
727 North Washington Street
Alexandria, Virginia 22314

United States Department of
  Agriculture
Food and Nutrition Office
500 12th Street, S.W.
G.H.I. Building
Washington, D.C. 20250

Regional USDA Food and Nutrition
  Offices:
Burlington, MA; Trenton, NJ;
  Atlanta, GA; Chicago, IL;
  Denver, CO; Dallas, TX; San
  Francisco, CA.

United States Department of
  Health and Human Services
Food and Drug Administration
Public Health Service
Office of Public Affairs
Washington, D.C. 20204

USEFUL READING

Adams, Catherine F., and Agricultural Research Service, United States Department of Agriculture, *Nutritive Value of American Foods: In Common Units, Handbook 456.* Washington, D.C.: U.S. Government Printing Office, 1975.

American Diabetes Association and American Dietetic Association, *The Family Cookbook.* Englewood Cliffs, N.J.: Prentice-Hall, Inc., 1980.

Ault, Ray, and Uraneck, Liz, *Kids Are Natural Cooks.* Boston: Houghton-Mifflin Co., 1974.

Bayrd, Ned, and Quilter, Chris, *Food for Champions.* Boston: Houghton-Mifflin Co., 1982.

Berko, Robert L., *Guide to Salt Content of Your Foods.* South Orange, N.J.: Consumer Education Research Center, 1983.

Brody, Jane, *Jane Brody's Nutrition Book: A Lifetime Guide to Good Eating for Better Health and Weight Control.* New York: W. W. Norton & Co., 1981.

Castle, Sue, *The Complete New Guide to Preparing Baby Foods.* New York: Bantam Books, Inc., 1981.

Clark, Nancy, R.D., *The Athlete's Kitchen: A Nutrition Guide and Cookbook.* Boston: CBI Publishing Co., Inc., 1981.

Cumming, Candy, R.D., and Newman, Vicky, R.D., *Eater's Guide: Nutrition Basics for Busy People.* Englewood Cliffs, N.J.: Prentice-Hall, Inc., 1981.

Hess, Mary Abbott, R.D., and Hunt, Anne Elise, R.D., *Pickles & Ice Cream: The Complete Guide to Nutrition During Pregnancy.* New York: McGraw-Hill Book Co., 1983.

Jacobson, Michael F., *The Complete Eater's Digest and Nutrition Scoreboard: The Consumer's Factbook of Food Additives and Healthful Eating.* Garden City, New York: Doubleday & Company, Inc., 1985.

Jacobson, Michael, Liebman, Bonnie F., and Moyer, Greg, *Salt: The Brand Name Guide to Sodium Content.* New York: Workman Publishing, 1983.

Katzen, Mollie, *Moosewood Cookbook*. Berkeley, California: Ten Speed Press, 1977.

La Leche League International, *The Womanly Art of Breastfeeding*. Franklin Park, Illinois: La Leche League International, 1981.

Lansky, Vicki, *Feed Me! I'm Yours*. New York: Bantam Books, 1981.

Lappé, Frances Moore, *Diet for a Small Planet*. New York: Ballantine Books, 1972.

Lawrence, Ruth A., *Breastfeeding, A Guide for the Medical Profession*. St. Louis: C.V. Mosby Co., 1980.

Pennington, Jean A.T., and Church, H.N., *Bowes and Church's Food Values of Portions Commonly Used*, Fourteenth Edition. Philadelphia: J.B. Lippincott Company, 1985.

Satter, Ellyn, R.D., *Child of Mine: Feeding with Love and Good Sense*. Palo Alto, California: Bull Publishing Co., 1983.

Sheedy, Charlotte Baum, and Keifetz, Norman, *Cooking for Your Celiac Child*. New York: The Dial Press, Inc., 1969.

White, Alice, *The Total Nutrition Guide for Mother and Baby: From Pregnancy through the First Three Years*. New York: Ballantine Books, 1983.

INDEX

THE BOSTON CHILDREN'S HOSPITAL

The Children's Hospital in Boston is the largest pediatric health-care institution in the United States and is the world's largest pediatric research center. Founded in 1869 as a 20-bed hospital for children, it is now an internationally renowned center for comprehensive pediatric health care.

Children's offers a complete range of health care services, including medical and surgical services for patients from birth through age 21 (and older in special cases). Approximately one-third of the hospital's patients are adolescents and young adults.

Children's is the primary pediatric teaching hospital of the Harvard Medical School, where most of its senior physicians hold faculty appointments. The staff includes more than 500 active physicians and dentists, 400 house staff members and fellows, and a nursing staff of approximately 800. The hospital employs nearly 4,000 people and is served by 700 volunteers.

Children's Hospital is committed to providing health information and has published several authoritative books for parents, including the best-selling *Child Health Encyclopedia*.